QT 3T

NHS Blood and Transplant

00006993

KV-325-921

RECEIVED
-? AUG 2003
DR C NAVARRETE

Please return this book on or before the date shown below

NHSBT Library and Learning Resources
Filton Blood Centre, 500 North Bristol Park, Northway,
Bristol BS34 7QH. Tel. 0117 9217345

WITHDRAWN
13 NOV 2024

NHSBT
LIBRARY

TISSUE ENGINEERING, STEM CELLS, AND GENE THERAPIES

ADVANCES IN EXPERIMENTAL MEDICINE AND BIOLOGY

Editorial Board:
NATHAN BACK, State University of New York at Buffalo
IRUN R. COHEN, The Weizmann Institute of Science
DAVID KRITCHEVSKY, Wistar Institute
ABEL LAJTHA, N. S. Kline Institute for Psychiatric Research
RODOLFO PAOLETTI, University of Milan

Recent Volumes in this Series

Volume 525
ADVANCES IN PROSTAGLANDIN, LEUKOTRIENE, AND OTHER BIOACTIVE LIPID RESEARCH: Basic Science and Clinical Applications
Edited by Zeliha Yazıcı, Giancarlo Folco, Jeffrey M. Drazen, Santosh Nigam, and Takao Shimizu

Volume 526
TAURINE 5: Beginning the 21st Century
Edited by John B. Lombardini, Stephen W. Schaffer, and Junichi Azuma

Volume 527
DEVELOPMENTS IN TRYPTOPHAN AND SEROTONIN METABOLISM
Edited by Graziella Allegri, Carlo V. L. Costa, Eugenio Ragazzi, Hans Steinhart, and Luigi Varesio

Volume 528
ADAMANTIADES-BEHÇET'S DISEASE
Edited by Christos C. Zouboulis

Volume 529
THE GENUS *YERSINIA*: Entering the Functional Genomic Era
Edited by Mikael Skurnik, José Antonio Bengoechea, and Kaisa Granfors

Volume 530
OXYGEN TRANSPORT TO TISSUE XXIV
Edited by Jeffrey F. Dunn and Harold M. Swartz

Volume 531
TROPICAL DISEASES: From Molecule to Bedside
Edited by Sangkot Marzuki, Jan Verhoef, and Harm Snippe

Volume 532
NEW TRENDS IN CANCER FOR THE 21ST CENTURY
Edited by Antonio Llombart-Bosch and Vicente Felipo

Volume 533
RETINAL DEGENERATIONS: Mechanisms and Experimental Theory
Edited by Matthew M. LaVail, Joe G. Hollyfield, and Robert E. Anderson

Volume 534
TISSUE ENGINEERING, STEM CELLS, AND GENE THERAPIES
Edited by Y. Murat Elçin

A Continuation Order Plan is available for this series. A continuation order will bring delivery of each new volume immediately upon publication. Volumes are billed only upon actual shipment. For further information please contact the publisher.

TISSUE ENGINEERING, STEM CELLS, AND GENE THERAPIES

Edited by

Y. Murat Elçin
Science Faculty and Biotechnology Institute
Ankara University
Ankara, Turkey

Kluwer Academic / Plenum Publishers
New York, Boston, Dordrecht, London, Moscow

Library of Congress Cataloging-in-Publication Data

International Symposium on Biomedical Science and Technology (9th : 2002 : Antalya, Turkey)
   Tissue engineering, stem cells and gene therapies / edited by Y. Murat Elçin.
     p. ; cm. -- (Advances in experimental medicine and biology, ISSN 0065-2598 ; v. 534)
   "Proceedings of BIOMED 2002, the 9th International Symposium on Biomedical Science
and Technology, held September 19-22, 2002, in Antalya, Turkey"--T.p. verso.
   Includes bibliographical references and index.
   ISBN 0-306-47788-2
   1. Biomedical engineering--Congresses. 2. Animal cell biotechnology--Congresses. 3.
Biomedical materials--Congresses. 4. Gene therapy--Congresses. 5. Stem
cells--Congresses. I. Elçin, Y. Murat. II. Title. III. Series.
   [DNLM: 1. Tissue Engineering--Congresses. 2. Gene Therapy--Congresses. 3. Stem
Cells--physiology--Congresses. QT 37 I615t 2003]
   R856.A21586 2002
   616'.027--dc21
                                                                                             2003051600

Proceedings of BIOMED 2002—The 9th International Symposium on Biomedical Science and Technology, held September 19–22, 2002, in Antalya, Turkey

ISSN 0065-2598

ISBN 0-306-47788-2

©2003 Kluwer Academic / Plenum Publishers, New York
233 Spring Street, New York, New York 10013

http://www.wkap.nl/

10 9 8 7 6 5 4 3 2 1

A C.I.P. record for this book is available from the Library of Congress

All rights reserved

No part of this book may be reproduced, stored in a retrieval system, or transmitted in any form or by any means, electronic, mechanical, photocopying, microfilming, recording, or otherwise, without written permission from the Publisher, with the exception of any material supplied specifically for the purpose of being entered and executed on a computer system, for exclusive use by the purchaser of the work.

Permissions for books published in Europe: *permissions@wkap.nl*
Permissions for books published in the United States of America: *permissions@wkap.com*

Printed in the United States of America

Preface

Recent years have seen an upsurge of significant interest in cell-based technologies. A range of productive and lively debate have taken place relating to tissue engineering, namely the construction of tissues and whole organs using molecularly-designed resorbable biomaterials to create tissue *de novo*, the potential use of human embryonic stem cells for transplantation and regenerative medicine, with similar potential for adult-derived stem cells, and gene therapy, in relation to cell transplantation. New findings in biomimetic materials, cell signalling pathways, extracellular matrix receptors and ligands, growth factors, and the human genome project, all present particularly motivating sources for the development of research in the evergrowing biomedical field.

The purpose of this book is to stimulate further the work in biomedicine and to make the issues of related scientific disciplines accessible to a wider readership by characterising the current state of research in the biomedical field. The lectures and a selection of the presentations from BIOMED 2002 - The 9th International Symposium on Biomedical Science and Technology, held in September 2002 in Turkey- constitute the basis for the volume. Tissue engineering, stem cells, cell and gene therapies were the major topics presented and discussed in the symposium. This book is intended to serve as an up-to-date synopsis of the major developments of our area through the work reflected in BIOMED 2002, though not covering all aspects of the topics, due to the natural restrictions within a volume of this kind.

The first part of the book is devoted to the studies which offer perspectives on the current status and the potential future of tissue engineering and stem-cell technologies. In the second part, the contributions based on experimental and clinical data are introduced. The discussions in this part concentrate mainly on the role of stem cells in liver tissue engineering, cell-based therapies in diabetes mellitus, chronic degenerative diseases of the central nervous system, and adult-derived stem cell therapies. In the third part, the focus is on the biomarkers for tissue-engineered products, namely for tissue-engineered skin. The fourth part deals with the novel biomaterials developed for various applications of tissue engineering on neural, vascular, aortic, bone, cartilage, endocrine-pancreas tissues. Finally, a coverage of the achievements in practical gene targeting, applications of controlled release in gene therapy and tissue engineering, antibodies in cancer, acute-phase genes and phage-displayed peptide libraries is presented in the last part.

The width and the depth of the contributions made by the prominent specialists from diverse backgrounds, such as materials science, chemistry, cell biology to engineering and medical sciences will, I believe offer the reader many an opportunity and challenge simultaneously. In the ordering of the chapters and the organizing of the sections, utmost attention has been accorded so as to minimise the possible difficulties that may arise from the interdisciplinary nature of the material at hand. The multiple authorship, inevitably, conditions a diversity according to the differing perspectives of the contributors, hence the obvious differences of emphasis and presentation as well as the theoretical approaches adopted. The editor's aim has not been to entirely resolve such problems but to allow differing perspectives to stand side by side. Nevertheless a certain harmonisation has been necessary.

The editor would like to acknowledge the cooperation of all the individual contributors and thank them most sincerely for their efforts. My particular appreciation is due to Ankara University Biotechnology Institute, and to E. Pişkin and V. Hasırcı, the BIOMED Series coordinators. Finally, I owe a great debt of gratitude to my family for their support throughout the project.

Y. Murat Elçin, Editor

Contents

I. PERSPECTIVES FOR TISSUE ENGINEERING AND STEM CELLS

1. Tissue engineering: confronting the transplantation crisis
   R. Nerem 1

2. Human embryonic stem cells- realising the potential
   J. McWhir, A. Thomson, and V. Sottile 11

3. Human embryonic or adult stem cells: an overview on ethics and perspectives for tissue engineering
   P. Henon 27

4. Stem cell biology and plasticity
   E. Kansu 47

II. STEM CELLS IN TISSUE ENGINEERING AND CELL - BASED THERAPIES

5. Liver tissue engineering: successes and limitations
   V. Dixit and Y. M. Elçin 57

6. Pancreatic islet and stem cell transplantation in diabetes mellitus: results and perspectives
   R. G. Bretzel 69

7. Cell based therapy of chronic degenerative diseases of the central nervous system
Ye. V. Pankratov, A. I. Ivanov, T. D. Kolokoltsova, Ye. A. Nechayeva, I. F. Radayeva, L. I. Korochkin, A. V. Revischin, S. A. Naumov, I. A. Khlusovi, and A. I. Autenshlus 97

8. CD 34+ cells in hematopoietic stem cell transplantation
T. Demirer 107

9. The effects of different growth factors on human bone marrow stromal cells differentiating into hepatocyte-like cells
Y.-S. Weng, H.-Y. Lin, Y.-J. Hsiang, C.-T. Hsieh, and W.-T. Li 119

III. BIOMARKERS FOR TISSUE-ENGINEERED PRODUCTS

10. Oxidative DNA damage biomarkers used in tissue-engineered skin
H. Rodriguez, P. Jaruga, M. Birincioglu, P. E. Barker, C. O'Connell, and M. Dizdaroglu 129

11. Biomarkers used to detect genetic damage in tissue-engineered skin
C. O'Connell, P. E. Barker, M. Marino, P. McAndrew, D. H. Atha, P. Jaruga, M. Birincioglu, M. Dizdaroglu, and H. Rodriguez 137

IV. BIOMATERIALS IN TISSUE ENGINEERING AND REPAIR

12. Design peptide scaffolds for regenerative medicine
S. Zhang and C. E. Semino 147

13. Progresses in synthetic vascular prostheses: toward the endothelialization
M. Crombez and D. Mantovani 165

14. Adhesion and growth of rat aortic smooth muscle cells on lactide-based polymers
L. Bacáková, M. Lapcíková, D. Kubies, and F. Rypácek 179

15. Biodegradable copolymers carrying cell-adhesion peptide sequences
    V. Proks, L. Machová, S. Popelka, and F. Rypáček 191

16. Polymer based scaffolds and carriers for bioactive agents from different natural origin materials
    P. B. Malafaya, M. E. Gomes, A. J. Salgado, and R. L. Reis 201

17. Preparation and characterization of natural/synthetic hybrid scaffolds
    G. Khang, S. J. Lee, C. W. Han, J. M. Rhee, and H. B. Lee 235

18. Polyhipe polymer: a novel scaffold for *in vitro* bone tissue engineering
    M. Bokhari, M. Birch, and G. Akay 247

19. Pancreatic islet culture and transplantation using chitosan and PLGA scaffolds
    Y. M. Elçin, A. E. Elçin, R. G. Bretzel, and T. Linn 255

V. GENE THERAPY AND OTHER APPROACHES

20. Challenges and prospects for targeted transgenesis in livestock
    M. M. Marques, A. J. Thomson, and J. McWhir 265

21. Controlled release of bioactive agents in gene therapy and tissue engineering
    D. Ş. Keskin and V. Hasırcı 279

22. Interleukin 1 (IL-1) induces the activation of stat3
    A. Arman and P. E. Auron 297

23. The use of antibodies in diagnosis and therapy of cancer
    A. Muvaffak and N. Hasırcı 309

24. Detection of phage displayed peptides with blocking ability in vascular endothelial growth factor (VEGF) model
    B. Erdağ, B. K. Balcıoğlu, A. Kumbasar, and B. Çırakoğlu 327

25. Index 335

TISSUE ENGINEERING: CONFRONTING THE TRANSPLANTATION CRISIS

Robert M. Nerem
Georgia Tech/Emory Center For the Engineering of Living Tissues, Parker H. Petit Institute for Bioengineering and Bioscience, Georgia Institute of Technology, Atlanta, Georgia, 30332-0363, U.S.A.

1. INTRODUCTION

There appears to be relatively wide agreement that in this 21st century advances in biology will define scientific progress. What is not often said, however, is that, not only will advances in biology define scientific progress, it also will revolutionize how we engineer products.

One example of this is the medical implant industry. With the advent of tissue engineering, these engineered implants will be revolutionized through tissue engineering. This term is used here in the broadest sense and is defined to include biological substitutes and/or the fostering of remodeling to repair, replace, regenerate, or enhance tissue/organ function.[1] This technology represents the interface between the biological revolution and the traditional medical implant industry. This industry is being reinvented and is becoming biology based. It is this incorporation of biology, in many cases living cells, that will result in next-generation medical implants which will be very different from those we have today.

This process already has started, and there is little question but that tissue engineering has a level of hype that far exceeds the current state of the art. One of the purposes of this article is thus to "paint" a more realistic "picture" of tissue engineering, while at the same time holding up the potential and promise of what might be considered a revolutionary approach to the engineering of medical implants.

2. THE TISSUE ENGINEERING INDUSTRY

Projections of the ultimate size of the tissue engineering industry have ranged up to and even in excess of $100 billion in annual sales. The industry today, however, is in a fledgling state, an industry still in the process of being born. Table 1 presents data[2] from a 2001 report. To this one must add annual sales and the best estimate for 2001 is less than $50 million.

Table 1. Present State of the Tissue Engineering Industry [2]

Number of Companies	66
Number of Employees	3100
Annual Investment	$580 Million
Annual Growth Rate	16%

An updated report will soon be out that will indicate that the industry is still growing; however, this really doesn't tell the whole story for the industry is going through a real "shake out." In this many of the small, startup companies are being severely challenged. One of the early pioneering companies, Organogenesis, is facing serious financial difficulties. This is a company that had the first living cell product, Appligraf, approved by the U.S. Food and Drug Administration.[3] This skin substitute, having both an epidermis and a dermis and made using collagen gel technology and allogeneic cells, was approved in 1997. Yet today Organogenesis' stock is down to a few cents and Novartis, a major partner, has pulled out. But it is particularly painful to see what they are going through since they were once a pioneering leader; however it is possible that they may be able to reorganize and survive.

Organogenesis is not the only tissue engineering company facing challenges as another early pioneer, Advanced Tissue Sciences (ATS) in La Jolla, California, is faring even worse. ATS has two skin substitute products, Transcyte which is acellular and was the first tissue-engineered product approved by FDA and Dermagraft which is a dermal equivalent made using allogeneic cells.[4] ATS has declared bankruptcy, sold approximately half of the company to Smith and Nephew, and the remainder is being closed. The good news is that the technology is not lost, as it has been transferred to Smith and Nephew, and both Transcyte and Dermagraft will continue to be sold. The rest of the company, however, appears to be lost.

Although the skin substitutes of ATS and Organogenesis have been a clinical success in that patients have been very much helped, they have not been the commercial success for that the companies, in fact the entire tissue engineering community had hoped there is some good news, and this is that in spite of the problems being faced by some of the smaller companies, several of the bigger companies are increasing their investment in tissue engineering. This includes both Smith and Nephew and Johnson and Johnson. For these companies there is a recognition that tissue engineering will be an important part of their future.

One final comment on the industry is as follows, and this is really a question, not a comment. Is it possible that for some of these tissue-engineering startups the technology moved too soon from benchtop research to the commercial world? Although one cannot answer this with any degree of assuredness, it is clear that once a concept moves to the commercial world the "clock is ticking."

3. CORE, ENABLING TECHNOLOGIES

As already noted, the skin substitute products, though not a commercial success, at least not as of yet, have been a clinical success. Furthermore, they have taught us much about what the critical issues are that must be addressed for the next tissue-engineered products.[5] These critical issues are listed in Table 2 and give rise to the core technologies that will enable the future.

Table 2. Critical Technical Issues in Bringing Tissue-Engineered Products to Market

Addressing issues of cell sourcing
Developing interactive biomaterials
Engineering 3D constructs/healing responses
Scaling up manufacturing processes
Preserving manufactured products
Controlling in vivo biological responses
Engineering immune acceptance
Assessing post-implantation viability

In fact, it was these critical issues which led to the establishment of the Georgia Tech/Emory Center for the Engineering of Living Tissues (GTEC), funded in 1998 with an Engineering Research Center Award from the National Science Foundation. The original strategy was developed with GTEC's industrial partners, seven at the time, 19 now. This has led to

GTEC's matrix strategy illustrated in Figure 1. In this there are three programmatic areas, and these are (1) cardiovascular substitutes, (2) metabolic, secretory organs, e.g. the pancreas and liver, and (3) orthopaedic tissue engineering. Within each of these programmatic areas, projects are grouped into one of three core technologies. These are cell technology, construct technology, and the technologies required for the integration into living systems. These are described next using examples from the cardiovascular substitutes program.

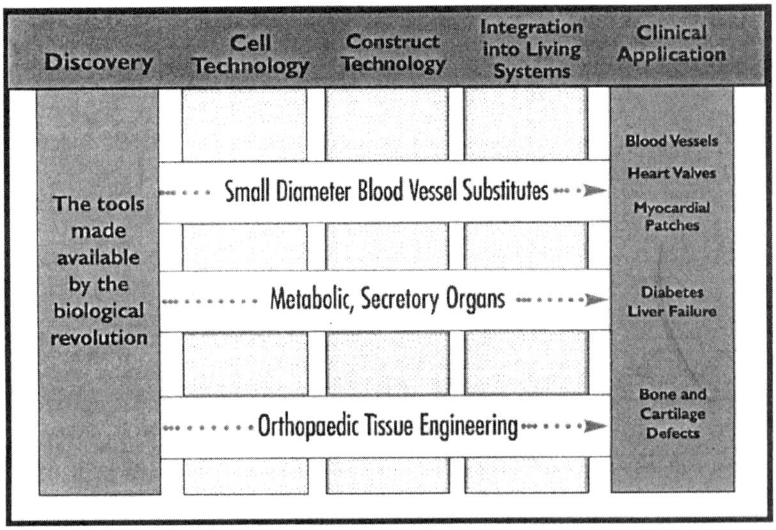

Integration of Enabling Core Technologies

Figure 1. The matrix strategy of the Georgia Tech/Emory Center for the Engineering of Living Tissues.

Cell Technology. Included in this first of the three core technologies is both cell source and the manipulation of cell function. It is the former which is a truly critical issue. Obviously, from the viewpoint of immune acceptance, it is autologous cells which would be the choice; however, these do not lend themselves to creating a tissue substitute which is available off the shelf.

In the case of the tissue engineering of a blood vessel substitute, it is the vascular endothelial cell which is the "show stopper" in terms of cell source. Here initial successes may be achieved with autologous cells, either derived from biopsied adipose tissue or from circulating endothelial cells, that are more like an endothelial progenitor cell. As already noted, the use of autologous cells does not provide for off-the-shelf availability. The one exception to this may be if one could implant a non-endothelialized blood vessel substitute and then recruit circulating endothelial cells from the flowing blood to form a confluent monolayer on its lumen.

Ultimately one would prefer to employ non-autologous endothelial cells; however, in general this will require using some type of strategy for the engineering of immune acceptance. This will be elaborated on somewhat later in this section. Another source would be either embryonic [6,7] or adult stem cells. Along with tissue engineering, this area also receives a lot of hype; however, there is much still to be learned before the use of stem cells becomes a practical alternative. Not only do we need to know more about the differentiation pathways and the associated signals, but we also need to better understand how to expand stem cells and issues related to process quality control.

The use of embryonic stem cells is quite controversial, and at this point it is unclear whether they will be needed in tissue engineering. What is clear, however, at least to this author, is that tissue engineering will greatly benefit from the harnessing of the developmental, biological processes. To achieve that we need to be able to do research using embryonic stem cells if we are to have the opportunity to fully understand development biology.

Construct Technology. Once one has cells with the appropriate functional characteristics, then the issue is how to incorporate them into a three-dimensional structure that mimics native tissue both in architecture and function. In this a scaffold can be used to create the architecture, where the scaffold either could be a synthetic material, a biological material, or some hybrid. Furthermore this is somewhat complicated by the fact that most tissues and organs are multi-cellular in nature. Furthermore, cells in a three-dimensional structure may have very different characteristics from those observed when cultured in monolayer.

Another part of construct technology are issues related to the manufacturing of a tissue substitute. This includes process scale up and the preservation of a product once manufactured. In regard to the former, it is one thing to make one of a kind on the benchtop of a research laboratory, it is quite different to make a 1000 per week with the reproducible quality that would be required for an FDA-approved product. Once manufactured, a critical issue is the preservation of a living cell product for off-the-shelf availability. Although seemingly everyone knows how to preserve cells, it is quite another matter to preserve a three-dimensional structure into which are incorporated living cells.

Integration into Living Systems. When a tissue-engineered construct, particularly one with living cells, is implanted into a living system, there are a variety of biological responses that may take place. No attempt will be made here to review the variety of effects which may be observed; however, there is one key issue that will be addressed. This is the issue of immune acceptance, an issue which is very much related to the source of cells used as discussed earlier. If non-autologous cells are to be used, then in general one will need to employ some type of strategy to engineer immune acceptance.

One strategy that GTEC has pursued is the use of co-stimulation blockade. This strategy is based on the understanding that not only must a foreign object be recognized as being non self, but there also must be present the co-stimulatory signal, sometimes called signal 2. If one can block this co-stimulation signal, then immune rejection can be prevented. Studies in rodents have demonstrated the feasibility of using such a strategy.[8] Unfortunately, a recent series of vascular allograft experiments in non-human primates indicate that, although short-term patency is improved, long-term acceptance or tolerance is not achieved. Thus the GTEC team has moved on to a chimeric strategy in which the donor of tissue or cells also provides bone marrow to be implanted in the host. The development of strategies for the engineering of immune acceptance thus remains an important research area.

4. THE TRANSPLANTATION CRISIS

In Table 3 is listed some of the tissues and organs to which tissue engineering is being applied. Those listed in the lefthand column are ones where some success is either being or is beginning to be achieved. This includes applications of skin substitutes and the area of orthopaedic tissue engineering, the latter including both soft tissues and bone. In the righthand column is listed the vital organs, *i.e.* the heart and its components and the kidney, liver, and pancreas. It is these vital organs for which there is a transplantation crisis, and it is here where tissue engineering has the potential to make a major impact.

Table 3. Some Tissue Engineering Applications

Severe Burns	Blood Vessels
Skin Ulcers	Heart Valves
Facial Reconstruction	Myocardial Patches
Cartilage	Heart
Tendons	Bioartificial Pancreas
Ligaments	Kidney
Bone	Liver

This transplantation crisis is due to the tremendous disparity between patient need and donor availability. In the U.S. alone there are in excess of 75,000 patients awaiting single or multiple organ transplants. Of these on the waiting list, more than 15 die each day. The patient need continues to increase, but not the availability of donor organs. Tissue engineering has the potential to dramatically increase the supply of organs for these patients. The challenge, however, is great and thus progress is slow. Table 4 summarizes where we are in the development of replacements for these organs. Some additional comments are in order.

This transplantation crisis is due to the tremendous disparity between patient need and donor availability. In the U.S. alone there are in excess of 75,000 patients awaiting single or multiple organ transplants. Of these on the waiting list, more than 15 die each day. The patient need continues to increase, but not the availability of donor organs. Tissue engineering has the potential to dramatically increase the supply of organs for these patients. The challenge, however, is great and thus progress is slow. Table 4 summarizes where we are in the development of replacements for these organs. Some additional comments are in order.

Table 4. Current State of Development in the Tissue Engineering of Vital Organs

Organ	State of Development
Heart Myocardial Repair	Myocardial cell transplantation in clinical trials, myocardial patches under development, at least 5 years away
Small-Diameter Blood Vessel Substitutes	A number of promising concepts, at least 10 years away
Heart Valves	Current prosthetic valves are reasonable effective, a tissue-engineered heart valve 15 years away
Kidney	Extracorporeal system in clinical trials
Liver	Extracorporeal systems in clinical trials, an implantable liver 20-30 years away
Pancreas	Human islet transplantation showing some success, but cannot handle the large patient need; an engineered bioartificial pancreas still only being tested in small animals

First, it should be noted that, if we could engineer myocardial repair and replacement blood vessels and heart valves, then we would have all the components of heart. With this and with further advances in diagnostic imaging so that one can detect diseases of the heart at an earlier stage, then this author believes that the need for total heart transplantation will decrease significantly.

Second, the heart may seem like a complicated organ; however, it is simple compared to the others with the liver perhaps being the most complex. It is because of the complexity of these vital organs that implantable units may be decades away. Furthermore, it will be impossible to engineer in all of the functions of the normal organ. In the case of a bioartificial pancreas, the goal is simply to provide insulin-secreting cells which are glucose responsive. Even with this simplified approach and with over $200 million invested, there is no product on the horizon. In fact nothing has gone beyond small animal studies.

5. CONCLUDING DISCUSSION

What has been attempted here is to present a realistic picture of tissue engineering including the technologies, the specific applications under development, and the state of the industry. This emerging industry is critical to the success of tissue engineering for if the technologies cannot be used to enable commercially successful products, then it will not be possible to address the wide patient need.

For tissue engineering to achieve its potential, researchers need to focus on the core, enabling technologies, and there must be multiple, parallel approaches. There also must continue to be a focus on functionality, and here a key question for any tissue or organ is what are the essential functions that must be captured?

What else is needed is a real success story. Although none of the products currently in clinical trials suggests a "blockbuster" product, tissue engineering has enormous potential and in addressing the replacement of vital organs, it offers the opportunity to confront the transplantation crisis.

REFERENCES

1. Nerem, R.M., and Sambanis, A., 1995, Tissue engineering: From biology to biological substitutes. *Tissue Engineering* **1**, 3-13.
2. Lysaght, M.J., and Reyes, J., 2001, The growth of tissue engineering. *Tissue Engineering* **7** (5), 485-493.
3. Parenteau, N., 1999, Skin: The first tissue-engineered products – the Organogenesis story. *Scientific American* **280** (4), 83-84.
4. Naughton, G., 1999, Skin: The first tissue-engineered products – the Advanced Tissue Sciences story. *Scientific American* **280** (4), 84-85, 1999.

5. Nerem, R.M., Ku, D.N., and Sambanis, A., 1998, Core technologies for the development of tissue engineering. In *Tissue Engineering for Therapeutic Use 2*. Elsevier, New York, pp. 19-29.
6. Solter, D., and Gearhart, J., 1999, Putting stem cells to work. *Science* **283**, 1468-1470.
7. Vogel, G., 1999, Harnessing the power of stem cells. *Science* **283**, 1432-1434.
8. Larsen, C.P., Elwood, E.T., Alexander, D.Z., Ritchie, S.C., Hendrix, R., Tucker-Burden, C., Cho, H.R., Aruffo, A., Hollenbaugh, D., Linsley, P.S., Winn, K.J., and Pearson, T.C., 1996, Long-term acceptance of skin and cardiac allografts by blockade of the CD40 and CD28 pathways. *Nature* **381**, 434-438.

HUMAN EMBRYONIC STEM CELLS – REALISING THE POTENTIAL

Jim McWhir, Alison Thomson, and Virginie Sottile
Department of Gene Expression and Development, Roslin Institute, Roslin, Midlothian, Scotland EH25 9PS, U.K.

1. INTRODUCTION

Murine embryonic stem (mES) cells are permanent tissue culture cell lines isolated from explanted blastocysts[1,2]. mES cells share an unusual set of properties with the stem cells of germ cell tumours (EC cells). Both cell types can be cultured under conditions in which they cycle indefinitely, or in which they terminally differentiate into a variety of specialised cells. When undifferentiated mES or EC cells are returned to the preimplantation embryo they resume a normal programme of development and give rise to chimaeric animals. However, only mES cells give rise to germ-line contributions. In mice the importance of mES cells has been predominantly as a tool to effect very precise genetic changes in transgenic animals by manipulating mES cells in vitro prior to blastocyst injection. The differentiation of mES cells in vitro also gives rise to a wide range of differentiated cell types[3-6], although this occurs in a much less organised manner than in the blastocyst. In vitro differentiation of mES cells suggests obvious therapeutic applications for ES cells in the treatment of degenerative and metabolic disease.

The potential role for ES cells in regenerative medicine was of largely academic interest until the isolation of the first human ES (hES) cell lines in 1998[3,4]. Much as followed earlier developments in assisted reproduction and organ transplantation, stem cell biology has become a matter of intense public debate. This debate is fuelled by three driving forces: (1) the potential power of hES cell technologies to cure human disease (2) the possibility that adult-derived stem cells may have similar potential, and (3) the controversial origin of embryonic stem cells. The purpose of this chapter is to critically examine the real potential for hES-derived regenerative medicine.

2. CHARACTERISTICS OF HUMAN ES CELLS

Human ES cells express markers characteristic of human embryonal carcinoma (EC cells) and of primate ES cells: SSEA-3, SSEA-4, Tra-1-60, Tra-1-81, telomerase and Oct4[3,5]. Unlike murine ES cells, hES cells are not responsive to exogenous leukemia inhibition factor (LIF), are feeder-dependant and require supplementation with basic fibroblast growth factor (bFGF) (complete protocols are provided in Lebkowski et al[5]). Early culture protocols required that hES cells be co-cultured on a feeder layer of inactivated murine embryonic fibroblasts (MEFs). More recently it has been shown that this requirement may also be met by culture in media conditioned by prior incubation with MEF cells[6]. This demonstrates that the factor or factors provided by the feeder layer are diffusible. Such xenosupport systems, even based upon conditioned medium, still run the risk of transfer of pathogens. We now know that human fetal and adult fibroblasts can also support the undifferentiated growth of hES cells[7].

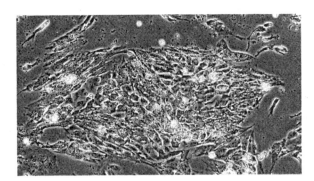

Figure 1. Human ES cells cultured in conditioned medium.

Human ES cells are sensitive to the method of disaggregation at passage and, at least in their early passages, are generally disaggregated mechanically. Established protocols provided by WiCell for the routine culture of the lines derived by Thomson et al[3], call for culture on a matrix of laminin, collagen IV and heparin sulphate (Matrigel) and for the use of collagenase at passage to separate cells into small clumps[3,6]. Other groups have successfully used trypsin for routine passage[4] and it remains unclear if passage protocols are transferable among cell lines. In our hands the H9 and H1 cell lines[3] are readily disaggregated in a solution of 0.25% trypsin plus EGTA (TEG), to yield robust cultures of undifferentiated cells and improved plating efficiency (see Figure 2). However, it remains to be seen if such treatments have long-term effects on pluripotentiality or on karyotype. Clearly it is critical at this still early stage, to better define the optimal conditions for hES culture.

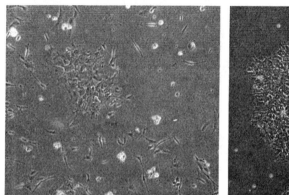 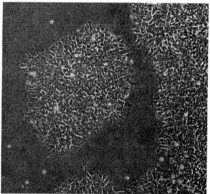

Figure 2. Human ES cells (H9) 90 hours after passage with collagenase (left panel) and trypsin/EGTA (right panel). The trypsin regime yields a greater proportion of undifferentiated cells and higher plating efficiency.

3. DIFFERENTIATION OF HUMAN ES CELLS

The promise of human ES cells lies in their potential to give rise to clinically relevant cell types for regenerative medicine. What evidence exists that this can be achieved? Cultivation to high density for extended periods or failure to replace a feeder layer leads to spontaneous differentiation of hES cells[4]. More systematic differentiation can be obtained by passaging onto non-adherent plastic in the absence of either conditioned medium or bFGF. Under these conditions H1, H9 and H7 hES lines[3] form aggregates known as 'embryoid bodies'. After 4-6 days of suspension culture embryoid bodies can be plated onto a tissue culture surface where they attach and differentiate into a broad range of cell types (Figure 3). However, all hES lines may not be equivalent. Reubinoff and colleagues[4] could not induce embryoid bodies in their hES lines, although these lines did differentiate spontaneously as monolayer cultures when switched into standard medium and allowed to grow to high density.

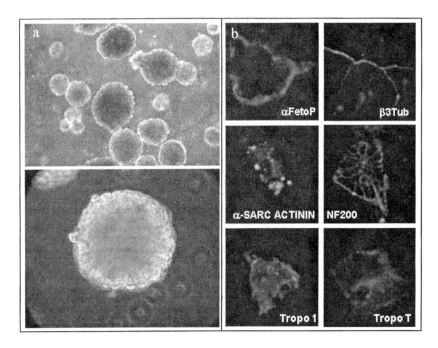

Figure 3. (a) Human ES cells induced to form embryoid bodies. (b) Embryoid bodies were then plated onto an adherent surface, cultured for 10 days and stained for α-feto protein (endoderm), β-tubulin and NF200 (ectoderm), α-sarcomeric actinin Tropo1 and tropoT (mesoderm).

While the undirected differentiation of hES cells from embryoid bodies (at least with some hES lines) is not difficult, this procedure gives rise to a complex and unpredictable pattern of cell types. The real challenge in regenerative medicine is to purify large numbers of functional cell types or their progenitors through directed differentiation. The holy grail in this field will ultimately be the specific induction of a single differentiation pathway in defined media. While we are some way from achieving that goal in any of the lineages of clinical interest, some early success has been achieved with directed differentiation for neural cells, cardiomyocytes and osteoblasts.

3.1 Neurogenesis

Three recent reports describe the generation of brain cells from hES cells. Zhang et al.,[8] have reported a stepwise progression from embryoid bodies to neural rosettes, which are subsequently harvested by selective dissociation as free-floating aggregates that generate both neurons and glia. Reubinoff et al.,[10] showed that simply maintaining hES cells in culture without passage or replenishment of feeders and in the absence of bFGF[9] gave rise to colonies expressing neural markers. These were then mechanically dissected and replated in serum-free medium to form free-floating spherical structures similar to neurospheres isolated from adult brain tissue. Both groups performed engraftment studies into the lateral ventricle of neonate rats and showed that transplanted cells migrated into many brain regions. However, it is not yet clear if these cells have integrated at a functional level. Neuronal subtype differentiation in both studies was limited to glutamatergic neurons and GABA-producing neurons. In a third study [11], a wide variety of ES-derived neural cell types were demonstrated in vitro and shown to have action potential. However, a present limitation of these techniques, like those for adult CNS-derived stem cells, is the absence of effective protocols for the derivation of enriched populations of the most clinically relevant cell types in the central nervous system (CNS) – dopaminergic neurons (Parkinson's disease), cholinergic neurons (Alzheimer's) and oligodendrocytes for repair of myelination defects.

3.2 Cardiogenesis

Human cardiomyocytes terminally differentiate soon after birth and therefore lack the ability to regenerate after ischaemic injury. This has prompted interest in identifying cell types capable of replenishing the injured myocardium with healthy cells and augmenting heart function. Beating cardiac muscle can be readily derived from hES cells following simple embryoid body formation, but under these circumstances cardiomyocytes form a small minority of cells within a mixed population. The challenge in this area is to derive sufficient numbers of pure cardiomyocytes to be clinically relevant and to achieve significant levels of engraftment.

Several groups have reported the enhanced generation of functional cardiomyocytes from hES cells after treatment with 5-aza-dC[12,13] (a de-methylation reagent), enrichment by Percoll gradient separation[12], and treatment with retinoic acid (RA)[14]. Cardiomyocytes can comprise between 8 and 70% of the differentiated population when the same protocol is repeated with a different cell line[12]. It seems that greater genetic variability among hES lines relative to that between mouse ES lines may complicate the development of directed hES differentiation over the corresponding murine protocols. Human ES cells may also use different signalling pathways to mES cells, thus complicating the transfer of mES protocols to the human system. For example, DMSO and RA have both been shown to enhance mEC[15] and mES[16] cardiogenesis but DMSO has no such effect on hES cells[12] and the effect of RA is observed in 1 report[13], but not in another[12].

3.3 Osteogenesis

Skeletal defects arising from developmental abnormalities, bone inflammation, tumours, degenerative diseases such as osteoarthritis and osteoporosis, and traumatic injury severely diminish the quality of life. These disorders are in principle, treatable by stem cell-based approaches. We have recently developed a procedure for the directed differentiation of hES cells to osteoblasts in which the majority of cells express osteogenic markers and are associated with calcification in vitro (Sottile and McWhir; unpublished data).

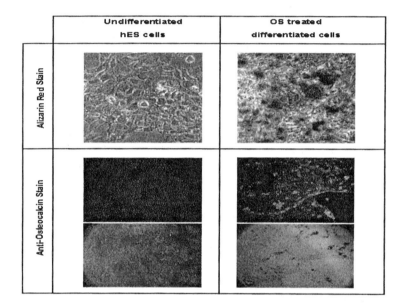

Figure 4. Human ES cells, left panel following 21 days differentiation without osteogenic factors, right panels following 21 days differentiation in osteogenic medium (OS). Top panels show staining for mineralisation, bottom panels are immunohistology for expression of the osteoblast-specific marker osteocalcin.

One of the surprises in hES-derived osteogenesis is that the time course of calcification parallels that from adult-derived mesenchymal stem (MSC) cells (data not shown). This implies either that hES cells make a very rapid commitment to a cell type analogous to the MSC, or that osteogenesis proceeds by a different pathway.

Although for some applications terminally differentiated cells may themselves be engrafted to good effect (eg. Dopaminergic neurons for

Parkinson's) in many cases applications will rely upon the short to medium term growth of the graft post transplantation, both to provide tissue mass and to integrate into host tissue. A general problem therefore, is to identify and amplify progenitor cells. For most lineages such cells are wholly uncharacterised. A great deal of work remains to be done in defining protocols, not so much for terminal differentiation in vitro, but rather for the proliferation of progenitor cells. Progenitor cells could then be either engrafted to proliferate in vivo or added to scaffolds in vitro prior to engraftment. There is a great deal of basic science to be done in the characterisation and isolation of progenitors cells in all clinically relevant lineages.

3.4 Other Lineages

There is now an extensive literature on the differentiation of mouse ES cells to a wide variety of cell types. With the exception of neurogenesis and cardiogenesis the human ES literature remains sparse. In spite of their therapeutic importance, little has yet been published on the derivation of islet cells from hES cells. This reflects the still early stage of development of hES differentiation technology as well as the concentration of much of this work within the commercial rather than academic research community. Assady et al.,[17] observed that spontaneous differentiation of hES cells included cells with characteristics of insulin-producing β-cells. Although this is an encouraging first step, these putative ES-derived islet cells remain small numbers of cells interspersed among a mixed population.

Hepatocyte differentiation from hES cells is important both in regenerative medicine and for drug and toxicity testing, and an expandable population of ES-derived cells with the features of hepatocytes has recently been observed following treatment with sodium butyrate[18]. Endothelial cells form the lining of the blood vessels. Such cells could in principle provide a source of human cells for engineering new blood vessels in ischaemic tissue and possibly for cotransplantation along with muscle cells for cardiac regeneration. Human ES-derived endothelial cells have been purified from differentiating hES cells using antibodies to platelet endothelial cell-adhesion molecule 1 (PECAM1)[19], and were seen to form vessel-like structures in matrigel.

One of the most clinically important lineages is the haematopoietic. Blood is the single tissue for which engraftment issues have largely been worked out in the development of routine transfusion procedures. Human ES cells have been shown to differentiate to haematopoietic precursor cells when co-cultured with the murine bone marrow cell line S17 or the yolk sac endothelial cell line C1620[20]. The challenge now is to further develop this procedure for the amplification and purification of haematopoietic stem cells. ES-derived haematopoietic cells may also have important applications in tolerisation (see section 4 below).

The response of hES cells to cytokines and chemical inducers of differentiation is difficult to analyse in complex populations and in medium which contains unknown and variable components. Schuldiner et al.,[21] have studied the effects of multiple factors on the differentiation of hES cells. Activin-A and TGFβ1 induced mesodermal cells. Retinoic acid, EGF, BMP4 and bFGF activated both endodermal and mesodermal markers and NGF and HGF led to derivatives of all three germ layers. The effects of some factors, however, vary depending upon the cell population on which they act. For example, bFGF, necessary for the undifferentiated growth of hES cells, under other conditions promotes their differentiation to mesoderm[22].

4. ADULT STEM CELLS

Public debate over the ethics of hES technology arises from the controversial origin of ES cells in the preimplantation embryo. The derivation of new lines from embryos surplus to the requirements of assisted reproduction programmes involves no new ethical issues over those already associated with superovulation/IVF/embryo transfer. Nevertheless, there is a degree of public disquiet about the use of hES cells in regenerative medicine. This is largely based upon the 'slippery slope' argument that progressive relaxation may eventually lead to reproductive cloning. The debate has become clouded by the simultaneous appearance of a number of reports suggesting multi- or pluri-potentiality for a variety of adult 'stem' cells previously thought to have restricted differentiation capacity. Although this possibility is not strictly relevant to the ethical arguments over hES cells, it has been argued that the potential of adult stem cells renders the further development of hES cells unnecessary. What evidence exists that adult stem cells do have equivalent potential to ES cells?

Adult stem cells are defined as self-renewing and able to repopulate the tissue in which they reside. Traditionally stem cells have been regarded as either uni-, multi- or pluri-potential and conventional wisdom held that the murine ES cell was the only example of the latter (able to give rise to all foetal and adult tissues). More recently, some have used the term 'adult stem cell' to imply pluripotentiality[eg. 23], although this is strictly unproven for any non-ES cell type, and indeed unlikely if we are to understand that pluripotentiality would include even germ cells. Nevertheless, the evidence for **multi**-potentiality of some adult stem cells is mounting.

4.1 Mesenchymal Stem Cells

Transplanted whole bone marrow or haematopoietic stem cells (HSCs) have been reported to give rise to skeletal muscle[23,24], heart muscle[25,26], endothelium[24-27], liver[28], lung, gut and skin epithelia[29] and neuroectoderm[30-33]. Human mesenchymal stem cells, (MSCs), are a multipotential subpopulation present in the adherent fraction of explanted bone marrow, which can be maintained in vitro for 4 to 15 cell doublings after freezing[34]. Like bone marrow and HSCs, cultured MSCs also produce multiple tissue contributions following transplantation[35]. It remains unclear which of the in vivo contributions from whole bone marrow transplants arise from HSCs from MSCs or indeed from another, as yet uncharacterised stem cell, resident within bone marrow. With the exception of the minority of reports in which clonal origin of all contributions can be rigorously established[eg31], most engraftment data can be equally well explained either by the presence of a multipotential stem cell or as a consequence of the engraftment of multiple stem cells, each with restricted potentiality. A third possible explanation is suggested by experiments from 3 labs, including our own, which show that spontaneous fusion can occur to give rise to stem cell-like cells with hybrid genotypes[36-38]. However, none of these data prove that such fusions actually occur following transplantation of adult stem cells and this remains a matter of some debate. Clinically, it is important to remember that although there is debate over the mechanism of engraftment, the fact that graft-derived cells do integrate into host tissue is not at issue. Adult-derived stem cells may have clinical applications regardless of the mechanism of their integration.

4.2 Multipotential Adult Progenitor Cells (MAPCs)

The primary disadvantage of MSCs for regenerative medicine is that their proliferation in culture is limited to a few passages[34]. Verfaillie and colleagues have described a rare subpopulation within marrow stromal cells[39-41], muscle[41] and brain[41] which can give rise to what seem to be permanent, multipotential stem cells (multipotential adult progenitor cells; MAPCs). If this result can be replicated in other labs, it promises to be an extremely powerful technology, although it remains to be seen if the potentiality of MAPCs is as wide as that of ES cells. For example, no contributions from bone marrow-derived MAPCs have yet been detected to skeletal or cardiac muscle. The emergence of MAPCs from multiple tissues raises the intriguing possibilities that pluripotential stem cells may either be circulating cells or that a resident stem cell population may be present in all tissues.

4.3 Other Adult Stem Cells

The central nervous system (CNS) has generally been thought to have limited capacity for self-repair. Recent evidence, however, suggests that cells that are capable of neurogenesis occur in both the subventricular zone and ventricular subependyma[42-44]. Most remarkably, cultures of cells taken from the CNS can give rise to in vitro structures known as neurospheres, cells from which apparently give rise to broad contributions in chimaeric mice[45,46]. Although CNS-derived stem cells are unlikely to be useful clinically, at least on a patient-derived basis, this unexpected plasticity has caused some of us to look again at the potentiality of other cell types. Stem cells also occur in the gut epithelium, hair follicle, liver, skeletal muscle and skin. It will be critical to establish if the apparent multipotentiality of cells resident in CNS and bone marrow can also be demonstrated within any of these other tissues.

5. IMMUNE TOLERANCE

The ultimate objective of regenerative medicine, to replace cells that have been lost as a consequence of disease, has been severely hampered by supply. Although adult stem cells can be derived from the patient, their number is limited. It is far more likely that regenerative medicine will depend upon the use of an allogeneic model in which banks of cells (probably derived either from ES cells or MAPCs) are supplied as allografts. What are the immunological consequences of such a model?

The long-term use of immunosupression would limit successful clinical application of stem cell therapy to only the most serious conditions. For others, the risk of immunosuppressive treatment would be greater than that associated with the condition itself. There are two ways in which this problem can be addressed. Stem cells can be genetically modified to include features that confer protection against the host immune system. Alternatively, the patient him(her)self can be treated in such a way as to generate long–term tolerance to the graft.

Subversion of the immune system by the expression of transgenes in hES cells could include the expression of certain viral genes which have evolved specifically for that purpose (reviewed in[47]) or possibly forced expression of HLA genes associated with immunotolerance (eg:HLA-G[47]). However, this general strategy suffers from an associated heightened risk of susceptibility to viral infection and/or tumorigenesis.

Graft rejection arises largely as the consequence of interactions between T-cells and antigen presenting cells (APCs). If the T-cell receives the appropriate signals from the APC, it becomes activated and destroys the graft. However, the immune system has also evolved methods to prevent T-cells becoming activated against 'self' antigens and considerable success has been reported in attempts to co-opt those mechanisms in order to engineer graft acceptance (reviewed in[48]).

Allogeneic haematopoietic engraftment in animals can lead to long-term chimaerism, which usually renders the host permanently tolerant of donor organ or tissue transplants[49]. Unfortunately chimaeras generated from bone marrow frequently suffer from host versus graft (HVG) disease due to co-transfer of active donor T-cells. Rat embryo-derived cells (putative rat ES cells) have recently been shown to have the same property of tolerance induction[50], but provide the additional advantage that co-transfer of T-cells and hence HVG disease is not an issue. This raises the possibility that hES cells could be used (either directly or following in vitro differentiation to haematopoietic cells) for the induction of tolerance. In a subsequent step the same ES line would then be used to generate a second cell type, which could be engrafted therapeutically.

Finally, is the immune rejection problem as serious as it first seems? Most of our knowledge of allograft rejection relates to organ transplantation in which complex tissues including blood vessels and residual haematopoietic cells from the donor are introduced surgically under traumatic conditions. Anecdotal reports suggest that MSCs are not rejected by the immune system and do not stimulate an immune or allergic response[eg.51]. Unfortunately these data are not available in the refereed literature and it is difficult to comment critically. Nonetheless, it is intriguing to speculate that stem cells from various sources may share similar properties of immuno-privilege.

6. CONCLUSION

The development of stem cell therapy is still at a primitive stage. Even the control of the undifferentiated growth of hES cells is not well understood. Directed hES differentiation protocols are few in number and are still unproven at the level of functional engraftment. At the same time adult stem cells also remain an unknown quantity. Although MAPCs seem to offer most of the advantages of ES cells with the additional advantage of certain immuno-acceptance, this work needs to be verified in an independent lab. With these uncertainties it is clearly not an appropriate time to make important strategic decisions about the restriction of effort to one cell type or another. The prudent way forward is to vigorously investigate all options. It seems most likely that different applications in regenerative medicine will favour stem cells of both adult and embryonic origin. The need for scale up suggests that for all but the most critical applications the only realistic model is allogeneic, and hence, the further development of tolerisation approaches must be considered a high priority.

There are several important considerations to keep in mind. (1) Differentiation from embryonic and adult stem cells may proceed by different pathways. This has the implication that the control of ES derived differentiation may be more readily understood and hence more quickly reduced to practice, as it is likely to be closer to the developmental model. A further implication is that functionality may differ among the progeny of stem cells from different sources. (2) One of the uncertainties surrounding the use of patient-derived MSC material is their response to the environment post engraftment, and the possible erosion of their repair potential due to an imbalanced host metabolism. For example, would patient-derived MSCs maintain a pro-osteogenic potential when transplanted into an osteoporotic bone whose hormonal environment has led to excessive adipogenesis and impaired osteogenesis of the endogenous cell pool[49]. If the differentiation products of ES and adult stem cells have different qualitative properties, we might expect a different outcome with hES-derived material. (3) ES cells have the advantage of providing 'off the shelf' treatment. With the possible exception of MAPCs, adult stem cells do not have the proliferative capacity to provide sufficient cell numbers to treat multiple patients. This potential of hES cells for scaling up is not a trivial advantage. Patient-derived stem cell treatment will require biopsy followed by the isolation under exacting conditions of cell lines for each individual. For many applications this will be justifiable. However, in some cases insufficient time will be available. In other cases the requirement for skilled technical staff and expensive equipment would effectively deny large-scale application, particularly to those without access to well funded and sophisticated medical treatment. (4) Human ES research may be essential in developing the full potential of adult stem cells. Human ES cells are readily amenable to genetic modification and can be grown in large numbers to provide material with which to study the control of differentiation - in particular the characteristics of the elusive progenitor cells.

ACKNOWLEDGEMENTS

The work from our laboratory was supported by grants from the biotechnology and biological sciences research council and from Geron Corporation.

REFERENCES

1. Evans, M.J., and Kaufman, M., 1981, Establishment in culture of pluripotential cells from mouse embryos. *Nature* **292**, 154-156.
2. Martin, G.R., 1981, Isolation of a pluripotential cell line from early mouse embryos cultured in medium conditioned by teratocarcinoma stem cells. *Proc. Natl. Acad. Sci USA* **78**, 7634-7638.
3. Thomson, J.A., Itskovitz-Eldor, J., Shapiro, S.S., Waknitz, M.A., Swiergiel, J.J., Marshall, V.S., and Jones, J.M. 1998, Embryonic stem cell lines derived from human blastocysts. *Science* **282**, 1145-1147.
4. Reubinoff, B.E., Pera, M.F., Fong, C., Trounson, A., and Bongso, A., 2000, Embryonic stem cell lines from human blastocysts: somatic differentiation *in vitro*. *Nature Biotechnology* **18**, 399-404.
5. Lebkowski, J.S., Gold, J., Xu, C., Funk, W., Chiu, C., and Carpenter, M., 2001, Human embryonic stem cells: culture differentiation, and genetic modification for regenerative medicine applications. *The Cancer J* **7** (suppl.2), S83-S93.
6. Xu, C., Inokuma, M.S., Denham, J., Golds, K., Kundu, P., Gold, J.D., and Carpenter, M., 2001, Feeder-free growth of undifferentiated human embryonic stem cells. *Nature Biotechnology* **19**, 971-974.
7. Richards, M., Fong, C., Chan, W., Wong, P., and Bongso, A., 2002, Human feeders support prolonged undifferentiated growth of human inner cell masses and embryonic stem cells. *Nature Biotechnology* **20** (9), 933-936.
8. Zhang S., Wernig, M., Duncan, I.D., Brustle, O., and Thomson, J.A., 2001, *In vitro* differentiation of transplantable neural precursors from human embryonic stem cells. *Nature Biotechnology* **19**, 1129-1133.
9. Reubinoff, B.E., Itsykson,P., Turetsky,T., Pera,M.F., Reinhartz,E.,Itzik,A. and Ben-hur,T. 2001, Neural progenitors from human embryonic stem cells. *Nature Biotechnology* **19**, 1134-1140.
10. Zhang, S-C., Ge, B., and Duncan I.D., 1999, Adult brain retains the potential to generate oligodendroglial progenitors with extensive myelination capacity. *Proc. Natl. Acad Sci. USA* **96**, 4089-4094.
11. Carpenter, M., Inokuma, M.S., Mujtaba, T., Chui, C.P., Rao, and M.S., 2001, Enrichment of neurons and neural precursors from human embryonic stem cells. *Exper. Neur.* **172**, 383-397.
12. Xu, C., Police, S., Rao, N., and Carpenter, M.K., 2002, Characterization and enrichment of cardiomyocytes derived from human embryonic stem cells. *Circ Res.* **91** (6), 501-508.
13. Kehat, I., Kenyagin-Karsenti, D., Snir, M., Segev, H., Amir, M., Gepstein, A., Livne, E., Binah, O., Itskovitz-Eldor, J., and Gepstein. L., 2002, Human embryonic stem cells can differentiate into myocytes with structural and functional properties of cardiomyocytes. *J. Clin. Invest.* **108**, 407-414.
14. Schuldiner, M., Yanuka, O., Itskovitz-Eldor, J., Melton, D.A., and Benvenisty, N., 2000, Effects of eight growth factors on the differentiation of cells derived from human embryonic stem cells. *Proc. Natl. Acad. Sci. USA.* **97** (21), 11307-11312.
15. Edwards, M.K., Harris, J.F., and McBurney, M.W., 1983, Induced muscle differentiation in an embryonal carcinoma cell line. *Mol Cell Biol* **3**, 2280-2286.
16. Wobus, A.M., Kaomei, G., Shan, J., Wellner, M.C., Rohwedel, J., Ji, G., Fleischmann, B., Katus, H.A., Hescheler, J., and Franz, W.M., 1997, Retinoic acid accelerates embryonic stem cell-derived cardiac differentiation and enhances development of ventricular cardiomyocytes. *J. Mol. Cell. Cardiol.* **29**, 1525-1539.

17. Assady, S., Maor, G., Amit, M., Itskovitz-Eldor, J., Skorecki, K.L., and Tzukerman, M., 2001, Insulin production by human embryonic stem cells. *Diabetes* **50**, 1691-1697.
18. Rambhatla, L., Chui, C-P., Kundu, P., Peng, Y., and Carpernter, M.K., 2003, Generation of hepatocyte-like cells from human embryonic stem cells. *Cell Transplantation* (in press).
19. Levenberg, S., Golub, J.S., Amit, M., Itskovitz-Eldor, J., and Langer, R., 2002, Endothelial cells derived from human embryonic stem cells. *Proc. Natl. Acad. Sci. USA.* **99** (7), 4391-4396.
20. Kaufman, D.S., Hanson, E.T., Lewis, R.L., Auerbach, R., and Thomson, J.A., 2001, Hematopoietic colony-forming cells derived from human embryonic stem cells. *Proc. Natl. Acad. Sci USA.* **19**, 10716-10721.
21. Schuldiner, M., Yanuka, O., Itskovita-Eldor, J., Melton, D., and Benvenisty, N., 2000, Effects of eight growth factors on the differentiation of cells derived from human embryonic stem cells. *Proc. Natl. Acad. Sci USA.* **97** (2), 11307-11312.
22. Bianchi, G., Muraglia, A., Daga,A., Corte,G., Cancedda, R., and Quarto R. 2001, Microenvironment and stem cell properties of bone marrow-derived mesenchymal cells. *Wound Repair and Regeneration.* **9** (6), 460-466.
23. Ferrari, G. 1998, Muscle regeneration by bone marrow-derived myogenic progenitors. *Science* **279**, 528-530.
24. Gussoni, E., 1999, Dystrophin expression in the mdx mouse restored by stem cell transplantation. *Nature* **401**, 390-394.
25. Jackson, K., 1999, Regeneration of ischaemic cardiac muscle and vascular endothelium by adult stem cells. *J. Clin. Invest.* **107**, 1395-1402.
26. Lin, Y., Weisdorf, D.J., Solovey, A., and Hebbel, R.P., 2000, Origins of circulating endothelial cells and endothelial outgrowth from blood. *J. Clin. Invest.* **105**, 71-77.
27. Asahara, T., 1999, Bone marrow origin of endothelial progenitor cells responsible for postnatal vasculogenesis in physiological and pathological neovascularisation. *Circ. Res.* **85**, 221-228.
28. Petersen, B.E. 1999, Bone marrow as a potential source of hepatic oval cells. Science 284 1168-1170.
29. Theise, N.D., 2000, Derivation of hepatocytes from bone marrow cells in mice after radiation-induced myeloablation. *Hepatology* **31**, 235-240.
30. Lagasse, E., 2001, Purified hematopoietic stem cells can differentiate into hepatocytes in vivo. *Nature Med.* **6**, 1229-1234.
31. Krause, D.S., 2001, Multi-organ, multi-lineage engraftment by a single bone marrow-derived stem cell. *Cell* **105**, 369-377.
32. Kawada, H., and Ogawa, M., 2001, Bone marrow origin of hematopoietic progenitors and stem cells in murine muscle. *Blood* **98**, 2008-2013.
33. Clarke, D.L., 2000, Generalized potential of adult neural stem cells. *Science* **288**, 1660-1663.
34. Digirolamo, C.M., Stokes, D., Colter, D., Phinney, D.G., Glass, R., and Prokop, D.J., 1999, Propoagation and senescence of human marrow stromal cells in culture: a simple colony-forming assay identifies samples with the greatest potential to propagate and differentiate. *Br. J. Haematol.* **107** (2), 275-281.
35. Pittenger, M.F., MacKay, A.M., Beck, S.C., Jaiswal, R.K., Douglas, R., Mosca, J.D., Moorman, M.A., Simonetti, D.W., Crqaig, S., and Marshak, D.R., 1999, Multilineage potential of adult human mesenchymal stem cells. *Science* **284**, 143-146.
36. Ying, Q.-L., Nichols, J., Evans, E.P., and Smith, A.G. 2002, Changing potency by spontaneous fusion. *Nature* **416**, 545-547; advance online publication, 13 March 2002 (DOI 10.1038/nature729).

37. Tarada, N., Hamazaki, T., Oka, M., Hoki, M., Mastalerz, D. M., Nakano, Y., Meyer, E. M., Morel, L., Petersen, B. E., and Scott, E. W., 2002, Bone marrow cells adopt the phenotype of other cells by spontaneous fusion. *Nature* **416**, 542-545; advance online publication, 13 March 2002 (DOI 10.1038/nature730).
38. Pells, S., Di Domenico, A.I., Gallagher, E.J., and McWhir, J., 2003, Multipotentiality of neuronal cells following spontaneous fusion with ES cells and nuclear reprogramming *In Vitro Stem Cells and Cloning* (in press).
39. Jiang, Y., Jahagirdar, B.N., Reinhard, R.L., Schwartz, R.E., Keene, C.D., Ortiz-Gonzalez, X., Reyes, M., Lenvik, T., Blackstad, M., Du, J., Aldrich, S., Lisberg, A., Low, W.C., Largaespada, D.A., and Verfaillie, C., 2002, Pluripotency of mesenchymal stem cells derived from adult marrow. *Nature* **418** (6893), 41-49.
40. Reyes, M., Lund, T., Lenvik, T., Aguir, D., Koodie, L. and Verfaillie, C.M., 2001, Purification and ex-vivo expansion of post natal human marrow mesodermal progenitor cells. *Blood* **98**, 2615.
41. Jiang, Y., Vaessen, B., Lenvik, T., Blackstad, M., Reyes, M., and Verfaillie, C.M., 2002, Multipotent progenitor cells can be isolated from postnatal murine bone marrow, muscle and brain. *Experimental Hematology* **30**, 896-904.
42. Alvarez-Buylla A., and Garcia-Verdugo, J.M., 2002, Neurogenesis in adult subventricular zone. *J. Neurosci.* **22**, 629-634.
43. Gage, F., 2002, Neurogenesis in adult brain. *J. Neurosci.* **22**, 612-613.
44. Seaberg, R.M., and van der Kooy, D., 2002, Adult rodent neurogenic regions: The ventricular subependyma contains neural stem cells but the dentate gyrus contains restricted progenitors. *J. Neurosci.* **22**, 1784-1793.
45. Clarke, D., Johansson, C., Wilbertz, J., Veress, B., Nilsson, E., Karlstrom, H., Lendahl, U., and Frisen, J., 2000, Generalized potential of adult neural stem cells *Science* **288**, 1660-1663.
46. Bjornson, C., Rietze, R., Reynolds, B., Magli, M., and Vescovi, A., 1999, Turning brain into blood: a hematopoietic fate adopted by adult neural stem cells *in vivo*. *Science* **283**, 534-537.
47. Tortella, D., Gewurz, B.E., Furman, M.H., Schust, D.J., and Ploegh, H.L., 2000, Viral subversion of the immune system. *Ann. Rev. Immunol.* **18**, 861-926.
48. Wekerle, T., Kurtz, J., Bigenzahn, S., Takeuchi, Y., and Sykes, M., 2002, Mechanisms of transplant tolerance induction using costimulatory blockade. *Curr. Opinion in Immunol.* **14**, 592-600.
49. Wekerle, T., and Sykes M., 2001, Mixed chimerism and transplantation tolerance. Annu. *Rev. Med.* **52**, 353-370.
50. Fandrich, F., Lin, X., Chai, G.X., Shulze, M., Ganten, D., Bader, M., Holle, J., Huang, D-S., Parwaresh, R., Zavazava, N., and Binas, B., 2002, Preimplantation-stage stem cells induce long-term allogeneic graft acceptance without supplementary host conditioning. *Nature Med.* **8** (2), 171-178.
51. OsirisTherapeuticsInc.website,www.osiristx.com/Technology/Technology_UniversalCell.ht
52. Verma, S., Rajaratnam, J.H., Denton, J., Hoyland, J.A., and Byers, R.J. 2002, Adipocytic proportion of bone marrow is inversely related to bone formation in osteoporosis. *J. Clin. Path.* **55**, 693-698.

HUMAN EMBRYONIC OR ADULT STEM CELLS: AN OVERVIEW ON ETHICS AND PERSPECTIVES FOR TISSUE ENGINEERING

Philippe R. Henon
Département d'Hématologie and Institut de Recherche en Hématologie et Transfusion, Hôpitaux de Mulhouse, 87 Avenue d'Altkirch, Mulhouse, France

ABSTRACT

Over the past few years, research on animal and human stem cells has experienced tremendous advances which are almost daily loudly revealed to the public on the front-page of newspapers. The reason for such an enthusiasm over stem cells is that they could be used to cure patients suffering from spontaneous or injuries-related diseases that are due to particular types of cells functioning incorrectly, such as cardiomyopathy, diabetes mellitus, osteoporosis, cancers, Parkinson's disease, spinal cord injuries or genetic abnormalities. Currently, these diseases have slightly or non-efficient treatment options, and millions of people around the world are desperately waiting to be cured. Even if not any person with one of these diseases could potentially benefit from stem cell therapy, the new concept of "regenerative medicine" is unprecedented since it involves the regeneration of normal cells, tissues and organs which could allow to treat a patient whereby both, the immediate problem would be corrected and the normal physiological processes restored, without any need for subsequent drugs.

However, conflicting ethical controversies surround this new medicine approach, inside and outside the medical community, especially when human embryonic stem cells (h-ESCs) are concerned. This ethical debate on clinical use of h-ESCs has recently encouraged the research on "adult" stem cells (ASCs) regarded as a less conflicting alternative for the future of regenerative medicine.

1. STEM CELL DEFINITIONS

Stem cells are unspecialized cells that can either self-renew indefinitely or differentiate into more mature cells with specialized functions.

Table 1. Stem Cell Definitions

Type of Stem Cells	Capacities and roles	Examples
TOTIPOTENT	Directly issued from the zygote divisions from the embryo, from day 0 to day 4	Zygote and immediate daughter cells
PLURIPOTENT	Give rise to all human tissue cells (about 200 cell types), but unable to form a human in his whole	♦Embryonic cells (ESC) in the blastocyte ♦Embryonic germ cells (EGS) in fœtus before the 8th week
MULTIPOTENT	Give rise to different cell lineages	♦Hematopoietic stem cells (HSC) ♦Mesenchymal stem cells (MSC)
UNIPOTENT	Can only give rise to one Differential cell lineage	♦Immature oligodendrocytes ♦Keratinocytes

In fact, the generic term "stem cells" covers a variety of cells with important morphological, biological and functional differences. These cell varieties are reported in Table 1.

Depending on their subtype, so-called stem cells can be identified in the inner mass of the blastocyt, in some of the fetus tissues, in umbilical cord and in placenta, and seemingly in several adult organs.

2. HUMAN EMBRYONIC STEM CELLS

2.1 Sources of h-ESCs

h-ESCs are found in the inner cell mass of the blastocyt which is the first organized stage of the embryo, lasting from the 4th to the 7th day after egg fertilization. From the 7th day, when *in utero* implantation occurs, ESCs are engaged in the formation of three embryonic layers: ectoderm, mesoderm, endoderm, and beside, the germinal cells (Fig. 1). However, at this point, they cannot produce a human in his whole.

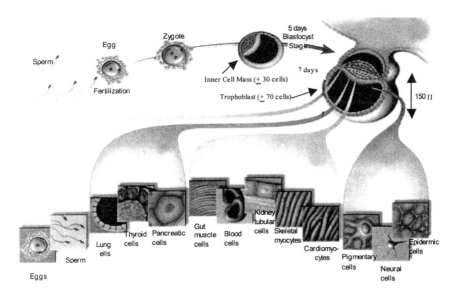

Figure 1. Schema of embryogenesis.

Recent technologies have been developed that now allow to extract h-ESCs from the inner cell mass, for their further *in vitro* culture under appropriate conditions[1]. In these conditions, ESCs have shown an indubitable ability to self-renew continuously, i.e. to produce more identical cells that are pluripotent. Sustained h-ESCs lines stemming from a single cell capable to proliferate through 300 to 400 population-doubling cycles can thus be established and propagated for more than 2 years now, without any apparent genetic change. Such h-ESCs lines could therefore constitute a permanent and convenient source of ESCs to be used for regenerative medicine.

Another possible source of h-ESCs would be to create embryos *de novo* using the same technique as that used for reproductive cloning in animals, the somatic cell nuclear transfer (SCNT) technique[2]: the nucleus of a donor's ovocyte (containing its DNA) is removed and replaced with the nucleus (and its DNA) of a somatic cell (ex. a skin or a blood cell) from the recipient. The ovocyte containing the transferred nucleus can then be engaged into the dividing cycle until it reaches the blastocyt stage, from which the inner cell mass can be removed and cultured as described above. The advantage of this technique is that it could allow to create histo-compatible h-ESCs, overcoming the problem of immune rejection in a given person.

2.2 Limitations and Risks of h-ESCs Culturing

These techniques would, ideally, provide potentially unlimited sources of cells capable *in vitro* of further differentiation in view of transplantation therapies. However, put aside the various divergent ethical opinions which will be examined later, these techniques could present some limitations and risks.

First, the culture conditions required so far to keep h-ESCs from differentiating include growing them on a layer of so-called "feeder cells" (mouse embryonic fibroblasts) in a medium containing fetal calf serum. Although these feeder cells are inactivated by irradiation so they cannot divide and expand, they can still produce various growth factors that sustain h-ESCs proliferation.[1] However, such an *in vitro* culturing, using animal-derived products, presents risks of spreading viruses or other infectious agents normally not found in humans, as prions for example. Thus it would be essential to establish feeder- and serum-independent culture conditions to both permit propagation on large scale of h-ESCs in culture and at the same time avoid the potential risk of animal infectious agents transfer to the ESCs[3].

Another important concern is that h-ESCs in tissue culture give rise, all at once, to a mixture of cell types[4]. When removed from feeder layers and transferred to suspension culture, ESCs form indeed multicellular aggregates of differentiated as well as undifferentiated cells called "embryonic bodies": cell differentiation is often anarchic and mostly variable from one embryonic body to another within the same culture[5].

But even once these technical obstacles will have been overcome, two crucial risks should be subject to a vigilant monitoring. The most hazardous, and not the least, is the possibility that transplantation of differentiated h-ESCs derivatives into human recipients may result in the formation of ESCs-derived tumors. In his original paper, J. Thomson has thus shown that h-ESCs injected into mice gave growth to teratomas. Although h-ESCs maintained undifferentiated in culture for more than 2 years have shown a stable and normal number of chromosomes[1], it does not mean that ESCs lines will not be subject to random mutations that affect all cell lines as they age. Keeping in mind that theoretically one mutation can occur every time a human or animal cell divides, a cell dividing approximately 200 times in culture could be expected to experience as many different mutations[6]. Even if it does not appear to be a significant malignant tumor formation in a small number of studies reporting on experimental transplantation of differentiated cells derived from murine ESCs in adult rodents[7,8], these studies, not specifically designed to address this question, lack of sufficient animal numbers and, overall, long-term surveillance to allow firm conclusions[3]. Therefore, one must be extremely vigilant on the long-lasting integrity of existing h-ESC lines and should favour the permanent development of new h-ESC lines in the future, which would furthermore allow to increase the genetic diversity of cells proposed for further transplantation.

However, immune rejection could be the most foreseeable and serious obstacle to successful transplantation of h-ESCs and their derived tissues. Major histo-compatibility (MHC) proteins that help the immune system identify an invader, have been claimed not to be expressed in ESCs. Therefore, it has been suggested that ESCs would provoke less immune reaction than a whole-organ transplant. But it is not clear whether this will be true for the regenerated tissues derived from h-ESCs. For example Drukker et al.[9] have measured the amount of fluorescence that showed up in 3 stages of ESCs development after their exposition to fluorescent-tagged antibody that attaches the MHC molecules: undifferentiated ESCs; so-called embryoid bodies that form as ESCs begin to differentiate; teratoma formed by differentiated ESCs. A non-embryonic stem cell line called HeLa was tested as control. The investigators have found very low, but consistant expression of MHC class I molecules on the undifferentiated ESCs; although the levels were not as high as in the teratomas and the HeLa cells, they were high enough to probably trigger an immune rejection.

Thus, it is likely that therapies preventing immunologic rejection will have to be systematically applied after h-ESCs transplantation. With the present knowledge, the easiest would be to still use immuno-suppressive drugs, as it has been done for decades in case of allogeneic hematopoietic stem cell or solid organ transplants. Unfortunately, those drugs currently available are associated with numerous complications, either immediate like GVHD or opportunistic infections, or delayed, such as secondary lymphomas. If such a risk can be acceptable in the treatment of fatal diseases as leukemia or heart failure, eventually curing a non-fatal (at least at short-term) although discomfortable disease, for example diabetes mellitus or

Parkinson's, at the expense of a new one likely more severe, would be difficult to justify.

Therefore, new methods limiting the immune response have to be developed. The most sophisticated one would consist in engineering h-ESCs to reduce their immunogenecity. Several techniques are already theoritically considered. For example, h- ESCs could be genetically altered to either eliminate foreign MHC genes or to replace them with others specifically matched to a particular transplant recipient[10,11] Another possibility would be to use the somatic cell nuclear transfer technology (see above) which would lead to h-ESC derived cells that are an exact genetic match to the recipient[2]. Establishing hematopoietic chimerism by non-myeloablative therapy followed by simultaneous or successive transplantation of hematopoietic stem cells and a second tissue derived from the same ESCs line, could avoid the rejection of the second tissue since it would be regarded as "self" by the induced chimeric system[12]; no long term treatment with immunosuppressive drugs would then be necessary.

However, all these techniques have still to be proven as actually feasible, efficient and safe in humans. Additional experimental researches using big animal models are thus previously required to determine which one(s) would be the most appropriate.

3. ETHICS

Evidently, as demonstrated above, it will still be a long way from the bench to the clinical use of h-ESCs or derived tissues. The development of transplantation therapies from h-ESC lines, once established pure cultures of specific cell type, will indeed require to test their physiologic function and methods to prevent rejection, and to demonstrate both their efficacy and their safety in non-human primate models. Despite the public's misunderstanding impression that clinical applications of such new therapies in humans are certain and imminent, one must in fact consider that stem cell research is still in its infancy.

But even though all technical problems could be rapidly resolved, a major obstacle to h-ESC research and clinical use is represented by strong oppositions from ethical, moral or religious groups. Particularly, the concept of therapeutic cell cloning, consisting in a deliberate *in vitro* procreation of human embryos with the sole goal to use them as tissue factories, prompts, all around the world, torrid and sometimes irrational discussions rising scientists against representatives of those religions who argue the premise that h-ESC research and further clinical use will inevitably destroy potential human lifes. Furthermore, the debate is largely polluted by the obsessive fear to implicitly open the way to human reproductive cloning, requiring basically the same technology and which is almost universally rejected (Table 2).

Table 2. ETHICS: Divergent Religons' View on Research and Clinical Use of ESC

Religions	ESC Research	Therapeutic Cell Cloning	Reproductive Cell Cloning
CATHOLIC	Prohibited (life begins at conception)	Prohibited	Prohibited
ORTHODOX	Prohibited (life begins at conception)	Prohibited	Prohibited
PROTESTANTS	Acceptable (if conducted reasonably and ethically)	Acceptable	Prohibited
MUSLIM	Acceptable (fœtus has moral existence only at the end of the 4th month)	Acceptable	Prohibited
JEWISH	Acceptable (embryo has no moral status until 40 days)	Acceptable	Acceptable (in case of sterility)
BUDDHIST	Prohibited (life begins at conception)	Prohibited	Acceptable (if no genomic modification)

The approach which proposes to dispose of, rather than destroy, supefluous cryopreserved embryos which will definitely not be reimplanted for reproductive purpose, could somewhat be better accepted for creation of new h-ESC lines. Arguing that it would be morally better to use these unumployed embryos as a gift and to participate this way in the perpetuation of our species by treating and perhaps curing debilitating diseases, would indeed be more easily receivable by many. Several governemental authorities have already accepted this approach, when others only hypocritically authorize importation of embryos or/and h-ESC lines conceived in other countries.

Other standpoints are most ambiguous. For example, the US government authorized, on August 2001, US public research to only use h-ESC lines already existing worldwide at this time (approximately 82 cell lines), when private groups are free to experiment any kind of h-ESC research, except reproductive cell cloning. Table 3 summarizes the policies which are presently defined all around the world. But things are evolving fast under the public pressure.

Table 3. Summary of Policies Presently Defined Around the World

Countries	Therapeutic Cell Cloning (=creating embryo)	Use of Stem Cell Lines	Use of Superfluous Embryos
France, Spain	Prohibited	Probably authorized in a near future	Authorized (with restrictions)
Italy, Austria, Ireland	Prohibited	Prohibited	Prohibited
U.K., Denmark	Authorized	Authorized	Authorized
Israel, Sweden, Belgium, India	Prohibited	Authorized	Authorized
Germany	Prohibited	Authorized (imported)	Prohibited
U.S.A	Prohibited (public) Free (Private)	Authorized under Restrictive conditions (Public) Free (Private)	Authorized (in most states)
Canada	Prohibited	under consideration	under consideration
Japan, Netherlands, Korea	Authorized last fall	Authorized last fall	Authorized last fall
Australia	Currently Prohibited but under consideration	Authorized	Authorized

On the other hand, the success story of bone marrow and since the mid-eighties, of blood stem cell transplant, has recently paved the way to transplantation of somatic stem cells which seemingly also exhibit developmental potential heretofore not considered possible. It is now conceivable that many erroneous functions can be corrected through transplantation of an appropriate amount of cultured or engineered "adult" stem cells. Ethical advantages of such an approach are evident, since adult stem cells would be collected either from volunteer adult donors in the allogeneic setting or, still even better, from the patient himself, which would furthermore avoid any deleterious immunologic reaction after transplantation. Of course, opponents of human embryos destruction warmly applaud this approach that they strongly encourage to develop.

4. ADULT STEM CELLS

4.1 Definition

So called "Adult Stem Cells" (ASCs) are undifferentiated cells that occur in differentiated tissues in theoritically the adult body but in fact from birth. They can renew themselves in the body, making identical copies of themselves for the lifetime of the organism, or become specialized to yield the cell types of the tissue of origin. Thus, they are presently considered as multipotent stem cells. They are rare, often difficult to identify and to purify, and when grown in culture, are difficult to maintain in the undifferentiated state. Sources of ASCs presently known include skin, brain, skeletal muscle, pancreas, liver, the eye, dental pulp, the limit of the grastro-intestinal tract and, maybe the most important, bone marrow and blood.

Bone marrow is a composite tissue that contains both an hematopoietic parenchyma and a stroma constituted of different cell types such as fibroblasts and endhotelial, fat, and smooth muscle cells. It is classically admitted that all these cell lineages derive from dedicated multipotent stem cells: hematopoietic stem cells for the hematopoietic tissue and mesenchymal stem cells for the stroma.

4.2 Hematopoietic Stem Cells (HSCs)

HSCs are among the very few stem cells to have been presently fully phenotypically identified and isolated in mice. If it is not so in humans, since their exact phenotype is still harmly debated, a small population of cells certainly containing those capable of long term repopulating of bone marrow is now identified. But it was a long story since Maximow postulated in 1909 that "lymphocyte act as a common stem cell and migrates through tissues to seed in appropriate microenvironments"[13], and Papenheim hypothesized in 1917 "the existence of an undifferentiated stem cell giving rise to all blood cells via an intermediate state of progenitor cells"[14]. After a long period of silence, different groups in the 1950's showed in experimental animals either that hematopoietic recovery could occur from transplanted bone marrow after irradiation damage[15-17], or that the shielding of part of the hematopoietic tissue during lethal total body irradiation resulted in the subsequent reconstitution of the marrow in the irradiation areas[18]. Therefore, the basic concept of bone marrow transplantation was born, rapidly reinforced by the identification in splenic mouse of the cell type responsible for BM-transplant success[19]. These experimental results were further exploited and applied in humans at the end of the 60's by Donnal Thomas and his group (Seattle,

USA) who first realized successful allogeneic bone marrow transplants on a large scale, making this technique uncirconvenable in the treatment of leukemias, inherited blood disorders and certain immune diseases. Almost 10 years later, G. Santos, (Baltimore, USA), N.C. Gorin (Paris, France) and others applied the same transplant technology in the autologous setting.

In parallel, other investigators evidenced during the sixties the presence in blood of either mice[20] or of dogs[21] of mononuclear cells capable to reconstitute bone marrow hematopoiesis, thus introducing the concept of "blood stem cell". But things progressed slowly until the Goldman's group demonstrated in the early 1980's that blood progenitor cells collected at the hypercytic phase of CML, before any treatment, could restore autologous hematopoiesis when reinfused after myeloablative therapy[22]. And while Civin discovered in 1984 the CD34 antigen as a marker of hematopoietic progenitor cells in human bone marrow[23], several groups in different parts of the world[24-28] carried out almost simultaneously in the mid 80's clinical experiments in humans, showing that reinfusion of mobilized autologous blood progenitor cells produced a satisfactory and permanent reconstitution of hematopoiesis.

And still more recently, Gluckman and Broxmeyer demonstrated in 1988 the feasibility of umbilical cord blood cell transplants[29].

4.3 Adult Stem Cell Plasticity

Therefore, the historical success of blood and bone marrow transplants, now performed by the thousands every year all around the world, both inspired the hope that many diseases could someday be treated with appropriate stem cell therapy and seemingly confirmed the long-standing biological dogma - that specific organic tissues always derived from dedicated multipotent stem cells. However, there is a growing body of evidence for a few years that these tissue-specific stem cells could, at least under certain circumstances, be reprogrammed and eventually match the versatility of ESC, thus differentiating into lineages other than their tissue of origin. Such a broader differentiation repertoire introduces the very new and provocative concept of adult stem cell "trans-differentiation" or "plasticity".

This dramatic reappraisal was triggered by a paper published in early 1999 which reported that, after transplantation into irradiated mice, genetically labeled neural stem cells were found to produce a variety of blood cell types including myeloid cells as well as early hematopoietic cells[30]. Thus, neural stem cells could have a wider differentiation potential than previously thought. But, the considerable and unusual engraftment across MHC barriers and the significantly delayed engraftment observed in this model, associated to the fact that another experiment using a population of neural stem cells derived from a *single* progenitor cell failed to generate any blood cells[31], put this work in the position of an isolated finding at this point of time.

However, further investigators have soon rushed into the gap thus open in the dogma of multipotent adult stem cells inalienably dedicated. Clarke et al.[32] showed that neural stem cells from the adult mouse brain could contribute to the formation of chimeric chick and mouse embryos and give rise to cells of all germ layers. This would demonstrate that an adult neural stem cell seemingly has a very broad developmental capacity and thus might potentially be used to generate a variety of cell types for transplantation in different diseases. But here again, the impact of this study is limited by the fact that the pups were allowed to survive only through embryonic day 11, which is too early to tell whether the brain-derived cells could really be functional.

Going back to HSCs, several groups have recently brought strong arguments on their transdifferrentiation capacities. For example, Jackson et al. transplanted first 2000 murine HSCs, phenotypically characterized as $CD34-/^{lo}$, $c-kit^+$, $Sca-1^+$, and isolated from males, into lethally irradiated female mice[33]. Once stable hematopoietic engraftment was achieved, these transplanted mice were rendered ischemic by transient coronary artery occlusion followed by reperfusion. Interestingly, the engrafted HSCs or their progeny spontaneously migrated into ischemic cardiac muscle and blood, where they differentiated both to cardiomyocytes, found primarily in the peri-infarct region at a prevalence of around 0.02%, or to endothelial cells found at a prevalence of around 3.3% in small vessels adjacent to the infarct. D. Orlic et al. also observed that $CD34^+$, Lin^-, $C-kit^{hi}$ enriched bone marrow cells, injected directly in the myocardium 48 hours after experimental ischemic damage, gave rise near the site of injection to cells exhibiting the markers and morphology of immature cardiomyocytes, endothelial cells and smooth muscle cells[34]. The injected hearts showed a 35% improvement of their function, with appearance of neo-angiogenesis into the injured zone. Kocher et al. also purified bone marrow $CD34^+$, Lin^-, $C-kit^{hi}$ cells, that contrarily to the above investigators, they injected into the bloodstream of mice 48 hours after experimental myocardium ischemic damage: they further saw an engraftment in both the neo-vasculature of the repairing myocardium and the improvement of post-infarct cardiac function[35]. Still more impressive, Lagasse et al. have injected in the bloodstream of 9 irradiated FAH-knockout mice, a model of fatal hereditary tyrosinemia - a lethal liver defect - as few as 50 $c-kit^{hi}$, Thy^{lo} $Sca-1^+$ Lin^- (KTSL) BM cells, purified at a rate of 95 - 98%[36]. The transplanted KTSL population first restored hematopoiesis in 4 of the 9 mice, but also seemed to secondarily cure them of their liver disease; effectively, when these mice were killed 7 months after the cell reinfusion, between a third and a half of their liver tissue were derived from KTSL population. The transfer of such small numbers of cells very carefully phenotypically characterized leading to the acquisition of a novel function, could constitute an almost equivocal demonstration of HSC transdifferentiaton (or plasticity).

However, once carried out the initial fit of enthusiasm that one can experience faced with such seemingly convincing and concordant data, the reality of defined types of stem cell transdifferentiation appears highly questionable. First, not one study showed a cell purification > 98%; it is easy to understand that a single alien cell in ostensibly purified cell concentrates could produce misleading results. Furthermore, multiple "purified" cells have been reinjected in all the above studies; but proving cell plasticity requires to demonstrate that a single well characterized donor cell is capable to create a "sole" population and not just a scattering of cells in the new tissue.

Therefore, Krause et al. have attempted to meet this requirement by performing a two stage study: they first injected dye-tagged male mouse blood stem cells into irradiated females, then they killed the recipients and pulled out tagged cells that had homed in BM. They secondly implanted a *single* of these tagged cells into each of a 2nd group of female mice which were killed 11 months later: their histochemical examination showed that some of the progeny of the transplanted single cell had been incorporated into various tissues, including lung (up to 20% pneumocytes), skin, intestine, liver, bone and blood. Thus, a proof that a single blood stem cell can actually give rise to multiple cell types seems to be clearly administered by this study, reinforcing the cell plasticity thesis[37].

However, two more recent studies, published at the same time in Nature challanged this thesis, both suggesting that what can appear as adult stem cell *reprogramming* might instead be *cell fusion*[38,39]. Indeed, when adult mice bone marrow or brain cells were cultivated together with ESCs, the two cell types occasionally formed hybrid cells that looked like ESCs but showed twice the normal number of chromosomes, being thus likely genetically instable. But the practical significance *in vivo* of such an *in vitro* phenomenon must be moderated as it implies to co-culture adult and embryonic stem cells, a situation which would not be encountered *in vivo* in case of adult stem cell transplantation alone. The fusion danger might rather result from a clinical reimplantation of ESCs in damaged tissues, which of course would represent a strong limitation of the method.

More disturbing is the study very recently reported by the Weissman's group, who generated chimeric animals by transplantation of a single green fluorescent protein-marked HSC into lethally irradiated non-transgenic recipients[40]. Such single HSCs robustly reconstituted peripheral blood leucocytes in these animals, but did not actually contribute to non-hematopoietic tissues, which would signify that spontaneous "transdifferentiation" of circulating HSCs and/or their progeny is an extremely rare event, if it occurs at all. In fact, two critical determinants should thus be required for transdifferentiation triggering: preliminary tissue damage and high level of circulating or reinfused HSCs.

4.4 Mesenchymal Stem Cells (MSCs)

MSCs are stem cell-like precursors that are known to physiologically give rise to collagen, muscle, cartilage and bone; they also act as support cells that are important in the differentiation and growth of HSCs[41]. Although representing a very small cell population into the bone marrow, MSC can be easily isolated and grown in *in vitro* cultures. Furthermore, when transplanted in an allogeneic setting, they seem not to be rejected by the recipient-immune system, nor to stimulate immune or allergic responses. These properties are being currently explored for regenerative medicine: MSCs are thus experimented as support for allogeneic HSCs transplantation, but overall, their injection in large animal models has been shown to participate in the regeneration of injured connective tissues such as bone, cardiac muscle or meniscus, and even, in appropriate conditions, of injured brain parenchyma[42].

However, not all MSCs could be actually subject to such a broad differentiation capacity. Indeed, C. Verfaillie and her group have recently identified in mice rare and tiny cells co-purified with MSCs and which can differentiate, at the single level, not only into MSCs but also into cells of the three germ layers[43]. They called these cells multipotent adult progenitor cells or MAPCs. When injected into a blastocyt, single MAPCs contribute functionally to most somatic tissues. Robust, early and persistent engraftment of hematopoietic lineages in addition to the epithelium of the liver, lung and gut occurred *in vivo* when MAPCs were transplanted into non-irradiated recipients. The same group has also demonstrated that MAPCs from post-natal human bone marrow were progenitors for angioblasts, thus contributing to angiogenesis[44] and also could differentiate into functional hepatocyte-like cells, even producing urea[45]. However, MAPCs do not seem capable to develop skeleton, heart or brain, at least in physiological situation; maybe they could spring into action in the heart or the brain in response to injury. Even it it would not be so, MAPCs might thus be adult stem cells that really do show plasticity, capable to dedifferentiate in culture to become pluripotent. As such, they might be an ideal source for therapy of numerous inherited or degenerative diseases. Reactions to the whole of this work are tremendously enthusiastic. But, similar results have now to be reproduced by other teams and extended to big animals before MAPCs could be used for clinical assays in humans.

4.5 Clinical Experimental Assays Using Autologous ASCs in Humans

Benefiting of experimental data from rodents' studies, several clinical investigators have overpassed the expected increment of knowledge and the big animal experimental-step highly recommended by many, and have started phase-I assays in humans suffering from post-ischemic cardiac failure. One group has used autologous myoblasts previously isolated from sketelal muscle and expanded *in vitro*, then reinjected directly around and inside the infarcted zone during by-pass surgery[46]. Although a significant improvement of the cardiac function was observed in 9 out of 10 patients, myoblasts are only capable to give rise to myocytes, but not to angioblasts and endothelial cells which are required for revascularisation of the infarcted zone. They are in fact only unipotent stem cells. Furthermore, it seems that the potential of contractility of the expanded myoblasts progeny was somewhat different from the own contractility of the cardiac muscle, which probably explain cardiac rythm troubles observed in several of the transplanted patients.

All other groups have used mononuclear cells "purified" from autologous whole bone marrow, which were rapidly reinjected either directly intra myocardium[47,48] or by intra-coronary catheterism[49]. All groups reported an improvement of the cardiac function. However, the scientific value and accuracy of these clinical assays are extremely weak as such "purified" mononuclear cells contain, in fact, HSCs as well as MSCs or other progenitors: it is thus impossible to determine which type of progenitor cell could be responsible for cardiac improvement.

In the full assurance of our huge expertise in the field of peripheral blood stem cells, we personally have started in cardiac patients a phase-I protocol exploiting the multipotent potential of $CD34^+$ cells harvested in the peripheral blood. Total $CD34^+$ cells are indeed reknown to contain, apart "true" hematopoietic progenitor cells programmed for permanent hematopoiesis self-renewal ($CD34^+38^-$), other subsets characterized either as angioblasts ($CD34^+133^+$) or endothelial progenitor cells ($CD34^+KDR^+$), both involved in the angiogenesis process, and also muscle cell progenitors. Once reinjected into the myocardic ischemic lesion, one can then expect that these $CD34^+$ subsets will reconstitute at least partially, a functional myocardic tissue.

5. CONCLUSION

Stem cell research would probably offer unprecedented opportunities in developing new treatments for debilitating diseases or tissue injuries for which there are few or no cure. The two main options focusing either on ESCs or ASCs, which scientifically are complementary, should certainly be pursued in parallel and substantially funded by public organisms. Both have their specific advantages and inconveniences.

Theoretically, h-ESCs research would open larger fields for further therapeutic developments. Studies from animals show that ESCs are clearly capable of developing into multiple tissue types and of long-term self renewal in culture and also *in vivo*, which have not yet been conclusively demonstrated for ASCs. But studies with human stem cells are essential to make progress in the development of therapies for human diseases. Although much can be learned using the few existing human cell lines, it still remains important concerns about the risks of long term genetic mutation or alteration of biologic properties of these cell lines, which could determine clinical aberrations once their progeny has been transplanted *in vivo*. The answers to these concerns should be brought by continued monitoring of the existing cell lines, but also by the continuous development of new cell lines in the near future. Furthermore, even if embryonic bodies derived from human cell lines are capable to produce *in vitro* cells featuring for various tissues (cardiomyocytes, pigmented and non-pigmented epithelial cells, neural cells, liver and pancreas cells...), they always occur among a mixture of other cell types, variable from an embryonic body to another. Overall, no one has yet demonstrated any *in vivo* reconstitution of an organ with its physiological function in its whole, with cells derived from ESCs in either humans or experimental animals. Thus, new biochemical, tissue culture, and molecular biology techniques are required to control and limit differentiation towards a specific organ. Also, scientific efforts, including manipulation of MHC genes or somatic cell nuclear transfer should be actively pursued in parallel to prevent posttransplant immune rejection, which still represent a substantial obstacle.

Thus, it is still far away from the bench to routine regenerative therapies from ESCs, all the more since the use of embryos as ESCs source is hotly controversial on ethical, moral, political or religious grounds.

On the contrary, ASCs do not raise such controverses especially in the autologous setting. For a long time now, $CD34^+$ HSCs, harvested either from bone marrow or peripheral blood, have proven to be multipotent adult stem cells capable to give rise to all blood lineages. Even if they are seemingly capable to also differentiate into few amounts of endothelial and muscle progenitors, it is not clear if it is actually through a phenomenon of transdifferentiation rather than due to a mixture of different types of progenitor cells, all bearing the CD34 antigen while already dedicated towards different tissues since embryonic or fetal stages. MAPCs might be better candidates as a proof for ASC plasticity, unless they can be in fact ESCs preserved at adult age. However it may be, the environment in which ASCs can grow or are placed to grow has certainly an important, but poorly understood effect on their fate. Their actual potential of migration to injured tissues, which might provide more flexibility in choosing where to transplant them and more predictability about where they will home after transplant, has to be precisely determined. Furthermore, activated ASCs themselves also secrete cytokines that can secondarily mobilize or protect other cells residing into the targeted-tissue and could increase even more the salutary effects of the transplant.

It is true that conclusive experiments establishing the exclusive role of ASCs to produce tissues different from those they are theoritically dedicated to are still lacking. However, it does not seem ethically shocking and scientifically irrational to conduct henceforth clinical pilot studies - while continuing developmental researches at the bench - during which autologous ASCs easily yielded in humans and purified at the highest possible rate (even still including a few other residual cells) will be implanted in severely diseased or injured organ in the hope that they will give rise to the mature functional cells needed by that organ. Any significant posttransplant improvement of the organ function would strongly emphasize such an approach and trigger new developments of the ASCs knowledge concerning for example their adhesion and homing mechanisms, their rate of differentiation into a new tissue, their potential of local persistence and survival in the injured organ. It could also encourage the improvement of adjuvant techniques as ASCs culture and expansion, allowing to then obtain enough cells from a small initial cell sample for a fast and safe transplantation. In a recent past, performing blood stem cell transplantation in a more or less empiric manner (at least at the beginning) had thus boosted researches on the phenotypic nature of HSCs and, more generally on hematopoiesis mechanisms, including cytokines, and had also largely facilitated the further development of gene therapy. It was a clear demonstration that combination of clinical and more fundamental research constitutes the two conniving arms of medical progress.

REFERENCES

1. Thomson, J.A., Itskovitz-Eldor J, Shapiro, S., Waknitz M.A., Swiergiel, J.J., Marshall, V.S., and Jones, J.M., 1998, Embryonic stem cell lines derived from human blastocysts. *Science* **282**, 1145-1147.
2. First, N.L., and Thomson, J., 1998, From cows stem therapies? *Nat. Biotechnol.* **16**, 620-621.
3. Odorico, J.S., Kaufman, D.S., and Thomson, J.A., 2001, Multilineage differentiation from human embryonic stem cell lines. *Stem Cells* **19**, 193-204.
4. Reubinoff, B.E., Per, M.F., Fong, C.Y., Trounson, A., and Bongso, A. 2000, Embryonic stem cell lines from human blastocysts: somatic differentiation *in vitro*. *Nat. Biotechnol* **18**, 299-404.
5. Itskovitz-Eldor, J., Schulding, M., Karesenti, D., Eden, A., Yanuka, O., Amit, M., Soreq, H., and Benvenisty, N., 2000, Differentiation of human embryonic stem cells into embryoid bodies comprising the three embryonic germ layers. *Mol. Med.* **5**, 88-95.
6. Kunkel, T.A., and Bebenek, K., 2000, DNA replication fidelity. *Annu Rev. Biochem.* **69**, 497-529.
7. Klug, M.G., Soonpaa, M.H., Koh, G.Y. *et al.*, 1996, Genetically selected cardiomyocytes from differentiating embryonic stem cells from stable intracardiac grafts. *J. Clin. Invest.* **98**, 216-224.
8. McDonald, J.W., Liu, X., Qu, Y. *et al.*, 1999, Transplanted embryonic stem cells survive, differentiate and promote recovery in injured rat spinal cord. *Nat. Med.* **5**, 1410-1412.
9. Drukker, M., Katz, G., Urbach, A. *et al.*, 2002, Characterization of the expression of MHC proteins in human embryonic stem cells. *PNAS* **99**, 9864-9865.
10. Westphal, C.H., and Leder, P., 1997, Transposon-generated « knock-out » and « knock-in » gene-targeting constructs for use in mice. *Curr. Biol.* **7**, 530-533.
11. Hardy, R.R., and Malissen, B., 1998, Lymphocyte development. The (knock) ins and outs of lymphoid development (Editorial). *Curr. Opin. Immunol.* **10**, 155-157.
12. Spitzer, T.R., Delmonico, F., Tolkoff-Rubin, N. *et al.* 1999, Combined histocompatibility leukocyte antigen-matched donor bone marrow and renal transplantation for multiple myeloma with end stage renal disease : the induction of allograft tolerance through mixed lymphohematopoietic chimerism. *Transplantation* **68**, 480-484.
13. Maximow, A., 1909, Der lymphozyt als gemeinsame Stammzelle der verschiedenen Blutelemente in der embryonalen Entwicklung und im postfetalen Leben der Saugetiere. *Folia Haemat* (Lpz), 8.
14. Pappenheim, A., 1917, Prinzipien der neueren morphologischen Haematozytologie nach zytogenetischer Grundlage. *Folia Haemat.* **99**, 21-91.
15. Lorenz, E. Uphoff, D., Reid, T.R., and Shelton, E., 1951, Modification of irradiation injury in mice and guinea pigs by bone marrow injections. *J Natl Cancer Inst*, **12**, 197-202.
16. Ford, C.E., Hamerton, J.L., Barnes, D.W.H., and Loutit, J.F., 1956, Cytological identification of radiation-chimeras. *Nature* **177**, 452-460.
17. Nowell, P.C., Cole, L.J., Habermeyer, J.G., and Roan, P.L., 1956, Growth and continued function of rat marrow cells in irradiated mice. *Cancer Res.* **16**, 258-265.
18. Micklem, H.S., Anderson, N., and Ross, E., 1975, Limited potential of circulating haemopoietic stem cells. *Nature* **256**, 41-44.
19. Till, J.E., and McCulloch, E.A., 1961, A direct measurement of the radiation sensitivity of normal mouse bone marrow cells. *Radiat. Res.* **14**, 213.

20. Goodman, J.W., and Hodgson, G.S., 1962, Evidence for stem cells in the peripheral blood of mice. *Blood* **19**, 702-14.
21. Cavins, J.A., Scheer, S.C., Thomas, E.D., and Ferrebee, J.W., 1964, The recovery of lethally irradiated dogs given infusions of autologous leukocytes preserved at −80°C. *Blood* **23**, 38-43.
22. Haines, M.E., Goldmann, J.M., Worsley, A.M. *et al.* 1984, Chemotherapy and autografting for patients with chronic granulocytic leukaemia in transformation : probable prolongation of life for some patients. *Br. J. Haematol.* **58**, 711-722.
23. Civin, C., Strauss, L.C., Brovall, C., Fackler, M.J., Schwartz, H., and Shaper, J.H., 1984, Antigenic analysis of hematopoiesis. III. A hematopoietic progenitor cell surface antigen defined by a monoclonal antibody raised against KG-Ia cells. *J.Immunol.* **133**, 157-165.
24. Juttner, C.A., To, L.B., Haylock, D.N., Brandford, A., and Kimber, R.J., 1985, Circulating autologous stem cells collected in very early remission from acute non-lymphoblastic leukaemia produce prompt but incomplete haematopoietic reconstitution after high-dose melphalan or supralethal radiotherapy. *Br.J.Haematol.* **61**, 739-745.
25. Reiffers, J., Bernard, Ph., and David, B., 1986, Successful autologous transplantation with circulating haemopoietic stem cells in a patient with acute leukaemia. *Exp.Hematol.* **14**, 312-315.
26. Körbling, M., Dorken, B., Ho, A.D., Pezzuto, A., Hunstein, W., and Fliedner, T.M., 1986, Autologous transplantation of blood-derived hemopoietic stem cells after myeloblative therapy in a patient with Burkitt's lymphoma. *Blood* **67**, 529-532.
27. Kessinger, A., Armitage, J.O., and Landmark, J.D., 1986, Use of autologous cryopreserved peripheral stem cells to shorten marrow aplasia after high dose therapy for patients with advanced breast cancer and bone marrow metastases. *Proc. Am. Soc. Clin. Oncol.* **5**, 245
28. Debecker, A., Hénon, Ph., Lepers, M., Eisenmann, J.C., Selva, J., 1986, Collection de cellules circulantes en sortie d'aplasie post-chimiothérapique dans les leucémies aigues. *Nouv. Rev. Fr. Hematol.* **28**, 287-292.
29. Gluckman, E., Broxmeier, H.E., Auerbach, A.D. *et al.*, 1989, Hematopoietic reconstitution in a patient with Fanconi's anemia by means of umbilical cord blood from an HLA-identical sibling. *N. Engl. J. Med,* **321**, 1174-1178.
30. Bjornson, C.R.R., Rietze, R.L., Reynolds, B.A., Magli, M.C., and Vescovi, A.L., 1999, Turning brain into blood : A hematopoietic fate adopted by adult neural stem cells in vivo. *Science* **283**, 534-537.
31. Morshead, C.M., Benveniste, R., Iscove, N.N. *et al.*, 2002, Hematopoietic competence is a rare property of neural stem cells that may depend on genetic and epigenetic alterations. *Nat. Med.* **8**, 268-273.
32. Clarke, D.L., Johansson, C.B., Wilbertz, J. *et al.*, 2000, Generalized potential of adult neural stem cells. *Science* **288**, 1660-1663.
33. Jackson, K.A., Majka, S.M., Wang, H. *et al.*, 2001, Regeneration of ischemic cardiac muscle and vascular endothelium by adult stem cells. *J.Clin.Invest.* **107**, 1395-1402.
34. Orlic, D., Kajstura, J., Chimenti, S. *et al.*, 2001, Bone marrow cells regenerate infarcted myocardium. *Nature* **410**, 701-705.
35. Kocher, A.A., Schuster, M.D., Szabolcs, M.J. *et al.*, 2001, Neovascularization of ischemic myocardium by human bone-marrox-derived angioblasts prevents cardiomyocyte apoptosis, reduces remodeling and improves cardiac function. *Nat. Med.* **7**, 430-436.
36. Lagasse, E., Connors, H., Al-Dhalimy, M. *et al.*, 2000, Purified hematopoietic stem cells can differentiate into hepatocytes in vivo. *Nat.Med.* **6**, 1229-1234.

37. Krause, D.S., Theise, N.D., Collector, M. *et al.*, 2001, Multi-organ, multi-lineage engraftment by a single bone marrow-derived stem cell. *Cell* **105**, 369-377
38. Terada, N., Hamazaki, T., Oka, M. *et al.*, 2002, Bone marrow cells adopt the phenotype of other cells by spontaneous cell fusion. *Nature* **416**, 542-545.
39. Ying, Q.Y., Nichols, J., Evans, E.P., and Smith, A.G., 2002 Changing potency by spontaneous fusion. *Nature* **416**, 545-548.
40. Wagers, A.J., Sherwood, R.I., Christensen, J.L., and Weissmann, I.L., 2002, Little evidence for developmental plasticity of adult hematopoietic stem cells. *Science* **297**, 2256-2259.
41. Prockop, D., 1997, Marrow stromal cells as stem cells for non-hematopoietic tissues. *Science* **276**, 71-74.
42. Jin, H.K., Carter, J.E., Huntley, G.W., and Schuchman, E.H., 2002, Intracerebral transplantation of mesenchymal stem cells into acid sphingomyelinase-deficient mice delays the onset of neurological abnormalities and extends their life span. *J.Clin.Invest.* **109**, 1183-1191.
43. Jiang, Y., Jahagirdar, B.N., Reinhardt, R.L. *et al.*, 2002, Pluripotency of mesenchymal stem cells derived from adult marrow. *Nature* **418**, 41-49.
44. Reyes, M., Dudek, B., Jahagirdar, B., Koodie, K., Marker, Ph., and Verfaillie, C.M., 2002, Origin of endothelial progenitors in human postnatal bone marrow. *J. Clin. Invest.* **109**, 337-346.
45. Schwartz, R.E., Reyes, M., Koodie, L. *et al.*, 2002, Multipotent adult progenitor cells from bone marrow differentiate into functional hepatocyte-like cells. *J.Clin.Invest.* **109**, 1291-1302.
46. Menasche, P., Hagege, A.A., Scorsin, M. *et al.*, 2001, Myoblast transplantation for heart failure. *Lancet* **357**, 279-280.
47. Hamano, K., Nishida, M., Hirata, K. et al., 2001, Local implantation of autologous bone marrow cells for therapeutic angiogenesis in patients with ischemic heart disease : clinical trial and preliminary results. *Jpn.Circ.J.* **65**, 845-847.
48. Porcellini, A., Reimers, B., Azzarello, G., Pascotto, P., and Vinante, O., 2002, Intramyocardial inoculation of autologous bone marrow cells in patients with refractory myocardial ischemia. *Blood*, **100** (suppl. 1), 217a (Abstract).
49. Strauer, B.E., Brehm, M., Zeus, T. *et al.*, 2002, Repair of infarcted myocardium by autologous intracoronary mononuclear bone marrow cell transplantation in humans. *Circulation* **106**, 1913-1918.

STEM CELL BIOLOGY AND PLASTICITY

Emin Kansu
Hacettepe University, Institute of Oncology, Ankara, Turkey

1. INTRODUCTION

Multipotent stem cells are found in mature tissues and are formed by the body to replace worn out cells in tissues and organs.[1,2] Stem cells in the bone marrow, called hematopoietic stem cells form the various kinds of blood cells. Neural stem cells form the brain and central nervous system. Mesenchymal stem cells form fat, bone, muscle and cartilage. Multipotent stem cells are sometimes called somatic or adult stem cells.[1-5]

Within last twenty years several in-vitro techniques have been developed to isolate, clone and grow stem cells in soft agar or methylcellulose-based media. Utilizing special Petri dishes into which the stem cells are seeded virtually all three hematopoietic lineages can be grown including erythroid, myeloid and megakaryocytic colonies.

2. TYPES AND FEATURES OF STEM CELLS

Hematopoietic stem cells (HSCs) are present in peripheral blood, bone marrow and cord-blood and are capable to give rise to blood and immune system cells. HSCs can be enriched using several techniques and can be cultured in clonogenic (colony-assay) or expansion culture-assays. The culture of choice will depend on the goal of the scientist to fully characterize the stem cells or simply increase the number of progenitors. Colony assays have been widely used for a wide variety of clinical and research applications. HSCs can be induced in-vitro to form stem cell colonies provided that the appropriate growth factors or colony-stimulating factors (CSFs) have been incubated and present in the culture media (Figure 1).

The potential uses of hematopoietic stem cells (HSCs) in the therapy of human diseases continue to progress very rapidly. In last three decades, HSCs are utilized to treat the chemotherapy or chemo-radiotherapy induced myelosuppression as well as in the treatment of hematologic malignancies, solid tumors and non-malignant diseases.

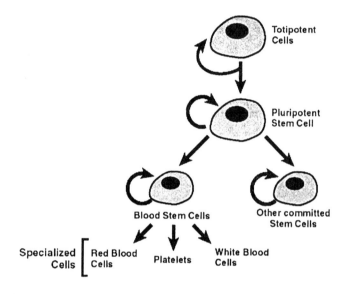

Figure 1. Stem cells (obtained from ref. no. 35; NIH Strategies for Implementing Human Embryonic Stem Cell Research. *NIH Report*, March 8, 2002).

2.1 Cord Blood Stem Cells

Umbilical cord blood contains neonatal and a rich concentration of stem cells. These cells are pluripotent and are capable of differentiating into various cell types such as hematopoietic cells (blood and immune system-forming cells). These properties of cord blood stem cells are similar to those shown by embryonic stem cells. However, unlike embryonic stem cells, umbilical cord blood stem cells are abundant, easily collected and are not highly immunogenic. This source is abundant, easily collected and is free from moral and ethical concerns. Stem cells from cord blood have been used in stem cell transplantation procedures in the treatment of life-threatening or debilitating diseases. Parents choose to preserve umbilical cord blood for many reasons. They may have an immediate family member who requires a stem cell transplant and their baby's cord blood may be an appropriate source of stem cells for treatment of the disease. Parents may decide to store cord blood because their family's medical history may indicate there is an increased risk of disease. Finally, some parents decide to preserve their child's cord blood as a protective precaution should it ever be needed as a stem cell source for the child from which it was obtained or another family member[6-10].

2.2 Embryonic Stem Cells

Embryonic stem cells (ESCs) are pluripotent cells derived from blastocysts that can be propagated indefinitely undifferentiated in vitro, can differentiate to all cell lineages in vivo and can be induced to differentiate to all cell lineages in vivo, and can be induced to differentiate to most cell types in vitro. ESCs are derived from the inner cell mass of the blastocyst that is the early developmental stage of the embryo prior to its implantation in the uterus wall. As well studied and widely recognized ESCs are able to differentiate into cells from all three embryonic germ layers that is defined as pluripotency. ESCs similar to other stem cell types are highly capable of self-renewal, maintain a full diploid karyotype and generate any tissue when introduced into an embryo (Figure 2)[4-8].

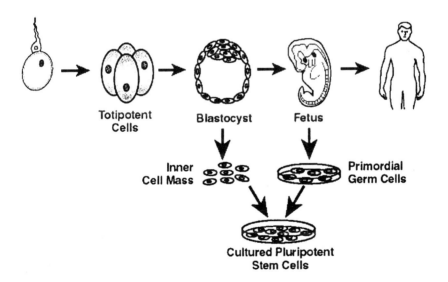

Figure 2. Embryonic stem cells (obtained from ref. no. 35; NIH Strategies for Implementing Human Embryonic Stem Cell Research. *NIH Report*, March 8, 2002).

ESCs are unrestricted in their pattern of differentiation mainly to the somatic and germ cell lineages. ESCs can also be manipulated to differentiate into a diversity of cell types. It is commonly practiced that ESCs be cultured on feeder cells and the cells pile up maintaining discrete colonies on top of the feeder layers. The ESC lines usually are maintained at relatively high densities to obtain high growth rate in order to minimize spontaneous differentiation. The initial choice of cells is from the blastocyst stage embryo. Blastocysts are grown in culture in standard tissue-culture media and usually do not require special reagents. The recovery of stem cells usually is in the range of 10 to 30%, and commonly many embryos are lost and wasted. Following the use of the best methods for the culture of blastocysts, pluripotential stem cell colonies have to be accurately identified using cellular morphology and careful observation of growth patterns.

Although ES cells have been isolated from humans, their use in research as well as therapeutics is encumbered by ethical considerations. The ability to purify, culture and manipulate multipotent stem cells from nonembryonic origin would provide investigators with an invaluable cell source to study cell and organ development. In addition, such cells could serve to develop replacement tissues for congenital or degenerative disorders. Stem cells have been identified in most organ tissues, including hematopoietic, neural, gastrointestinal, epidermal, hepatic and mesenchymal stem cells (MSCs)[5-8,10-12,17-19].

2.3　Mesenchymal Stem Cells

Mesenchymal Stem Cells (MSCs) were identified and it was shown that when bone marrow (BM) is plated in fetal calf serum (FCS) containing medium, colonies of adherent fibroblast like cells develop that differentiate into bone and adipocytes. Since then, several investigators have shown that these cells can also differentiate into chondrocytes, adipocytes and at least in rodents, skeletal myocytes. MSCs can be purified on the basis of their ability to adhere to plastic. Expansion of cells from postnatal BM that can differentiate at the single-cell level not only into MSCs, but also into cells of visceral mesodermal origin, such as endothelium, which are defined as mesodermal progenitor cells (MPCs)[20-22].

Embryonic stem cells have been utilized in applied research to provide a source of stem cells for the amelioration and treatment of human diseases that cannot be treated by conventional techniques and modalities. In view of their pluripotency many investigators initiated very promising research projects exploring theurapeutic potentials of ESCs. It was soon reported that when ESCs are exposed to appropriate "cocktail" of growth factors, and "inducers" in the in-vitro cultures, they were able to differentiate into myocytes, neural cells, hepatocytes, endothelial cells and even to adipocytes (Figure 3)[15,16].

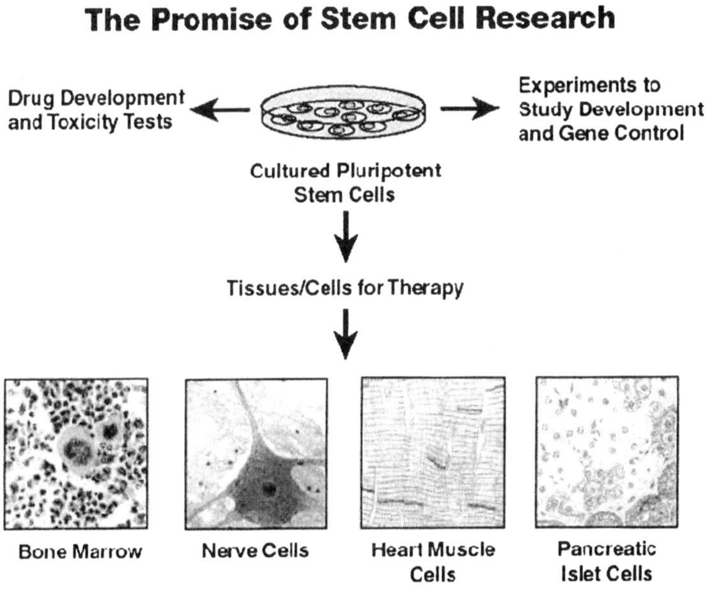

The Promise of Stem Cell Research

Drug Development and Toxicity Tests ← Cultured Pluripotent Stem Cells → Experiments to Study Development and Gene Control

↓

Tissues/Cells for Therapy

↓

Bone Marrow | Nerve Cells | Heart Muscle Cells | Pancreatic Islet Cells

Figure 3. Stem cell plasticity (obtained from ref. no. 35; NIH Strategies for Implementing Human Embryonic Stem Cell Research. *NIH Report*, March 8, 2002).

In principle, ECSs can make every cell in the body and they can make a differentiated cell. Researchers at the Columbia University showed directed differentiation of mouse ESCs into spinal progenitor cells and motor neurons. In recent experiments it has been demonstrated that working with ESCs have advantages over adult stem cells in which researchers can use normal developmental patterns as a guide in developing strategies for controlled differentiation.

The high potential of stem cells for generating non-hematopoietic cells for tissue repair and in regenerative medicine several studies are underway to explore these issues.

3. DEFINITION OF STEM CELL PLASTICITY

The ability of tissue –specific stem cells to differentiate to cell types different from the tissue of origin has been defined as *"stem cell plasticity"*.

Some explanations have been proposed for stem cell plasticity; a) persistence of multipotent stem cells in post-natal life, b) de-differentiation and re-differentiation of stem cells, c) presence of multiple tissue specific stem cells in different organs, and d) fusion of donor cells and resident cells[29-31].

Most studies of adult stem cell plasticity have used mouse models. Using (immune-deficient) SCID/beige mice, human adult stem cells derived from bone marrow or cord blood when injected in various tissues human donor cells repopulated both the bone marrow and liver tissue of recipient mice. Recent research studies have demonstrated that adult stem cells can exhibit a much wider potential for development and differentiation.

The extensive capacity of HSCs to maintain their numbers by self-renewal mechanisms clearly support the notion that stem cell population do not go through senescence process. Adult HSCs that constitute approximately 0.01% of the bone marrow population are long-lived cells.

4. APPLICATIONS OF STEM CELLS

In last five years it has been demonstrated that adult stem cells can differentiate in various lineages. Mouse ESCs were noted to have the ability to produce new strains of animals with specific genetic changes, and their capacities to differentiate into multiple lineages in in-vitro cultures. When the differentiation of embryoid bodies continues, a variety of cell types including endothelial, muscle, neuronal, hematopoietic and hepatic with high potential of adult and embryonic features[15-21].

Nowadays most clinicians and basic scientists are trying to develop techniques for application of human ESCs in cell-based replacement therapies. This type of approach can replace diseased or "damaged" tissue or cell populations. Although, the research in this area is in its infancy, long-term outcome of such experiments could be highly revolutionary in regenerative medicine[20-24].

The notion of using adult stem cells in some therapies is very attractive. Methods for transplanting stem cells need to be developed. It will be crucial to ensure that the transplanted cells are located in the tissues and function properly in heart, neural tissues and other organs. Studies done last four years provided the evidence that transplanted mouse ESCs can relieve Parkinson's disease and partially restore neural function in animals with spinal-cord injuries.

5. REGULATORY ISSUES IN STEM CELL RESEARCH

The use of embryonic stem cells in regenerative medicine raises ethical, legal and social concerns among the public. Regenerative medicine to overcome various chronic diseases will involve the implantation of normal tissue cells in patients with damaged organs. These stem cell-based therapies can be broadly implemented for diseased individuals with Parkinson's disease, Alzheimer's disease diabetes mellitus, spinal cord-injuries, osteoarthritis. These new approaches may also offer another advantage of overcoming the problem of tissue rejection in transplantation. Somatic-cell nuclear transfer technique could produce a lineage of stem cells that are genetically identical to the donor[24-27].

The wide spectrum of social, political, legal, economical, philosophical and ethical topics must be discussed in detail by the policy makers and specially formed administrative bodies. When President Bush announced their federal policy in 2001, it became quite clear that embryonic stem cell lines will be restricted for research and a national advisory or regulatory committee should be established to oversee policies in stem cell research[23,28-30].

In the United States, the NIH is implementing a policy permitting Federal funding of research on ongoing and existing human embryonic stem cell lines that fulfill President Bush's eligibility criteria:
1) NIH will not fund derivation of embryonic stem cells,
2) Embryonic stem cells will only be obtained from in-vitro fertilization embryos which are in excess of clinical need,
3) No profit is to be made by donors or clinics on the donation of embryos, and
4) Documentation of full informed consent by the donors is necessary.

The Canadian Institutes of Health Research (CIHR) released guidelines allowing publicly funded stem cell research on "surplus" embryos created at fertility clinic and donated with informed written consent of the donors. In 2001, United Kingdom became the first country clearly to allow the creation of embryos as a source of stem cells. Regulations were approved in 2001, enabled scientists to use embryonic stem cells for practical uses other than reproduction[31-35].

The American Society of Hematology (ASH) published a report urging that therapeutic cloning techniques and research avenues not to be limited to ban human reproductive cloning. Given the potential of stem cells United States Congress and the administration should allow scientists to pursue research in animals and in cultured cells[36,37].

REFERENCES

1. Jouneau, A., and Renard J.P., 2002, Cellules souches embryonnaires et clonage therapeutique. *Medecine et Sciences* **18**, 169-180.
2. Weissman, I.L., 2000, Stem cells: units of development, units of regeneration and units in evolution. *Cell* **100**, 157-168.
3. Thompson, E.M., Legouy, E., and Renard, J.P. 1998, Mouse embryos do not wait for the BMT: chromatin and RNA polymerasere modeling in genome activation at the on set of development. *Dev. Genet.* **22**, 31-42.
4. Cibelli, J.B., Kiessling, A.A., Cunniff, K., Richards, C., Lanza, R., and West, M. 2001, Somatic cell nuclear transfer in humans: Pronuclear and early embryonic development. *Regen. Med.* **2**, 25-31.
5. Moore, K.A., *et al.*, 1997, In-vitro maintenance of highly purified, transplantable hematopoietic stem cells. *Blood* **89**, 4337-4347.
6. McDonald, J.W., *et al.*, 1999, Transplanted embryonic stem cells survive, differentiate and promote recovery in injured spinal cord. *Nature Med* **5**, 1410-1412.
7. Jackson, K.A., *et al.*, 1999, Hematopoietic potential of stem cells isolated from murine skeletal muscle. *Proc. Natl. Acad. Sci. USA* **96**, 14482-14486.
8. Keller, G., and Snodgrass, H.R., 1999, Human embryonic stem cells. The future is now. *Nature Med.* **5**, 151-153.
9. Annas, G.J., *et al.*, 1999, Stem cell politics, ethics and medical progress. *Nature Med.* **5**, 1339-1341.
10. Phillips, R.L., *et al.*, 2000, The genetic program of hematopoietic stem cells. *Science* **288**, 1635-1640.
11. Lagasse, E., *et al.* 2000, Purified hematopoietic stem cells can differentiate into hepatocytes *in vivo*. *Nature Med* **6**, 1229-1234.
12. Orkin, S.H., 2000, Stem cell alchemy. *Nature Med* **6**, 1212-1213.
13. Stem cell research and therapeutic cloning: an update. The Royal Society publication. Policy Document / November 2000.
14. Mieth D. Going to the roots of the stem cell debate. The ethical problems of using embryos for research. *EMBO Reports* **1**, 4-6, 2000. Silver LM. Reprogenetics : Third millenium speculation. The consequences for humanity when reproductive biology and genetics are combined. *EMBO Reports* **1**, 375-378, 2000.
15. The use of embryonic stem cells in therapeutic research. Report of the International Bioethics Committee on the ethical aspects of human embryonic stem cell research. April 2000.
16. Odorico, J.S., *et al.*, 2001, Multilineage differentiation from human embryonic stem cell lines. *Stem Cells* **19**, 193-204.
17. Orlic, D., *et al.*, 2001, Bone marrow cells regenerate infarcted myocardium. *Nature* **410**, 701-705.
18. Theise, N.D., *et al.*, 2001, Liver from bone marrow in humans. *Hepatology* **32**, 11-16.
19. Lebkowski, J.S., *et al.*, 2001, Human embryonic stem cells : culture, differentiation, and genetic modification for regenerative medicine applications. *Cancer J.* **7** (Suppl. 2), 583-594.
20. Bianco, P., *et al.*, 2001, Bone marrow stromal cells: nature, biology, and potential applications. *Stem Cells* **19**, 180-192.
21. Yoder, M.C., 2001, Spatial origin of murine hematopoietic stem cells. *Blood* **98**, 3-5.
22. Hao, Q-Lin, *et al.*, 2001, Identification of a novel human multilymphoid progenitor in cord blood. *Blood* **97**, 3683-3690.

23. Vogel, G., 2001, Rumors and trial balloons precende Bush's funding decision. *Science* **293**, 186-187.
24. Report of the Committee on the Biological and BioMedical Applications of Stem Cell Research. National Academy of Sciences USA Washington, D.C. June 2001.
25. Colman, A., and Burley, J.C., 2001, A legal and ethical tightrope. Science, ethics and legislation of stem cell research. *EMBO Reports* **2**, 2-5.
26. Cibelli, J.B., Lanza, R.P., West, M.D., and Ezzell, C., 2001, The first human cloned embryo. *Scientific American*, November 24.
27. Lachmann, P., 2001, Stem Cell Research Second Update. The Royal Society Policy Document. September 2001. Stem cell research-why is it regarded as a threat ? An investigation of the economic and ethical arguments made against research with embryonic stem cells. *EMBO Reports* **2**, 165-168.
28. Bush draws a stem cell line. Newsweek, August 20, 2001.
29. Stem cells and future of regenerative medicine. Committee on the Biological and Biomedical Applications of Stem Cell Research, Board on Life Sciences-National Research Council and Board on Neuroscience and Behavioral Health-Institute of Medicine. Washington, D.C. National Academy Press, 2002.
30. Panel on Scientific and Medical Aspects of Human Reproductive Cloning. Scientific and medical aspects of human reproductive cloning. Washington, D.C. Natural Academy Press, 2002.
31. Weissman, I.L., 2002, Stem cells-scientific, medical and political Issues. *New Engl. J. Med.* **346**, 1576-1579.
32. Evers, K., 2002, European perspectives on therapeutic cloning. *New Engl. J. Med.* **346**, 1579-1582.
33. Körbling, M., Katz, R.L., Khanna, A., Ruifrok, A.C., *et al*. 2002, Hepatocytes and epithelial cells of donor origin in recipients of peripheral-blood stem cells. *New Engl. J. Med.* **346**, 738-746.
34. Jlang, Y., Jahagirdar, B.N., Reinhardt, R.L., Schwartz, R.E., *et al*. 2002, Pluripotency of mesenchymal stem stem cells derived from adult marrow. *Nature*, 20 June 2002, 1-8.
35. *NIH Report*, NIH Strategies for Implementing Human Embryonic Stem Cell Research. March 8, 2002.
36. *ASH Report,* Hematology advocates urge congress to keep stem cell research avenues open. April 25, 2002.
37. Regulation of embryonic stem cell research update. *ISCT Newsletter* **9** (1), 17, March 2002.

LIVER TISSUE ENGINEERING: SUCCESSES & LIMITATIONS

Vivek Dixit[1] and Y. Murat Elçin[2]
[1]*Division of Digestive Diseases, Department of Medicine, David Geffen School of Medicine, University of California - Los Angeles, Los Angeles, California 90095-7019, U.S.A.;* [2]*Ankara University, Faculty of Science, Tissue Engineering and Biomaterials Laboratory, and Biotechnology Institute, Ankara 06100, Turkey*

1. INTRODUCTION

Tissue engineering is an emerging, multidisciplinary, biotechnology that combines the principles of Engineering and Cell Biology to facilitate the formation *de novo* tissues and organs[1]. This new scientific discipline is primarily targeted towards the creation of functional biological substitutes as opposed to inert implants. Barely two decades in existence, tissue engineering has recently emerged as a viable alternative approach to treat the loss, or malfunction of a structural tissues or organ such as skin, cartilage, bone and small blood vessels[2]. Liver tissue engineering, however, represents a more daunting challenge because, unlike the aforementioned structural organs, the liver is a highly complex metabolic organ and comprises of many components and cell types. Successful creation of functional liver tissue requires a precisely orchestrated synthesis of the vascular system, the liver's biliary system, and the liver's parenchymal, stellate and other structural cells to form liver tissue.

The liver is a unique organ in that it has the extraordinary capacity to regenerate following injury. It is well known that the liver fabricates new tissue and functional structures by processing signals which are pre-programmed into cells[3]. In this regard, stem cells are known to play a crucial role during embryonic development and organogenesis. Recently, liver stem cells have also been implicated in liver regeneration following severe injury to the liver[4]. Thus, by exploiting the regenerative capacity of liver cells, and the body's own reservoir of stem cells, and using appropriate biomaterials, it may be possible to create *de novo* liver tissue for replacement of diseased tissue.

2. EARLY STRATEGIES FOR LIVER TISSUE ENGINEERING

Initial strategies for liver tissue engineering involved the development of suitable polymeric biomaterials scaffolds or constructs for culturing liver tissue. Several synthetic and natural polymers have since been used with varying success[5]. Early approaches involved the culture of liver cells on specially prepared biomaterials that were chemically or biologically modified to support cell growth[6]. These early studies successfully demonstrated that modified synthetic, or natural, polymers could be enabled to support enhanced hepatocyte growth.

Freshly isolated hepatocytes or established cell lines were grown *ex vivo* within predesigned scaffolds made up of exogenous three-dimensional extracellular matrices (ECMs) (Figure 1). The scaffold is eventually resorbed, leaving only transplanted cells and the stroma.

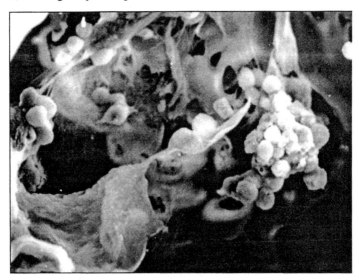

Figure 1. Freshly isolated hepatocytes can be seen growing on a polymeric scaffold composed of an extracellular matrix analogue.

It is well known that dissociated liver cells will re-assemble *in vitro* into structures that resemble the original tissue when provided with an appropriate environment. This approach may be used to engineer liver tissue growth, if the suitable ECMs can be incorporated into the scaffolds so as to bring isolated hepatocytes into contact with each other in an appropriate three-dimensional environment. Such scaffolds can provide sufficient mechanical support until the newly formed liver tissue, or liver organoids, are structurally stabilized, and can convey specific signals that will guide the expression of genes to form new liver tissue[7].

ECMs are important for localization and delivery of cells to specific body sites and maintenance of a three-dimensional space for new tissue formation. Synthetic ECMs can be designed as an attachment substrate and a delivery device for transplanted cells at specific sites of the body. To allow the delivery of a high density of cells, a large surface area-to-volume ratio is desirable. The ECM should maintain a potential space for tissue development and provide temporary mechanical support to withstand *in vivo* shear forces until the engineered tissue has sufficient mechanical integrity to support itself. Cell surface receptors interacting with the support material, interactions with the surrounding cells and the present growth factors of the environment can strongly effect the function of the seeded cells. Cell-adhesion peptides and growth factors can be incorporated into the synthetic ECM, or mechanical stimulation can be used to manipulate these factors[8].

2.1 Selection of Biodegradable Polymers Scaffolds

Biodegradable polymers with large surface area-to-volume ratio have been used in liver tissue engineering studies for more than a decade[9]. The chemical composition of the biomaterial and the biomechanics of the cell adhesion surface needs to be considered in developing such supports. To enhance cell adhesion the scaffold design can incorporate signaling peptides that affect hepatocyte regulation, function and reorganization. Ideally, the reorganization and expansion of transplanted cells should start during biomaterial degradation to yield in the formation of the uniform liver tissue organoids.

Homo- and heteropolymers of poly(glycolic acid) (PGA) and poly(lactic acid) (PLA) have been evaluated as synthetic ECM scaffolds for hepatocyte growth and reorganization. PGA-PLA blends were found to be suitable to extended hepatocyte culture and the cells retained differentiated function as measured by the rate of albumin and DNA syntheses[10]. Filamentous PGA sheets seeded with hepatocytes were transplanted into the mesentery of UDP-glucuronyl transferase-deficient Gunn rats; the specific hepatocyte function was then observed by determining bilirubin conjugates in bile[11]. We have also similarly reported the presence of conjugated bilirubin in the bile of Gunn rats when hepatocytes were transplanted in a Matrigel matrix within an alginate-poly L-lysine co-polymer microcapsule system[12].

Carbohydrate-modified poly(ethylene oxide) has been evaluated as a hepatocyte support and has exhibited sugar-specific attachment through the unique asialoglycoprotein receptors with considerable albumin production of the hepatocytes[13]. Heparin and lactose have also been similarly used to promote hepatocyte attachment and function on porous foams[14]. Hepatocytes on these substrates showed increased P450 monooxygenase activity and albumin production compared to their counterparts on collagen surfaces.

Hydrogel hollow fibers loaded with hepatocytes were transplanted intraperitoneally to Gunn rats without immunosuppression[15]. These encapsulation devices showed bilirubin conjugation in subjects and lowered the serum bilirubin levels, with minimal fibrosis. Chitosan, a glycoaminoglycan analogue, has been evaluated as an attachment substrate for rat and fetal porcine hepatocytes[7,16,17]. Modification of chitosan with collagen or albumin enhanced the biocompatibility, surface roughness and cell attachment characteristics of the glycosaminoglycan analogue polymer. The differences in attachment properties perhaps depends on the variable identification of surface receptors that recognize and bind specific amino acid sequences present in ECM molecules. Protein-modified chitosan surfaces provided a suitable environment for the metabolic activity of rat and fetal porcine hepatocytes, in terms of total protein and urea synthesis.

2.2 Cell Seeding

One of the major limitations in liver tissue engineering studies has been the insufficient survival of an adequate mass of transplanted cells. This problem has largely been related to seeding conditions that are sub-optimal. By pre-conditioning hepatocytes *in vitro* on degradable polymer scaffolds in a flow bioreactor prior to implantation, cell spheroids can be obtained with increased cell mass and function[18]. Thus, by using specifically designed flow perfusion systems, the cell survival, seeding efficiency and culture conditions (*e.g.* oxygen uptake) of hepatocytes can be improved significantly. The hepatocyte spheroids thus formed have shown liver-like morphology and preserved specific metabolic function, in terms of a high rate of albumin synthesis compared to static seeding conditions[19].

2.3 Hepatocyte Co-Culture Models

Several groups have developed co-culture and co–transplantation models based on hepatocytes and other types of cells, to improve the survival and function of the liver parenchymal cells.

Kneser et al.[20] have evaluated hepatocyte and pancreatic islet co-transplantation in polymeric matrices as an alternative non-invasive approach to hepatotrophic stimulation. Findings demonstrated the migration of alpha cells into the islet-surrounding hepatocytes, whereas beta cells remained immobile and the hepatocytes engrafted well. This procedure did not interfere with recipient glucose metabolism and did not induce hyperproliferative premalignant foci within the transplanted hepatocytes. This technique may be an attractive approach to hepatotrophic stimulation of bioartificial liver equivalents.

Naughton et al.[21] transplanted co-cultures of hepatocytes and liver stromal cells or bone marrow cells on three-dimensional polymer constructs to rats. The findings showed that association with stroma and the ECM and other products of these cells promotes the growth of hepatocytes in a stereotypic manner, with the generation of hepatic structures such as sinusoids.

2.4 Need for Angiogenesis

Although various groups have developed several specialized polymeric biomaterials that can sustain a high density of hepatocyte growth *in vitro*, a major challenge in liver tissue engineering has been the need to provide adequate nutrients and supply of oxygen to the newly formed liver organoids post-transplantation. Thus, several protocols developed for liver tissue engineering require liver cells to be grown on suitable biomaterials prior to transplantation in animals[22]. We have also utilized such procedures and realized that transplanted cells quickly die off unless the scaffolds bearing the hepatocytes are transplanted to sites that are highly vascularized prior to transplantation[23]. It is now apparent that a vascular network of dense capillaries is essential to support the survival and function of the liver organoids.

We have developed slow release methodologies for tissue angionenesis for such purposes[23]. Angiogenesis is the cellular assembly that results in growing of new blood vessels from a preexisting microvascular bed[24]. This event is controlled by autocrine and paracrine signals, in natural (*i.e.* wound healing, ischemia and female reproductive system) and pathologic conditions (*i.e.* tumor neovascularization, psoriasis and diabetic retinopathy).

2.5 Delivery of Angiogenic Factors

Studies in the last decade have shown that localized, site-specific delivery of angiogenic growth factors from degradable or nondegradable polymer devices can efficiently stimulate neovascularization[22,23]

Poly(lactide-co-glycolide), poly(anhydride), poly(ethylene-co-vinyl acetate), chitosan, alginate and collagen matrices have been developed for the delivery of angiogenic factors, *i.e.* vascular endothelial cell growth factor (VEGF), basic fibroblast growth factor (b-FGF), platelet-derived growth factor (PDGF), transforming growth factor-E (TGF-E), angiopoietins (Ang1 and Ang2) and coctails of endothelial cell growth factors.

2.6 Vascularization of Engineered Liver Organoid

The maintenance of tissue engineered liver organoids is a major issue in liver engineering. Previously, liver, spleen, lungs, mesentery, omentum and the peritoneal cavity were evaluated as vascular hepatocyte transplantation sites because of their high degree of vascularity. We have explored the possibility of transplanting hepatocytes attached to degradable scaffolds after vascularizing specific subcutaneous tissue flaps[22,23,25]. Using this approach, *ex vivo*-grown fetal porcine hepatocytes on chitosan scaffolds survived and exhibited differentiated function at the subcutaneous tissue flap of rats following neovascularization of the transplantation site and formed liver tissue-like structures from dissociated cells[7].

3. A NOVEL STRATEGY FOR LIVER TISSUE ENGINEERING

Our previous *in vitro* studies have successfully demonstrated the feasibility of creating liver tissue organoids from freshly isolated adult and fetal hepatocytes. However, these liver organoids could only survive for periods ranging from several days to weeks. Furthermore, by previously creating a vascularized bed prior to transplantation, liver organoids could be made to survive for slightly longer periods of time. However, these rudimentary liver tissue organoids could not be sustained indefinitely since they were created from isolated differentiated hepatocytes that had a limited lifespan. A major drawback with this approach was also the failure of the liver organoids to successfully integrate with the body's vascular system[7,22].

In an attempt to create *de novo* liver tissue *in vivo,* we have recently developed a novel strategy for liver tissue engineering that involved the use of putative liver stem cells[26]. This approach involves the use of a novel modified collagen-polypropylene (C-PP) composite scaffold, in a cone shaped configuration, that can be inserted into the liver with minimal bleeding and no mortality. Recently, we have also successfully tested this scaffold in a cylindrical configuration for multiple implants in larger animals.

Figure 2 below illustrates a scheme of the implantation procedure. Briefly, the C-PP scaffold was inserted into the medial lobe of the liver and secured to the organ using stabilizing disks as shown in the illustration.

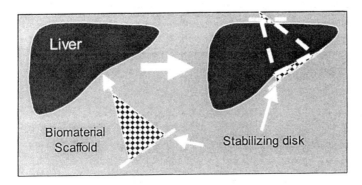

Figure 2. Scheme of scaffold implantation. C-PP scaffold is inserted into the medial lobe of the liver and secured in place with stabilizing disks.

Such implants can remain in place in the liver for more than 1 year, if necessary. Furthermore, such scaffolds can incorporate specialized polymer-immobilized biologically active factors (*e.g.*, hepatocyte growth factors and angiogenic factors) to stimulate tissue growth and enhance the proliferation of blood vessels within the implant.

The animals implanted with C-PP scaffolds were followed for up to one year post implantation. Selected preliminary morphological and histological evaluations are presented in Figures 3-5 below. Seven to 10 days following implantation of the C-PP scaffold extensive tissue growth inside the scaffold was seen. Control scaffold containing only the polypropylene skeleton structure component revealed a hollow dense connective tissue capsule around the scaffold wall (Figure 3).

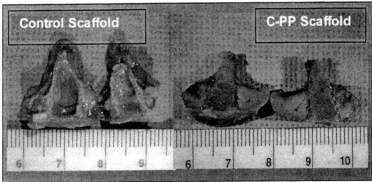

Figure 3. Extensive tissue growth inside the scaffold was seen 1 week following implantation of the C-PP scaffold. The control scaffold consisting only of the polypropylene skeleton component revealed a hollow dense connective tissue capsule around the scaffold wall.

Histological evaluation of the tissue within the C-PP scaffold revealed extensive neovascularization inside the scaffold. Interestingly, due to the thick connective tissue layer around the outside of the capsule, no liver tissue was in direct contact with the scaffold. Microscopic findings at 7-14 days after implantation showed loose network of connective tissue can be seen inside the C-PP scaffold (Figure 4).

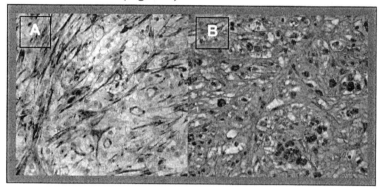

Figure 4. Immunohistochemical staining showing desmin-positive Stellate Cells (A) and OV-6 monoclonal rat antibody staining showing Oval Cells (B) inside the C-PP scaffold.

Approximately 3 months after implantation immunohistochemical staining of the tissue structure inside the C-PP scaffold revealed desmin-positive staining cells (Figure 4 A). These cells (brown staining) were identified as hepatic stellate cells because desmin is a known marker this cell type. Figure 4 B shows cells that stained brown with monoclonal anti-OV-6 antibody (Figure 4B). OV-6 is a well-known marker for hepatic oval cells (*or hepatic stem cells*), that can differentiate into hepatocytes and bile duct cells.

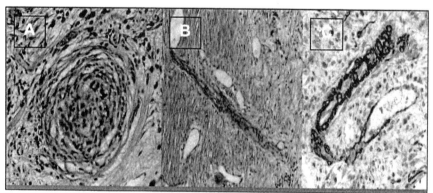

Figure 5. After 6-8 months following C-PP scaffold implantation rudimentary *de novo* liver tissue can be seen scattered throughout the inside of the scaffold. These liver structures can be seen as circular nodules (A), hepatic cylinders (B), and bile duct-like structures (C) that stained positive with OV-6 monoclonal rat antibodies.

After 6-8 months the cells inside the scaffold had differentiated into rudimentary nodules that may have contained both mature and immature hepatocytes (Figure 5 A and B). Some of these cells also revealed a large number of alpha-fetoprotein positive cells as well as cells that stained positive with OV-6 rat monoclonal antibody (*this data is not presented here*). At this time, these rudimentary nodules were scattered throughout the scaffold and appeared like rudimentary liver tissue with bile ducts, and juxtaposed to blood vessels, and bile duct-like cells (Figure 5 C).

These studies are the first reported observations of early stages of *de novo* liver tissue formation using the C-PP scaffold. The C-PP scaffold is a suitable tissue engineering scaffold supporting the development of *de novo* liver tissue growth *in vitro*. Thus, it is possible that the C-PP scaffold, or other similar scaffolds modified with hepatocyte growth factors and angiogenic growth factors, can play an important role in studying the biology of liver organogenesis in the adult animal.

4. FUTURE STRATEGIES IN LIVER TISSUE ENGINEERING

The field of liver tissue engineering is barely in its infancy. However, with the ongoing development of new natural and synthetic biomaterials for scaffolds, and their subsequent modification with hepatotrophic growth factors it may be possible to create sufficient mass of *de novo* liver *in vivo*. Current technology is able to produce only small amounts of liver tissue. Furthermore, this is a slow process taking as much as 8-12 months for new liver tissue to develop. This is a very long period and may not be appropriate for practical application at this time. The need for optimization of such scaffolds using liver specific and angiogenic growth factors will be necessary to shorten the time to create new liver tissue. Furthermore, the identification and characterization of hepatic stem cells involved in new liver tissue formation will also be necessary. Finally, liver tissue engineered with this technology needs to be tested in suitable models of liver disease such as cirrhosis and metabolic liver diseases. Such studies should allow for better "engineering" of the scaffold for optimal liver tissue formation. Such studies are currently ongoing in our laboratory.

ACKNOWLEDGEMENTS

This work was supported in part by a seed grant to Vivek Dixit, Ph.D., from the Stein-Oppenhiemer Foundation. Y. Murat Elçin, Ph.D., acknowledges the support of the Turkish Academy of Sciences, in the framework of the Young Scientist Award Program (EA-TÜBA-GEBİP/ 2001-1-1), and Ankara University Biotechnology Institute, Ankara, Turkey. The authors would also like to thank Professor Stewart Sell, Department of Pathology and Laboratory Medicine Division of Experimental Pathology, Albany Medical College, New York, for supplying the antibody OV-6, and Ms. Adrianna Hekiert, for excellent technical assistance.

REFERENCES

1. Griffith, L., and Naughton, G., 2002, Tissue engineering -- Current challenges and expanding opportunities. *Science* **295**, 1009-1014.
2. Lanza, R.P., Langer, R., and Chick, W.L., 1997, *Principles of Tissue Engineering.* Academic Press, Austin, TX.
3. Michalopoulos, G.K., and DeFrances, M.C., 1997, Liver regeneration. *Science* **276**, 60-66.
4. Petersen, B.E., Bowen, W.C., Patrene, K.D., Mars, W.M., Sullivan, A.K., Murase, N., Boggs, S.S., Greenberger, J.S., and Goff, J.P., 1999, Bone marrow as a potential source of hepatic oval cells. *Science* **284**, 1168-1170.
5. Elçin, Y.M., Dixit, V., and Gitnick, G., 1998, Hepatocyte attachment on biodegradable modified chitosan membranes : In vitro evaluation for the development of liver organoids. *Artif. Organs* **22**, 837-846.
6. Dixit, V., Piskin, E., Arthur, M., Denizli, A., Tuncel, S., Denkbas, E., and Gitnick, G., 1992, Hepatocyte immobilization on PHEMA microcarriers and its biologically modified forms. *Cell Transplantation* **1**, 391-399.
7. Elçin, Y.M., Dixit, V., Lewin, K., and Gitnick, G., 1999, Xenotransplantation of fetal porcine hepatocytes in rats using a tissue engineering approach. *Artif. Organs* **23**, 146-152.
8. Elçin, Y.M., 1998, Tissue engineering of liver: review. In *Biomedical Science and Technology*, (Hincal and Kas, Eds.), Plenum Press, NY, USA, pp. 109-116.
9. Mooney, D.J., Park, S., Kauffmann, P.M., Sano, K., McNamara, K., Vacanti, J.P., and Langer, R., 1995, Biodegradable sponges for hepatocyte transplantation. *J. Biomed. Mater. Res.* **29**, 959-965
10. Cima, L.G., Ingber, D.E., Vacanti, J.P., and Langer, R, 1991, Hepatocyte culture on biodegradable polymer substrates. *Biotech. Bioeng.* **38**, 145-152.
11. Johnson, L.B., Aiken, J., Mooney, D., Schloo, B.L., Cima, L.G., Langer, R., and Vacanti J.P., 1994, The mesentery as a laminated bed for hepatocyte transplantation, *Cell Transplantation* **3**, 273-280.
12. Dixit, V., Arthur, M., and Gitnick, G., 1992, Repeated transplantation of microencapsulated hepatocytes for sustained correction of hyperbilirubinemia in Gunn rats. *Cell Transplantation* **1**, 275-279.
13. Lopina, S.T., Wu, G., Merrill, E.W., and Cima, L.G., 1996, Hepatocyte culture on carbohydrate-modified star poly(ethylene oxide) hydrogels. *Biomaterials* **17**, 559-566.
14. Gutsche, A.T., Lo, H., Zurlo, J., Yager, J., and Leong, K.W., 1996, Engineering of a sugar-derivatized porous network for hepatocyte culture. *Biomaterials*, **17**, 387-392.

15. Gomez, N., Balladur, P., Calmus, Y., Baudrimont, M., and Honiger, J., 1997, Evidence of survival and metabolic activity of encapsulated xenogeneic hepatocytes transplanted without immunosuppression in Gunn rats. *Transplantation* **63**, 1718-1723.
16. Elçin, Y.M., Dixit, V., and Gitnick, G., 1998, Hepatocyte attachment on Biodegradable modified chitosan membranes: *In vitro* evaluation for the development of liver organoids. *Artif. Organs* **22**, 837-846.
17. Elçin, Y.M., Dixit, V., and Gitnick, G., 1995, Hepatocyte attachment on modified chitosan membranes. *Int. J. Artif. Organs* **18**, 464.
18. Kim, S.S., Sundback, C.A., Kaihara, S., Benvenuto, M.S., Kim, B.S., Mooney, D.J., and Vacanti, J.P., 2000. Dynamic seeding and *in vitro* culture of hepatocytes in a flow perfusion system, *Tissue Eng.* **6**, 39-44.
19. Torok, E., Pollock, J.M., Ma, P.X., Vogel, C., and Dandri, M., 2002, Hepatic tissue engineering on 3-dimensional biodegradable polymers within a pulsatile flow bioreactor. *Dig. Surg.* **18**,196-203.
20. Kneser, U., Kaufmann, P.M., Fiegel, H.C., Pollok, J.M., and Rogiers, X., 1999, Interaction of hepatocytes and pancreatic islets cotransplanted in polymeric matrices. *Virchows Archiv- Int. J. Pathol.* **435**, 125-132.
21. Naughton, B.A., Roman, J.S., Sibanda, B., Weintraub, J.P., and Kamali, V., 1994. Stereotypic culture systems for liver and bone marrow: Evidence for the development of functional tissue *in vitro* and following transplantation *in vivo*. *Biotech. Bioeng.* **43**, 810-825.
22. Elçin, Y.M., Dixit, V., and Gitnick, G., 1996, Controlled release of endothelial cell growth factor from chitosan-albumin microspheres for localized angiogenesis: *In vitro* and *in vivo* studies. *Artif. Cells Blood Subs. Immob. Biotech.* **24**, 257-271.
23. Elçin, Y.M., Dixit, V., and Gitnick, G., 2001, Extensive *in vivo* angiogenesis following controlled release of human vascular endothelial cell growth factor: Implications for tissue engineering and wound healing. *Artif. Organs* **25**, 558-565.
24. Folkman, J., 1996, What is the evidence that tumors are angiogenesis dependent? *J. Natl. Cancer Inst.* **82**, 4-6.
25. Elçin, Y.M., 2002, Angiogenesis in tissue engineering. *Int. J. Health Care Eng.* **16**, 114-115.
26. Takimoto, Y., Dixit, V., Arthur, M., and Gitnick, G., 2000, Direct evidence of *de novo* tissue engineered liver in rats transplanted with a collagen-based polypropylene composite scaffold. *Gastroenterology* **118**, 2405.

PANCREATIC ISLET AND STEM CELL TRANSPLANTATION IN DIABETES MELLITUS: RESULTS AND PERSPECTIVES

Reinhard G. Bretzel
Third Medical Department and Policlinic, University Hospital Giessen, Rodthohl 6, D-35392 Giessen, Germany

1. INTRODUCTION

Long-term studies strongly suggest that tight control of blood glucose achieved by conventional intensive insulin treatment, self-blood glucose monitoring and patient education can significantly prevent the development and retard the progression of chronic complications of type 1 diabetes mellitus[1,2]. However, the expense for this benefit was a threefold increase of the number of severe hypoglycemic episodes, a significant increase of the body weight, and dietary and other life-style restrictions affecting the quality of life[3].

By contrast, replacement of a patient's islets of Langerhans either by pancreas transplantation or by isolated islet transplantation (Fig. 1) is the only treatment of type 1 diabetes mellitus to achieve an insulin-independent, constant normoglycemic state and avoiding hypoglycemic episodes[4,5]. The expense of this benefit is the need for immunosuppressive treatment of the recipient with all its potential risks.

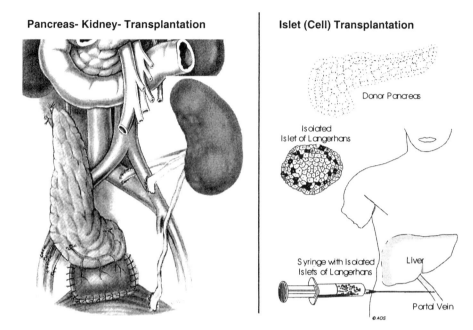

Figure 1. Pancreas-kidney transplantation into the pelvis with pancreatic duct drainage into the bladder (left). Islet transplantation into the portal venous system (right).

Results of pancreas transplantation have continued to improve, especially in the combined pancreas and kidney graft category. Results in this group are approaching those of other solid organs, but results of solitary pancreas grafting in non-uremic diabetic patients have been slow to follow and this method is still restricted to special centers. It has been demonstrated that successful pancreas transplantaton exerts beneficial effects on secondary complications of diabetes and improves quality of life. However, despite significant progress, pancreas transplantation is still associated with peri-operative mortality and significant morbidity[6-8].

In contrast, islet cell transplantation offers the advantage of being able to be performed as a minimally invasive procedure, in which islets can be perfused percutaneously into the liver via the portal vein[9]. Since about three decades, islet cell transplantation has been proposed for the scientific community and promised to patients and their families. However, the most convincing results in small animal studies did not as successfully translate to the clinical setting. Nonetheless, a few case reports of insulin independence achieved by intraportal islet allotransplants in type 1 diabetic recipients do exist[5, 10-14]. Recent data analysis from the International Islet Transplant Registry based at our institution showed that insulin independence after one year was achieved in only 11% of the patients[15].

The concept of islet cell transplantation is, however, most attractive since it offers many perspectives[16]: (1) In contrast to pancreas organ transplantation islet cell availability could become unlimited, when strategies such as the use of xenogenic islets, engineered beta-cell lines or in-vitro stem cell expansion and differentiation into insulin producing cells reach the stage of clinical applicability. (2) Islet cells may be transplanted without chronic immunosuppressive treatment of the recipient by making use of donor-specific tolerance induction strategies or immunoisolation systems. This unique set of characteristics could finally allow to offer islet transplants alone to adults and even adolescents and children with type 1 diabetes prior to the development and with the prospect of preventing such devastating diabetic secondary complications like end-stage renal disease, lower limb ischemia and amputations or blindness.

This review will summarize the current status and the perspectives of islet and stem cell transplantations in patients with type 1 diabetes mellitus.

2. ISLET TRANSPLANTATION

2.1 The History of Islet Cell Transplantation

It was Rudolf Virchow (1821-1902) who first suspected an incretory capacity of the pancreatic organ in addition to its known excretory capacity. Virchow's student, Paul Langerhans, first described in his doctoral thesis (1869) clusters of cells later named after him as islets of Langerhans. However, Paul Langerhans had no idea about the function of these cell clusters.

In April 1889, Joseph von Mering was working in Hoppe Seyler's Institute at the University of Strasbourg when Oskar Minkowski visited. Following one of their discussions on the metabolic role of the pancreatic gland, they began an investigation of the surgical removal of the pancreas from a dog. They found that diabetes mellitus develops after total pancreatectomy, providing final evidence that this disease is located in the pancreas[17]. Two years later, Oskar Minkowski gave a lecture on December 18, 1891 at the Strasbourg Society of Natural Science and Medicine which was published in the Berliner Klinische Wochenschrift[18]. He informed the audience that his and von Mering's series of experimental studies provided further evidence that diabetes mellitus develops after pancreatectomy as well as demonstrated for the first time that pancreatectomy-induced diabetes can be prevented by autografting pancreatic fragments under the skin. Furthermore, Minkowski concluded that something seems to be delivered by the pancreatic gland which facilitates sugar consumption by the peripheral tissue. Today, of course, we all know that this "something" is the hormone insulin, which 30 years later was extracted from pancreatic tissue and successfully injected in patients with insulin-requiring diabetes[19].

The pioneering work by Oskar Minkowski and Joseph von Mering, in particular their experimentation with the autotransplantation of pancreatic fragments paved the way toward clinical islet transplantations. Almost exactly two years after Minkowski's lecture, the first recorded human pancreatic fragment transplant was performed on December 20, 1893. Dr. P. Watson Williams and his colleague, Mr. Harsant, treated a 15-year old boy in the Bristol Royal Infirmary in Great Britain with the subcutaneous implantation of three pieces of freshly slaughtered sheep's pancreas, each "the size of a Brazil nut"[20]. They observed that glycosuria was lowered, however, the patient died after a few days.

2.2 Current Status of Clinical Islet Transplantation

As of August 2002, a total of 583 human islet cell transplantations performed between 1974 and 2002 in patients with type 1 diabetes mellitus have been reported to the International Islet Transplant Registry (ITR) established in 1989 and maintained at our department of Giessen University, Germany. An annual updated newsletter has been published[15]. The introduction of an automated method has permitted retrieval of a sufficient number of islets even from a single human donor pancreas to allow reversal of diabetes after allotransplantation in a type 1 diabetic patient and has made insulin independence more likely[21].

With this method available, a new era of clinical islet transplantation, either simultaneous with (SIK) or after kidney transplantation (IAK) started in the early nineties and a total of 493 islet allotransplants in type 1 diabetes mellitus have been performed between 1990 and August, 2002. There are only 8 institutions worldwide, 5 in North America and 3 in Europe, to have performed more than 10 cases (Table 1).

Data analysis has shown that at one year after islet transplantation the patient survival rate was 97%, the islet graft maintained function in 45% of the cases, and in 14% of the patients the ultimate goal, insulin independence, was achieved (Table 2). The longest insulin independence observed is now for more than 6 years (Table 2).

Table 1. Summary of Adult Islet Allografts in Type 1 Diabetic Recipients According to Institution and Year From 1990 Through August, 2002

Institution (Transplantation/Isolation)	1990	1991	1992	1993	1994	1995	1996	1997	1998	1999	2000	2001	2002	6
1. Giessen	-	-	1	5	5	12	11	17	6	4	5	8	7	81
2. Milan	4	3	2	4	4	4	1	-	5	5	12	4	7	55
3. Minneapolis	1	3	5	5	2	10	5	1	-	-	5	4	8	49
4. Miami	4	2	1	1	1	6	2	-	3	5	6	11	5	47
5. Edmonton	2	-	1	-	1	1	-	-	-	6	9	15	7	42
6. Geneva	-	-	-	-	-	-	4	2	4	5	4	1	6	26
7. Pittsburgh	7	5	3	3	4	3	1	-	-	-	-	-	-	26
8. St. Louis	3	3	2	4	2	-	-	-	-	-	-	-	3	17
9. Brussels	-	-	-	-	1	3	3	3	?	?	?	?	?	10
10. Indianapolis	-	-	-	-	-	-	4	5	1	-	-	-	-	10
11. Stockholm/Giessen	-	-	-	-	-	-	2	2	1	2	-	2	1	10
12. Grenoble/Geneva (Gragil)	-	-	-	-	-	-	-	-	-	2	3	1	2	8
13. Madrid	-	-	2	1	1	2	2	-	-	-	-	-	-	8
14. Oxford	-	1	1	1	1	2	-	1	1	-	-	-	-	8
15. Bethesda (NIH)	-	-	-	-	-	-	-	-	-	-	1	5	-	6
16. Zurich	-	-	-	-	-	-	-	-	-	-	1	4	1	6
17. Boston (Harvard)	-	-	-	-	-	-	-	-	-	-	1	1	3	5
18. Chicago (NWH)	-	-	-	-	-	-	1	-	-	-	-	1	3	5
19. Odense/Milan	-	-	-	-	-	5	-	-	-	-	-	-	-	5
20. Philadelphia	-	-	-	-	-	-	-	-	-	-	-	5	-	5
21. San Francisco/LA (UCLA-VA)	-	-	-	1	1	1	-	-	-	2	-	-	-	5
22. Strasbourg/Geneva (Gragil)	-	-	-	-	-	-	-	-	-	1	1	-	3	5
23. Buenos Aires	-	-	-	-	-	1	1	2	-	-	-	-	-	4
24. Cincinatti	-	-	-	-	-	-	-	-	-	-	-	-	4	4
25. London (Ontario)/St. Louis	2	1	1	-	-	-	-	-	-	-	-	-	-	4
26. Perugia	1	1	-	-	2	-	-	-	-	-	-	-	-	4
27. Houston/Miami	-	-	-	-	-	-	-	-	-	-	-	3	-	3
28. Innsbruck/Milano	-	-	-	-	-	2	1	-	-	-	-	-	-	3
29. Leicester	-	2	1	-	-	-	-	-	-	-	-	-	-	3
30. Lille	-	-	-	-	-	-	-	-	1	1	1	-	-	3
31. Los Angeles (UCLA-VA)	-	-	2	-	-	-	1	-	-	-	-	-	-	3
32. Lyon (Gragil)	-	-	-	-	-	-	-	-	-	-	1	1	1	3
33. Paris	3	-	-	-	-	-	-	-	-	-	-	-	-	3
34. Seattle	-	-	-	-	-	-	-	-	-	-	-	-	3	3
25. Memphis	-	-	-	-	-	-	-	-	-	-	-	-	2	2
35. Nantes	-	-	-	-	-	-	1	-	-	1	-	-	-	2
35. Worcester/Harvard	-	-	-	-	-	-	-	-	-	-	-	-	2	2
36. Baltimore	-	-	-	-	-	-	-	-	-	-	-	-	1	1
37. Berlin	-	-	-	-	-	-	-	-	-	-	1	-	-	1
38. Charlestown	-	1	-	-	-	-	-	-	-	-	-	-	-	1
39. Chicago University	-	-	-	-	-	-	-	-	-	-	-	1	-	1
39. Homburg (Saar)	-	-	-	1	-	-	-	-	-	-	-	-	-	1
40. Omaha	-	-	-	-	1	-	-	-	-	-	-	-	-	1
41. Seoul (Asan)	-	-	-	-	-	-	-	-	-	-	1	-	-	1
42. Seoul (Samsung)	-	-	-	-	-	-	-	-	-	1	-	-	-	1
	6	27	22	22	26	26	52	40	33	22	35	52	67	69	493

Total number of Adult Islet Allografts from 1974 -1989: 90

6 | 583

?Cases no longer reported to the Registry.

Table 2. Adult Simultaneous-Islet-Kidney (SIK) or Islet-After-Kidney (IAK) Transplantation in Type 1 Diabetic Patients in the Era 1990-08/2002: Results One Year Post Transplantation in 270 pre-Tx C-peptide Negative Recipients. *Patients with post-Tx basal C-peptide ≥ 0.5 ng/ml.

• Patient Survival	97%
• Islet Function	45%
• Off Insulin	14%
• Longest Insulin Independent Follow-Up	6 Years

As seen in previous ITR analyses, establishment of insulin independence was largely facilitated if (1) islets were isolated from pancreata with a mean preservation time ≤ 8 hours, (2) ≥ 6,000 islet equivalents (IEQ) per kg bodyweight of the recipient were transplanted, (3) islets were implanted into the liver via the portal vein, and (4) induction immunosuppression comprised monoclonal or polyclonal antibodies. These four factors could predict full success (in terms of insulin independence) with a high likelihood. Factors determined not to influence insulin independence at one year included patient age and body mass index, duration of diabetes, pretransplant HbA1c and daily insulin requirements, donor age, cold storage time of donor pancreas, and islet equivalent per kg bodyweight of the recipient.

Furthermore, the analyses may underscore the notion that intrinsic characteristics of the islet preparation (e.g. viability, apoptosis cascades triggered during islet isolation, purification and storage procedures) of the immediate post-transplant engraftment period (e.g. inflammatory and other response of the recipient toward an intravascular islet graft, "effective" engraftment), and factors during long-term islet survival (e.g. immune-mediated allo- and autoresponse of the recipient, susceptibility of islet grafts toward adverse diabetogenic effects of current immunosuppressive drugs, and functional exhaustion) may determine clinical success.

Undoubtedly, full (metabolic) success of islet transplantation is characterized by insulin independence. Partial success may be defined as islet endocrine function characterized by basal C-peptide secretion not accompanied by insulin independence in a specific recipient with type 1 diabetes mellitus. Nevertheless, patients with partially successful islet transplants may benefit from the long-run since basal serum C-peptide levels with a threshold of 0.5 ng/ml exerts significant biological effects[22-25](Fig. 2). Translated to the clinical situation, significant basal C-peptide levels after partially successful islet allotransplantation was followed by a decrease of daily insulin requirements, led to a stable metabolic control and was accompanied by less frequent or no hypoglycemic episodes[67]. Even in cases with partial success progression of diabetic secondary complications might be halted for the long run.

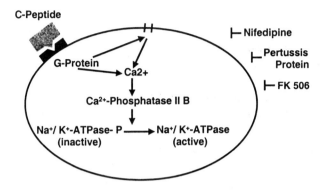

Figure 2. Proposed mechanism of C-peptide action. Adapted from references 22 and 23.

2.3 Islet Transplantation at Giessen University Center

The above mentioned detailed analysis of the ITR demonstrated that detectable graft function was lost in about 50% of the cases during the initial 3 months following transplantation (Fig. 3). Several reasons for this early graft loss have been discussed (Fig. 4).

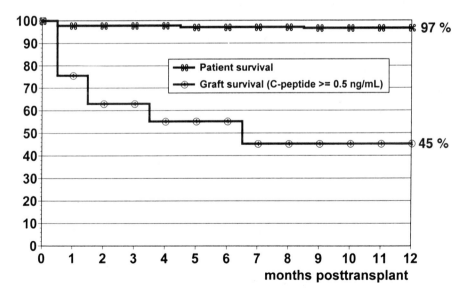

Figure 3. Cumulative one-year patient and graft survival in 270 pretransplant C-peptide negative type 1 diabetic recipients, transplanted in the era 1990-2000.

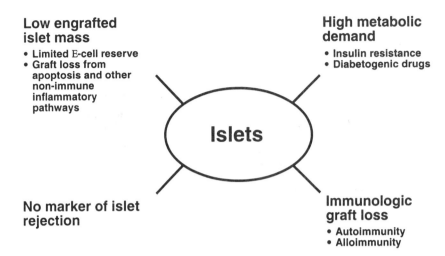

Figure 4. Possible reasons for early and late islet graft failure and obstacles to the success of clinical islet cell transplantation.

Therefore, after more than ten years of experience in islet isolation from the pancreas of large mammals and humans[27], we implemented into our clinical islet transplant protocol at Giessen University Center strategies to facilitate human islet isolation, purification and storage and a refined peritransplant management, in order to promote early islet engraftment and to make insulin independence more likely[28](Table 3). Islet transplantation into the liver through portal vein access was performed under local anesthesia by percutaneous-transhepatic catheterization of the portal vein[9](Fig. 5 and 6).

Table 3. The Giessen Protocol for Islet Allotransplantations in Type 1 Diabetic Subjects of the Recipient Categories Simultaneous-Islet-Kidney (SIK) and Islet-After-Kidney (IAK), respectively.

• *Islet Preparation*	Endotoxin-free-reagents
• *Pre-Tx*	ATG / ALG
• *Peri-Tx*	Total Parenteral Nutrition (TPN)
• *Post-Tx*	Prednisolone
	CYA (300 - 400 ng/mL WB trough level)
	Azathioprine or MMF
	IV insulin
	Nicotinamide
	Verapamil
	Pentoxifylline
	Antioxidants

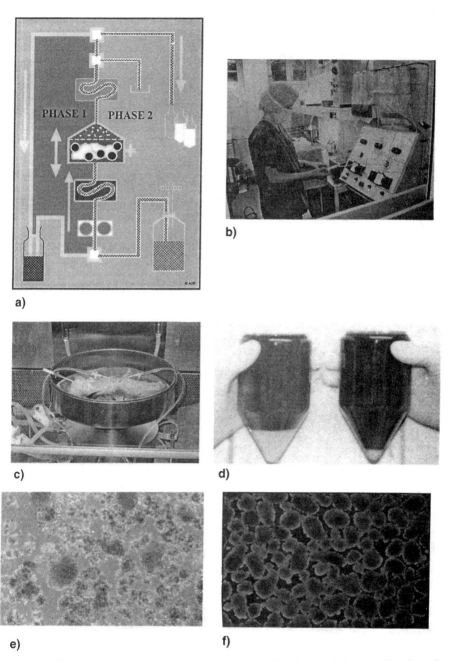

Figure 5. The Giessen Protocol: Islet isolation and purification. a) Schematic drawing of enzyme-digestion of the pancreas and islet isolation (modified acc. to Ricordi et al, 1988 (ref. 21); b) view at the clean rooms; c) retrieved human pancreatic organ (70-100 g) with ductal system cannulated for perfusion; d) beta cell mass after collagenase (enzyme) digestion (left) and consecutive purification on a density gradient system (right); e) crude preparation showing isolated islets contaminated with exocrine tissue; f) highly purified islet preparation.

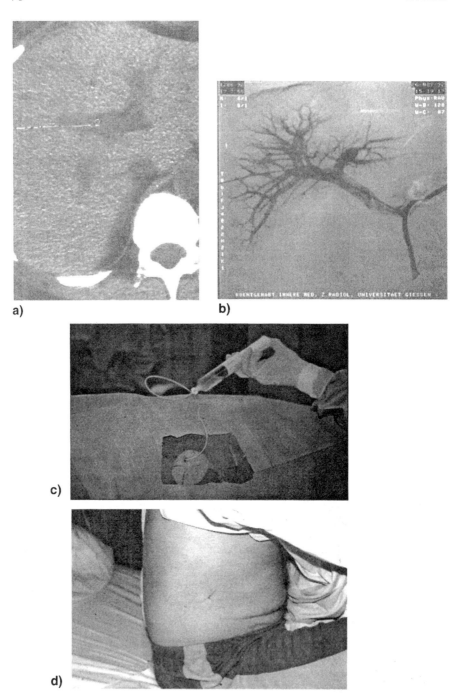

Figure 6. The Giessen Protocol: Islet (cell) implantation by percutaneous-transhepatic catheterization of the portal venous system in local anesthesia. a) CT-guided imaging of the portal venous system; b) fluoroscopy-guided localization of the catheter; c) infusion of the islet (cell) suspension; d) closure of the small cutaneous incision.

Almost all recipients received only one islet preparation yielded from a single donor pancreas. Using this protocol, we recently reported a markedly improved 3 months islet cell function rate of 100% for simultaneous-islet-kidney (SIK) recipients and 75% for islet-after-kidney (IAK) recipients, respectively[29].

A follow-up in our first 56 consecutive cases (SIK / n=35 and IAK / n=21) illustrates a significantly improved one-year islet allograft survival of 86% for SIK cases and 47% for IAK cases, respectively (Table 4). The comparative numbers for non-Giessen SIK and IAK cases are 38% and 34%, respectively (Table 5).

Table 4. Adult Simultaneous-Islet-Kidney (SIK)- or Islet-After-Kidney (IAK)-Transplantation in Type 1 Diabetic Patients at Giessen University Hospital Center: One-year Results. For Comparison Results of Non-Giessen Centers (ITR data) Given in Brackets.

	SIK (n=35)	IAK (n=21)
• Patient survival	35/35	19/21
• Islet function	86% *(38%)*	47% *(34%)*
• Insulin independence	17% *(7%)*	21% *(7%)*
• Kidney function	97%	100%

Table 5. Some Principles of Transplant Tolerance Induction.

- **Induction of micro- or macro-chimerism**
  deletion of mature T-cells by immunotoxin / irradiation + donor antigen (graft or bone marrow)
- **Modifying signal 1**
  anti-CD4 monoclonal antibody (lck56)
- **Blocking signal 2**
  blocking CD28/B7 (CTLA4Ig) or CD40L (CD154)/CD40 (anti-CD40LmAb)
- **Donor antigen (activation induced apoptosis ?)**
  donor specific blood transfusion; dendritic cells (vIL-10 etc.); soluble MHC molecules

2.4 Islet Transplants Alone (ITA) in Non-Uremic Type 1 Diabetic Subjects

The ultimate aim of islet cell transplantation and the most appealing aspect of this treatment concept is to achieve long-term function of the grafted tissue in non-uremic type-1 diabetic patients early in the course of the disease, before significant microvascular, macrovascular and neurological complications are developed (Fig. 7).

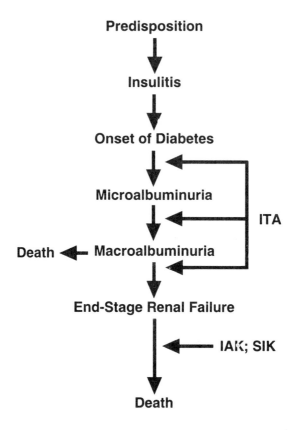

Figure 7. Indications and timing of islet (cell) transplantations in the natural course of type 1 diabetes mellitus. ITA Islet Transplants Alone; IAK Islet After Kidney Transplants; SIK Simultaneous Islet-Kidney Transplants.

We have recently performed for the first time islet transplants alone (ITA) in non-uremic patients with long-standing type-1 diabetes mellitus and hypoglycemia-associated syndrome, suffering from hypoglycemia unawareness, defect counterregulation and experiencing recurrent episodes of severe hypoglycemia[26]. We found that intraportal islet transplantation did not restore hypoglycemia-induced glucagon secretion, but it significantly improved the responses of most counterregulatory hormones and re-established both autonomic and neuroglucopenic hypoglycemia warning symptoms even in long-standing type-1 diabetes (Fig. 8). However, we were permitted by the local ethics committee to treat these recipients by a monoclonal anti-CD4 mouse antibody together with cyclosporine A only for four weeks. After drug withdrawal all patients consecutively lost islet graft function over the following three months, indicating that no permanent immunotolerance state was established.

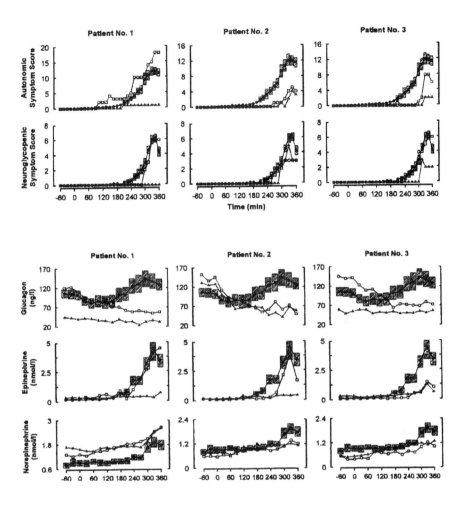

Figure 8. Islet Transplants Alone (ITA) in patients with long-standing type 1 diabetes and hypoglycemia-associated syndrome. Six-hours insulin-induced hypoglycemia clamp-tests performed before (Δ) and after (□) islet transplantation. Upper panels: Autonomic and neuroglycopenic symptom score in response to hypoglycemia. Lower panels: Response of counterregulation hormones glucagon, epinephrine, and norepinephrine to hypoglycemia. Shaded boxes indicate test responses of age-matched healthy control subjects (n=10). Adapted from reference 26.

2.5 New Strategies for Circumventing the Obstacles to the Success of Clinical Islet Cell Transplantation

In Figure 4, the major obstacles to the success of islet transplantation in subjects with type 1 diabetes mellitus have been illustrated. First, the imbalance between the islet mass engrafted and the metabolic demand determines the clinical outcome. From animal experiments, it was calculated that approximately 50 percent of the islets transferred will not engraft and primary non-function may be the result of low functional capacity of beta cells after the isolation procedure, of local inflammatory and apoptotic mechanisms, cytokines, clotting elements of the blood and hypoxia before revascularization of the islets in the hepatic microenvironment[30-36]. A high metabolic demand imposed on the islet graft results from the insulin resistance in diabetic recipients as well as from diabetogenic and probably toxic effects of high portal vein concentrations of conventional immunosuppressive agents (cyclosporine A, tacrolimus, glucocorticoids)[37,38]. Second, isolated islet grafts seem to be more prone to destruction by autoimmune recurrence and allograft rejection than whole pancreatic organ allotransplants[39-45].

These factors of islet graft failure have been targeted in new strategies to promote islet cell transplants. Some of these promising novel strategies will be described here.

2.5.1 Sequential islet transplants and steroid-free immunosuppression

Recently, the Islet Transplant Center of the University of Alberta in Edmonton, Canada, reported an increased success rate of islet allotransplantations[46]. They developed a novel protocol of sequential islet allotransplants prepared from two or more pancreases performed 2 - 10 weeks apart in order to achieve an adequate mass of (engrafted) islets. In order to overcome the problems with conventional immunosuppressives, these patients were given a glucocorticoid-free immunosuppressive regimen that included an interleukin 2 receptor antibody (daclizumab), sirolimus (rapamycin), and low-dose tacrolimus. Seven consecutive patients with type 1 diabetes and a history of severe hypoglycemia and metabolic instability ("Brittle-Diabetes") underwent islet transplants alone (ITA). All seven recipients quickly attained sustained insulin independence after transplantation of a mean ($\pm$SD) islet mass of 11,547 $\pm$ 1,604 islet equivalents (basis: diameter of 150 µm) per kilogram of body weight[46]. HbA1c concentrations were normal. More importantly, the recipients did no longer experience hypoglycemic episodes and severe adverse side effects were not observed in any of the recipients. Meanwhile, the authors have extended their experience with the Edmonton Protocol on a higher number of recipients with presently 100% graft survival and 75% insulin independence rates[47].

Meanwhile, several centers reported islet transplants alone in patients with hypoglycemia-associated syndrome. This previously rare indication seems to be now the main indication for clinical islet transplant trials. From

120 islet-transplant-alone cases reported to the International Islet Transplant Registry since the year 2000, 119 cases (99%) have functioning islet grafts and 74 recipients (89%) are reported off insulin (Figure 9).

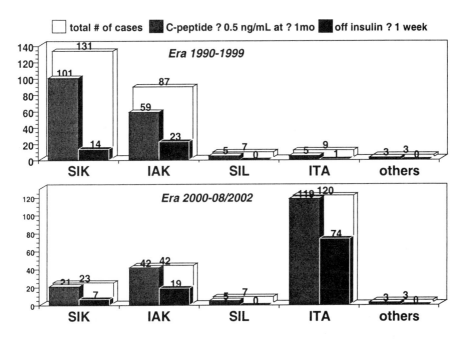

Figure 9. Insulin independence and basal C-peptide after adult islet allotransplantation in pre-transplant C-peptide negative type 1 diabetic recipients according to recipient category and era. SIK Simultaneous Islet-Kidney; IAK Islet-After-Kidney; SIL Simultaneous Islet-Liver; ITA Islet Transplants Alone.

The Immune Tolerance Network (ITN), one of the clinical research projects of the US National Institutes of Health together with the Juvenile Diabetes Research Foundation, has now started a multicenter controlled trial to coordinate implementation of the Edmonton Protocol. Seven centers in the USA / Canada and three centers in Europe (Geneva, Giessen, Milan) have been selected to participate.

2.5.2 New immunosuppressive agents - immunotolerance induction - encapsulation of islets

Several strategies for prevention of autoimmune recurrence following islet transplantation have been proven in the "preclinical" model of type 1 diabetes, the spontaneously diabetic NOD mouse. Among the few effective strategies (possibly through the regeneration of immunoregulatory T cells) are immunotherapy with antilymphocyte serum weeks before islet transplantation, Complete Freund's Adjuvant (CFA) and Bacille-Calmette-Guerin (BCG) adjuvant immunotherapy, (FCR)-non-binding anti-CD3 antibodies, combined therapy with IL-4 and IL-10, GAD65-based immunotherapy and combined administration of vitamin D3 analogue and cyclosporine (for overview see reference 48). A combination therapy with low-dose sirolimus and tacrolimus was recently described as synergistic in preventing recurrent autoimmune diabetes in non-obese diabetic (NOD) mice[49]. It has been suggested to overcome the problem of autoimmune diabetes recurrence by transplanting human islets rendered glutamat-decarboxylase (GAD)-less through introduction of an antisense transgene in vitro[50]. Indeed, it has been shown that NOD knockout mice or GAD antigene do not develop autoimmune diabetes[51].

The next step on the way to better outcomes in clinical islet transplantation is to develop effective protocols for stemming the thide of rejection. Immunosuppressive regimens are likely to undergo significant improvements with the advent of more selective and less toxic agents such as humanized interleukin-2-receptor antibodies which proved effective with no adverse effects on islet function and glucose metabolism in animal experiments[52-55].

Finally, tolerance induction is central to the thesis of islet transplantation. Meanwhile, the mechanisms of islet allograft rejection are better understood. At least, three levels of cell-to-cell crosstalk, between the antigen-presenting cells (APCs) and the recipient's T cells have to be taken into account (Fig. 9). Blockage of the co-stimulatory signal (signal 2) for T cell activation, and induction of hematopoietic chimerism are the two main and most promising strategies for tolerance induction[56, 57] (see also Table 5). Recent studies in non-human primates demonstrated that immunotolerance toward islet cells can be established by CD40-CD40 ligand (CD154) blockade[58, 59]. Pre-implantation-stage stem cells surprisingly were capable to induce long-term allogeneic graft acceptance with supplementary host conditioning[60]. However, most strategies that successfully induce transplant tolerance in murine models have failed upon translation into clinical therapies so far[61] and all clinical trials with a humanized anti-CD154 (CD40 ligand) antibody were completely halted due to unexpected high rates of thromboembolic complications in kidney transplant recipients[62, 63].

Therefore, the Immune Tolerance Network (ITN) is committed to supporting clinical research focussing on the following points: (1) novel immunotherapeutic strategies aiming at early withdrawal of immunosuppression with a suggested 40 patients as control group transplanted in the 10 centers according to the Edmonton protocol; (2) therapeutic establishment of hematopoietic chimerism, with emphasis on depletion- and irradiation-free conditioning protocols.

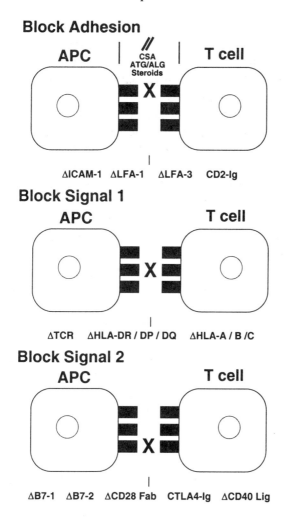

Figure 10. Crosstalk of donor antigen-presenting cells (APC) and recipient T cells on different levels and principles of blocking (immunosuppressive) agents.

Another approach to avoid life-long immunosuppressive treatment of the recipient would be to immunoisolate islets by means of macroencapsulation or microencapsulation prior to transplantation[64-67]. Porcine encapsulated islets have been reported to induce normoglycemia without immunosuppression in spontaneously diabetic monkeys for more than 800 days[68]. But, successful studies in several animal models were not followed by clinical studies. So far, a single case in whom the authors claimed full success in terms of insulin independence after transplantation of microencapsulated islets in a patient with previous kidney graft was reported in 1994[69]. However, the case was not well documented and there was no consecutive report on the follow-up of this recipient. The main problems with microencapsulation are the limited biocompatibility of the membranes, a lack of nutrients and oxygene supply of the islets, and small molecules, such as cytokines and other pro-inflammatory mediators can still enter and exit the protective membranes and impair the function of the encapsulated islets or exert fibrotic membrane overgrowth on the outer layer. Even a combination of islet pretreatment and islet encapsulation in barium alginate membranes did not establish long-lasting islet function in animal studies[70]. Very recently, at the 19th International Congress of the Transplantation Society, held in Miami / USA, August 25-30, 2002, a consortium of Mexican, Canadian and New Zealand researchers described their studies with neonatal porcine islet xenografts to type 1 diabetic children. The islets together with sertoli cells were inserted into neovascularized collagen tribes created by implanting a closed stainless steel mesh containing an inner Teflon stent subcutaneously 8 weeks prior to transplantation (Valdes-Gomzalaez RA et al., Transplantation 74, supplement 4, Abstract No. 246, 2002). No immunosuppression was given. The authors reported a one-year, insulin-free status achieved in one child. A second child of the 12 recipients in the study was off insulin for six months and currently requires 75 percent less insulin than before transplantation. Six of the 12 patients have functioning grafts. However, the scientific community at large may be sceptical until more data is available and more patients are studied. Whether these results can be duplicated by another center remains to be seen.

2.5.3 Xenotransplants - stem cell therapy - gene therapy

Provided, the problems with islet autoimmune destruction and allogeneic rejection are solved and the indication for islet allotransplants is extended to non-uremic type 1 diabetic patients, a further problem may suddenly emerge: huge amounts of donor islet tissue are needed. But, where should the islets come from? (Table 6)

Table 6. Possible Beta Cell Sources Beyond Cadaveric Donor Tissue.

- **Xenogeneic (porcine) islets**
- **Differentiation and expansion of embryonic or adult stem cells**
- **Genetically engineered artificial beta-cell lines**
- **Gene therapy for in-vivo or ex-vivo / in-vitro converting patient cells to beta-cells**

The pig is considered the primary alternative donor species for islet xenografts to humans due to ethical considerations, breeding characteristics, infectious disease concerns and its compatible size and physiology[71]. Porcine insulin has been widely used in humans and the pig insulin molecular structure differs from human insulin in only one aminoacid position.

A major barrier to progress in pig-to-human transplants is the presence of the terminal carbohydrate epitope, Δ-1,3-galactosyl (gal) on the surface of pig cells[72]. Humans (and Old World monkeys) have lost their corresponding galactosyl transferase activity in the course of evolution and therefore produce preformed natural antibodies against the epitope that are responsible for hyperacute rejection of porcine organs. Measures like temporary removal of natural antibodies through affinity absorption, expression of complement regulators, competitive inhibition of galactosyl transferase or blocking the expression of gal epitopes, resulted in only partial reduction in epitope numbers but failed to significantly extend xenograft survival in primate recipients[73]. There is also no clear-cut advantage of isolated islet xenografts over that of a whole pancreatic organ. CD40+ T cells of the recipient seem to play a major role in xenoislet rejection and conventional immunosuppressive agents allowed only a modest if any prolongation of islet xenograft survival in most pig-to-rodent models[74-78]. However, with the production of Δ-1,3-galactosyl transferase knockout pigs by nuclear transfer as very recently reported, there is now hope to overcome at least major problems with adult porcine islet xenograft hyperacute rejection[79].

Another source for islet xenograft tissue might be the fetal pancreas[80]. The cultured fetal porcine pancreas bears several potential advantages: (1) it contains a larger proportion of endocrine tissue; (2) the exocrine tissue undergoes atrophy during culture; (3) the fetal tissue inherits a considerable growth potential; and (4) it might be less immunogeneic. It should be noted that cell aggregates ("fetal porcine islet-like cell clusters"; FPCC's) do not trigger a hyperacute rejection when transplanted to rodents and it is likely that they are revascularized from the surrounding tissues thus containing recipient endothelial cells[81]. This would make such cultured fetal islet tissue ideal for clinical trials with xenotransplantations.

Fetal pig proislets can be easily produced at large-scale, further differentiate, mature and grow in culture or in vivo after grafting, may be stored long-term in liquid nitrogene and can be persistently reverse diabetes after xenografting and may be more resistant to diabetogenic agents than adult islet tissue[82-88]. However, preliminary experience with fetal pig proislets in a pre-clinical xenograft model using cynomolgus monkeys as recipients is not very promising[89].

The first clinical experience of fetal porcine pancreatic microfragment xenotransplantation into a conventionally immunosuppressed type 1 diabetic patient was reported more than two decades ago[90]. During 40 days after transplantation, insulin requirements did not change, but C-peptide appeared (at very low concentrations) in the urine, suggesting at least low function of the transplanted tissue[90]. Finally, the same group transplanted a total of 10 diabetic patients with porcine fetal pancreatic fragments, but again, no reduction in insulin requirement was observed in any of these patients[91].

However, the use of pigs as a source for organs and cells to be xenografted to humans has provoked ethical and epidemiological controversies[92]. Transfer of Porcine Endogenous Retroviruses (PERV) from porcine cells to human cells has been demonstrated in vitro and in vivo after xenotransplantation into immuno-incompetent and immunodeficient SCID mice[93-96]. However, there is until now no evidence of infection with PERV in those Swedish patients who were treated with porcine islet cell xenografts or in patients treated with living pig tissue[97, 98]. Another option to prevent recipient affection might be the use of specially breeded PERV-free pigs.

Stem cell therapy, the use of either embryonic or adult progenitor cells differentiated and expanded under special conditions to fully functional, insulin-producing beta cells is a second approach to overcome the problems with limited tissue supply for clinical islet transplantation in diabetes mellitus[99].

It is generally accepted that the pancreatic endocrine cells are of endodermal origin. The pathway from precursor cells to distinguished cell types, the genes and transcription factors involved, and the spatial and sequential temporal order meanwhile has become clear[100-104] (see also Fig. 10). Recent reports on the in-vitro differentiation and expansion of embryonic stem cells of murine or human origin to insulin-producing beta cells are very promising[105-107]. Transplanted into diabetic animals, these cells normalized blood glucose of the recipients[105, 106].

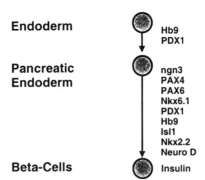

Figure 11. Relevant genes and transcription factors for the development of insulin-producing beta cells.

However, ethical concerns with the research on human embryonic material brought up the question as to whether adult ("old") cells can learn new tricks, i.e. may differentiate to insulin-producing cells. So-called Nestin-positive cells in the pancreatic duct or within the islets of Langerhans may be relevant progenitor cells[108]. By in-vitro cultivation of ductal epithelial cells from adult mice, islets could be obtained which responded in-vitro to glucose stimulation and reversed diabetes when transplanted into diabetic NOD mice[109]. A method to yield islets through in-vitro cultivation of adult human pancreatic ductal cells was described recently[110].

A third approach to overcome the problems with limited donor tissue supply is to make use of Gene Therapy for engineering pancreatic islets (for overview see reference 111). The principal advantage of this approach is that autologous tissue and cells can be used and the problems with graft rejection and disease recurrence would probably no longer exist. For example, gut, liver or muscle cells have been successfully targeted for transfection with the insulin-/pro-insulin gene[112-115]. A group in Israel recently described expression of insulin genes in the liver and amelioration of hyperglycemia in mice after viral transfection of the hepatocytes with the pancreatic and duodenal homeobox (PDX)-1 gene[116]. This is proof-of-principle for converting hepatocytes to beta cells[117].

3. CONCLUSION

Islet cell transplantation has raised hope for a cure of diabetes for over three decades. The failure to quickly reach this goal has been enormous disappointment to scientists, clinicians and patients. But, the field of islet transplantation has evolved and matured tremendously, it has witnessed significant progress and the results of recent human islet allotransplantations in patients with type 1 diabetes mellitus are encouraging. At the dawn of the millenium, with the synergy of a number of important innovative tools, including stem cell expansion, immunomodulation, and gene therapy, it is my believe that we enter this new century with a solid foundation for expanding fundamental research and for translating basic knowledge into clinical applications. The challenges will still be many, but the potential benefit for patients with type 1 diabetes will be extraordinary. Finally, it is necessary that the importance, potential, and feasibility of islet transplantation be better appreciated so that the need to develop this urgently needed therapy be more accepted[118].

ACKNOWLEDGEMENTS

We gratefully acknowledge grant support by JDRF (large individual grant), NIH-NIDDK (R01-DK56962-01 and ITN-Trial), and BMBF (FKZ07024806).

REFERENCES

1. The Diabetes Control and Complications Trial Research Group, 1993, The effect of intensive treatment of diabetes on the development and progression of long-term complications in insulin-dependent diabetes mellitus. *N. Engl. J. Med.* **329**, 977-986.
2. Wang, P.H., Lau, J., and Chalmers, T.C., 1993, Meta-analysis of effects of intensive blood-glucose control on late complications of type-1 diabetes. *Lancet* **341**, 1306-1309.
3. The Diabetes Control and Complications Trial Research Group, 1997, Hypoglycemia in the Diabetes Control and Complications Trial. *Diabetes* **46**, 271-286
4. Sutherland, D.E., Gores, P.F., Farney, A.C., Wahoff, D.C., Matas, A.J., Dunn, D.L., Gruessner, R.W., and Najarian, J.S., 1993, Evolution of kidney, pancreas, and islet transplantation for patients with diabetes at the University of Minnesota. *Am. J. Surg.* **166**, 456-491.
5. Bretzel, R.G., Browatzki, C.C, Schultz, A., Brandhorst, H., Klitscher, D., Bollen, C.C., Raptis, G., Friemann, S., Ernst, W., Rau, W.S., and Hering, B.J., 1993, Clinical islet transplantation in diabetes mellitus - report of the Islet Transplant Registry and the Giessen Center experience. *Diab. Stoffw.* **2**, 378-390.
6. Gruessner, R.W.G., Sutherland, D.E.R., Troppmann, C., Benedetti, E., Hakim, N., Dunn, D.L., and Gruessner, A.C., 1997, The surgical risk of pancreas transplantation in the cyclosporine era: an overview: *J. Am. Coll. Surg.* **185**, 128-144.
7. Manske, C.L., 1999, Risks and benefits of kidney and pancreas transplantation for diabetic patients. *Diabetes Care* **22**, B114-B120.
8. Humar, A., Kandaswamy, R., Granger, D. et al., 2000, Decreased surgical risks of pancreas transplantation in the modern era. *Ann. Surg.* **231**, 342-344.
9. Weimar, B., Rauber, K., Brendel, M.D., Bretzel, R.G., and Rau, W.S., 1999, Percutaneous transhepatic catheterization of the portal vein: a combined CT- and fluoroscopy-guided technique. Cardiovasc. *Intervent. Radiol.* **22**, 342-344.
10. Scharp, D.W., Lacy, P.E., Santiago, J.V., McCullough, C.S., Weide, L.G., Falqui, L. et al., 1990, Insulin independence after islet transplantation into type I diabetic patient. *Diabetes* **39**, 515-518.
11. Socci, C., Falqui, L., Davalli, A.M., Ricordi, C., Braghi, S., Bertuzzi, F. et al., 1991, Fresh human islet transplantation to replace pancreatic endocrine function in type 1 diabetic patients. Report of six cases. *Acta Diabetol.* **28**, 151-157.
12. Warnock, G.L., Kneteman, N.M., Ryan, E.A., Rabinovitch, A., and Rajotte, R.V., 1992, Long-term follow-up after transplantation of insulin-producing pancreatic islets into patients with Type 1 (insulin-dependent) diabetes mellitus. *Diabetologia* **35**, 89-95.
13. Gores, P.F., Najarian, J.S., Stephanian, E., Lloveras, J.J., Kelley, S.L., and Sutherland, D.E.R., 1993, Insulin independence in type I diabetes after transplantation of unpurified islets from single donor with 15-deoxyspergualin. *Lancet* **341**, 19-21.
14. Alejandro, R., Lehmann, R., Ricordi, C., Kenyon, N.S., Angelico, M.C., Burke, G. et al., 1997, Long-term function (6 years) of islet allografts in type 1 diabetes. *Diabetes* **46**, 1983-1989.

15. Brendel, M.D., Hering, B.J., Schultz, A.O., and Bretzel, R.G., 2001, International Islet Transplant Registry Newsletter No. 9: 1-20.
16. Bretzel, R.G., 1999, Biological alternatives to insulin therapy. *Exp. Clin. Endocrinol. Diabetes* 107, S39-S43.
17. Mering, J. von, and Minkowski, O., 1890, Diabetes mellitus nach Pankreasexstirpation. *Arch. Exp. Pathol. Pharmakol.* 26, 37.
18. Minkowski, O., 1892, Weitere Mittheilungen über den Diabetes mellitus nach Exstirpation des Pankreas. *Berliner Klin. Wochenschr.* 29, 90-94.
19. Banting, F.G., and Best, C.H., 1922, The internal secretion of the pancreas. *J. Lab. Clin. Invest.* 7, 251-266.
20. Williams, P.W., 1894, Notes on diabetes treated with extract and by grafts of sheep's pancreas. *Brit. Med. J.* 2, 1303.
21. Ricordi, C., Lacy, P.E., Finke, E.H., Olack, B.J., and Scharp, D.W., 1988, Automated method for isolation of human pancreatic islets. *Diabetes* 37, 413-420.
22. Johansson, B.L., Borg, K., Fernqvist-Forbes, E., Odergren, T., Remahl, S., and Wahren, J., 1996, C-peptide improves autonomic nerve function in IDDM patients. *Diabetologia* 39, 687-695.
23. Wahren, J., and Johansson, B.L., 1998, New aspects of C-peptide physiology. *Horm. Metab. Res.* 30, A2-A5.
24. Steiner, D.F., and Rubenstein, A.H., 1997, Proinsulin C-peptide - biological activity? [comment]. *Science* 277, 531-532.
25. Ido, Y., Vindigni, A., Chang, K., Stramm, L., Chance, R., Heath, W.F., DiMarchi, R.D., Di Cera, E., and Williamson, J.R., 1997, Prevention of vascular and neural dysfunction in diabetic rats by C-peptide. *Science* 277, 563-567.
26. Meyer, C., Hering, B.J., Grossmann, R., Brandhorst, H., Brandhorst, D., Gerich, J., Federlin, K., and Bretzel, R.G., 1998, Improved glucose counterregulation and autonomic symptoms after intraportal islet transplants alone in patients with type I diabetes mellitus. *Transplantation* 66, 233-240.
27. Brandhorst, D., Brandhorst, H., Hering, B.J., Federlin, K., and Bretzel, R.G., 1995, Islet isolation from the pancreas of large mammals and humans: 10 years of experience. *Exp. Clin. Endocrinol. Diabetes* 103 (suppl 2), 3-14.
28. Hering, B.J., Bretzel, R.G., Hopt, U.T., Brandhorst, H., Brandhorst, D., Bollen, C.C., Raptis, G., Helf, F., Grossmann, R., Mellert, J., Ernst, W., Scheuermann, E.H., Schoeppe, W., Rau, W., and Federlin, K., 1994, New protocol toward prevention of early human islet allograft failure. *Transplant. Proc.* 26, 570-571.
29. Bretzel, R.G., Brandhorst, D., Brandhorst, H., Eckhard, M., Ernst, W., Friemann, S., Rau, W., Weimar, B., Rauber, K., Hering, B.J., and Brendel, M.D., 1999, Improved survival of intraportal pancreatic islet cell allografts in patients with type 1 diabetes mellitus by refined peritransplant management. *J. Mol. Med.* 77, 140-143.
30. Vargas, F., Vives-Pi, M., Somoza, N., Armengol, P., Alcalde, L., Marti, M., Costa, M., Serradell, L., Dominguez, O., Fernandez-Llamazares, J., Julian, J.F., Samarti, A., and Pujol-Borrell, R., 1998, Endotoxin contamination may be responsible for the unexplained failure of human pancreatic islet transplantation. *Transplantation* 65, 722-727.
31. Kaufman, D.B., Platt, J.L., Rabe, F.L., Dunn, D.L., Bach, F.H., and Sutherland, D.E.R., 1990, Differential roles of Mac-1+ cells and CD4+ and CD8+ T lymphocytes in primary nonfunction and classical rejection of islet allografts. *J. Exp. Med.* 172, 291-302.
32. Bottino, R., Fernandez, L.A., Ricordi, C., Lehmann, R., Tsan, M.F., Oliver, R., and Inverardi, L., 1998, Transplantation of allogeneic islets of Langerhans in the rat liver. Effects of macrophage depletion on graft survival and microenvironment activation. *Diabetes* 47, 316-323.

33. Menger, M.D., Vajkoczy, P., Leiderer, R., Jager, S., and Messmer, K., 1992, Influence of experimental hyperglycemia on microvascular blood perfusion of pancreatic islet isografts. *J. Clin. Invest.* **90**, 1361-1369.
34. Berney, T., Molano, R.D., Cattan, P. et al., 2001, Endotoxin-mediated delayed islet graft function is associated with increased intra-islet cytokine production and islet cell apoptosis. *Transplantation* **71**, 125-132.
35. Bennet, W., Sunberg, B., Groth, C.G. et al., 1999, Incompatibility between human blood and isolated islets of Langerhans: a finding with implications for clinical intraportal islet transplantation? *Diabetes* **48**, 1907-1914.
36. El-Ouaghlidi, A., Jahr, H., Pfeiffer, G., Hering, B.J., Brandhorst, D., Brandhorst, H., Federlin, K., and Bretzel, R.G., 1999, Cytokine mRNA expression in peripheral blood cells of immunosuppressed human islet transplant recipients. *J. Mol. Med.* **77**, 115-117.
37. Shapiro, A.M., Gallant, H., Hao, E., Wong, J., Rajotte, R., Yatscoff, R., and Kneteman, N., 1997, Portal vein immunosuppressant levels and islet graft toxicity. *Transplant. Proc.* **30**, 641.
38. Drachenberg, C.B., Klassen, D.K., Weir, M.R., Wiland, A., Fink, J.C., Bartlett, S.T., Cangro, C.B., Blahut, S., and Papadimitriou, J.C., 1999, Islet cell damage associated with tacrolimus and cyclosporine: morphological features in pancreas allograft biopsies and clinical correlation. *Transplantation* **68**, 396-402.
39. Jaeger, C., Hering, B.J., Dyrberg, T., Federlin, K., and Bretzel, R.G., 1996, Islet cell antibodies and GAD65 antibodies in IDDM patients undergoing kidney and islet after kidney transplantation. *Transplantation* **62**, 424-426.
40. Jaeger, C., Brendel, M.D., Hering, B.J., Eckhard, M., and Bretzel, R.G., 1997, Progressive islet graft failure occurs significantly earlier in autoantibody positive than in autoantibody negative IDDM recipients of intrahepatic islet allografts. *Diabetes* **46**, 1907-1910.
41. Jaeger, C., Brendel, M.D., Eckhard, M., and Bretzel, R.G., 2000, Islet autoantibodies as potential markers for disease recurrence in clinical islet transplantation. *Exp. Clin. Endocrinol. Diabetes* **108**, 328-333.
42. Braghi, S., Bonifacio, E., Secchi, A., di Carlo, V., Pozza, G., and Bosi, E., 2000, Modulation of humoral islet autoimmunity by pancreas allotransplantation influences allograft outcome in patients with type 1 diabetes. *Diabetes* **49**, 218-224.
43. Tyden, G., Reinholt, F.P., Sundkvist, G., and Bolinder, J., 1996, Recurrence of autoimmune diabetes in recipients of cadaveric pancreatic grafts. *N. Engl. J. Med.* **335**, 860-863.
44. Halloran, P.F., Homik, J., Goes, N., Lui, S.L., Urmson, J., Ramassar, V., and Cockfield, S.M., 1997, The "injury response": a concept linking nonspecific injury, acute rejection, and long-term transplant outcomes. *Transplant. Proc.* **29**, 79-81.
45. Roep, B.O., Stobbe, I., Duinkerken, G., van Rood, J.J., Lernmark, A., Keymeulen, B., Pipeleers, D., Claas, F.H.J., and de Vries, R.R.P., 1999, Auto- and alloimmune reactivity to human islet allografts transplanted into type-1 diabetic patients. *Diabetes* **48**, 484-490.
46. Shapiro, A.M., Lakey, J.R., Ryan, E.A., Korbutt, G.S., Toth, E., Warnock, G.L., Kneteman, N.M., and Rajotte, R.V., 2000, Islet transplantation in seven patients with type 1 diabetes mellitus using a glucocorticoid-free immunosuppressive regimen. *N. Engl. J. Med.* **343**, 230-238.
47. Ryan, E.A., Lakey, J.R.T., Rajotte, R.V. et al., 2001, Clinical outcomes and insulin secretion after islet transplantation with the Edmonton protocol. *Diabetes* **50**, 710-719.
48. Hering, B.J., and Ricordi, C., 1999, Results, research priorities, and reasons for optimism: Islet transplantation for patients with type 1 diabetes. *Graft* **2**, 12-27.
49. Shapiro, A.M.J., Suarez-Pinzon, W.L., Power, R., and Rabinovitch, A., 2002, Combination therapy with low dose sirolimus and tacrolimus is synergistic in preventing

spontaneous and recurrent autoimmune diabetes in non-obese diabetic mice. *Diabetologia* **45**, 224-230.
50. Boehmer, H. von, and Sarukhan, A., 1999, GAD, a single autoantigen for diabetes. [comment]. *Science* **384**, 1135-1137.
51. Yoon, J.W., Yoon, C.S., Lim, H.W., Huang, Q.Q., Kang, Y., Pyun, K.H., Hirasawa, K., Sherwin, R.S., and Jun, H.S., 1999, Control of autoimmune diabetes in NOD mice by GAD expression or suppression in beta cells. *Science* **284**, 1183-1187.
52. Yakimets, W.J., Lakey, J.R.T., Yatscoff, R.W., Katyal, D., Ao, Z., Finegood, D.T., Rajotte, R.V., and Kneteman, N.M., 1993, Prolongation of canine pancreatic islet allograft survival with combined rapamycin and cyclosporine therapy at low doses. *Transplantation* **56**, 1293-1298.
53. Kneteman, N.M., Lakey, J.R., Wagner, T., and Finegood, D., 1996, The metabolic impact of rapamycin (sirolimus) in chronic canine islet graft recipients. *Transplantation* **61**, 1206-1210.
54. Guo, Z., Chong, A.S., Shen, J., Foster, P., Sankary, H.N., McChesney, L., Mital, D., Jensik, S.C., Gebel, H., and Williams, J.W., 1997, In vivo effects of leflunomide on normal pancreatic islet and syngeneic islet graft function. *Transplantation* **63**, 716-721.
55. Guo, Z., Chong, A.S., Shen, J., Foster, P., Sankary, H.N., McChesney, L., Mital, D., Jensik, S.C., and Williams, J.W., 1997, Prolongation of rat islet allograft survival by the immunosuppressive agent leflunomide. *Transplantation* **63**, 711-716.
56. Waldmann, H., 1999, Transplantation tolerance: where do we stand? *Nat. Med.* **11**, 1245-1248.
57. Acholonu, I.N., and Ildstad, S.T., 1999, The role of bone marrow transplantation in tolerance: organ-specific and cellular grafts. *Curr. Opin. Organ Transplant.* **4**, 189-196.
58. Kenyon, N.S., Chatzipetron, M., Masetti, M., Ranuncoli, A., Oliveira, M., Wagner, J.L., Kirk, A.D., Harlan, D.M., Burkly, L.C., and Ricordi, C., 1999, Long-term survival and function of intrahepatic islet allografts in rhesus monkeys treated with humanized anti-CD 154. *Proc. Natl. Acad. Sci. USA* **96**, 8132-8137.
59. Kenyon, N.S., Fernandez, L.A., Lehmann, R., Masetti, M., Ranuncoli, A., Chatzipetron, M., Iaria, G., Han, D., Wagner, J.L., Ruiz, P., Berho, M., Inverardi, L., Alejandro, R., Mintz, D.H., Kirk, A.D., Harlan, D.M., Burkly, L.C., and Ricordi, C., 1999, Long-term survival and function of intrahepatic islet allografts in baboons treated with humanized anti-CD 154: *Diabetes* **48**, 1473-1481.
60. Fändrich, F., Lin, X., Chai, G.X., Schulze, M., Ganten, D., Bader, M., Holle, J., Huang, D.-S., Parwaresch, R., Zavazava, N., and Binas, B., 2002, Preimplantation-stage stem cells induce long-term allogenic graft acceptance without supplementary host conditioning. *Nat. Med.* **8**, 171-178.
61. Chong, A.S., Yin, D., and Boussy, I.A., 2002, Transplantation tolerance: of mice and men. *Graft* **5**, 27-33.
62. Kawai, T., Andrews, D., Colvin, R.B., Sachs, D.H., and Cosimi, A.B., 2000, Thromboembolic complications after treatment with monoclonal antibody against CD40 ligand. *Nat. Med.* **6**, 114.
63. Kirk, A.D., and Harlan, D.M., 2000, Thromboembolic complications after treatment with monoclonal antibody against CD40 ligand (reply). *Nat. Med.* **6**, 114.
64. Zekorn, T., Horcher, A., Siebers, U., Federlin, K., and Bretzel, R.G., 1995, Islet transplantation in immunoseparating membranes for treatment of insulin-dependent diabetes mellitus. *Exp. Clin. Endocrinol. Diabetes* **103** (suppl 2), 136-139.
65. Siebers, U., Horcher, A., Bretzel, R.G., Federlin, K., and Zekorn, T., 1997, Alginate-based microcapsules for immunoprotected islet transplantation. In: *Bioartificial Organs: Science, Medicine and Technology* (A. Prokop, D. Hunkeler, A.D. Cherrington, eds.), Annals of the New York Academy of Sciences Vol. 831, pp. 304-312.

66. Siebers, U., Horcher, A., Brandhorst, H., Brandhorst, D., Hering, B., Federlin, K., Bretzel, R.G., and Zekorn, T., 1999, Analysis of the cellular reaction towards microencapsulated xenogeneic islets after intraperitoneal transplantation. *J. Mol. Med.* **77**, 215-218.
67. de Vos, P., Hamel, A.F., and Tatarkiewicz, K., 2002, Considerations for successful transplantation of encapsulated pancreatic islets. *Diabetologia* **45**, 159-173.
68. Sun, Y., Ma, X., Zhou, D., Vacek, I., and Sun, A.M., 1996, Normalization of diabetes in spontaneously diabetic cynomolgus monkeys by xenografts of microencapsulated porcine islets without immunosuppression. *J. Clin. Invest.* **98**, 1417-1422.
69. Soon-Shiong, P., Heintz, R.E., Merideth, N., Yao, Q.X., Yao, Z., Zheng, T., Murphy, M., Moloney, M.K., Schmehl, M., Harris, M., et al., 1994, Insulin independence in a type 1 diabetic patient after encapsulated islet transplantation. *Lancet* **343**, 950-951.
70. Zekorn, T.D., Horcher, A., Siebers, U., Federlin, K., and Bretzel, R.G., 1999, Synergistic effect of microencapsulation and immunoalteration on islet allograft survival in bioartificial pancreas. *J. Mol. Med.* **77**, 193-198.
71. Evans, R.W., 2001, In: *Xenotransplantation* (J.L. Platt, ed.), ASM Press, Washington, pp. 29-51.
72. Good, A.H., Cooper, D.K.C., and Malcolm, A.J. et al., 1992, Identification of carbohydrate structures which bind human anti-porcine antibodies: implications for discordant xenografting in man. *Transplant. Proc.* **24**, 559-562.
73. Miyagawa, S., Murakami, H., Takahagi, Y., Nakai, R., Yamada, M., Murase, A., Koyota, S., Koma, M., Matsunami, K., Fukuta, D., Fujimura, T., Shigehisa, T., Okabe, M., Nagashima, H., Shirakura, R., and Taniguchi, N., 2001, Remodeling of the major pig xenoantigen by N-acetylglucosaminyltransferase III in transgenic pig. *J. Biol. Chem.* **27**, 39310-39319.
74. Wennberg, L., Wallgren, A.C., Sundberg, B., Rafael, E., Zhu, S., Tibell, A., Karlsson-Parra, A., Groth, C.G., Korsgren, O., 1995, Efficacy of immunosuppressive drugs in islet xenotransplantation: a study in the pig-to-rat model. *Xenotransplantation* **2**, 222-229.
75. Wennberg, L., Karlsson-Parra, A., Sundberg, B., Rafael, E., Liu, J., Zhu, S., Groth, C.G., and Korsgren, O., 1997, Efficacy of immunosuppressive drugs in islet xenotransplantation. *Transplantation* **63**, 1234-1242.
76. Friedman, T., Smith, R.N., Colvin, R.B., and Iacomini, J., 1999, A critical role for human CD4+ T-cells in rejection of porcine islet cell xenografts. *Diabetes* **48**, 2340.
77. Jahr, H., Brandhorst, D., Brandhorst, H., Brendel, M., Eckhardt, T., El-Ouaghlidi, A., Hussmann, B., Lau, D., Nahidi, F., Wacker, T., Zwolinski, A., and Bretzel, R.G., 1998, Abstossungsreaktionen bei der tierexperimentellen xenogenen Transplantation von isolierten Langerhansschen Inseln des Schweins. *Zentralbl. Chir.* **123**, 823-829.
78. Lau, D., Hering, B.J., El-Ouaghlidi, A., Jahr, H., Brandhorst, H., Brandhorst, D., Vietzke, R., Federlin, K., and Bretzel, R.G., 1999, Isokinetic gradient centrifugation prolongs survival of pig islets xenografted into mice. *J. Mol. Med.* **77**, 175-177.
79. Lai, L., Kolber-Simonds, D., Kwang-Wook, P., Cheong, H.-T., Greenstein, J.L., Im, G.-S., Samuel, M., Bonk, A., Rieke, A., Day, B.N., Murphy, C.N., Carter, D.B., Hawley, R.J., and Prather, R.S., 2002, Production of Δ-1,3-galactosyltransferase knockout pigs by nuclear transfer cloning. *Science* **295**, 1089-1092.
80. Brown, J., Danilovs, J.A., Clark, W.R., and Mullen, Y.S., 1984, Fetal pancreas as a donor organ. *World J. Surg.* **8**, 152-157.
81. Korsgren, O., 1991, Xenotransplantation of fetal porcine islet-like cell clusters in diabetes mellitus: an experimental and clinical study. *Acta Univ. Upsal.* **295**, 1-40.
82. Korsgren, O., Sandler, S., Landström, A., Jansson, L., Andersson, A., 1988, Large-scale production of fetal porcine pancreatic islet-like cell clusters. An experimental tool for studies of islet cell differentiation and xenotransplantation. *Transplantation* **45**, 509-514.

83. Korsgren, O., Jansson, L., Eizirik, D., and Andersson, A., 1991, Functional and morphological differentiation of fetal porcine islet-like cell clusters after transplantation into nude mice. *Diabetologia* **34**, 379-386.
84. Liu, X., Federlin, K.F., Bretzel, R.G., Hering, B.J., and Brendel, M.D., 1991, Persistent reversal of diabetes by transplantation of fetal pig proislets into nude mice. *Diabetes* **40**, 858-866.
85. Liu, X., Brendel, M.D., Hering, B.J., Bretzel, R.G., and Federlin, K., 1992, Comparison of the potency of fetal pig pancreatic proislets and fragments to reverse diabetes. *Transplant. Proc.* **24**, 987.
86. Liu, X., Brendel, M.D., Brandhorst, H., Klitscher, D., Hering, B.J., Federlin, K.F., and Bretzel, R.G., 1993, Successful cryopreservation of fetal porcine proislets. *Cryobiology* **30**, 262-271.
87. Liu, X., Brendel, M.D., Brandhorst, D., Brandhorst, H., Hering, B.J., Federlin, K., and Bretzel, R.G., 1994, Reversal of diabetes in nude mice by transplantation of cryopreserved fetal porcine proislets. *Transplant. Proc.* **26**, 707-708.
88. Bretzel, R.G., Liu, X., Hering, B.J., Brendel, M., and Federlin, K., 1995, Cryopreservation transplantation and susceptibility to diabetogenic agents of fetal porcine proislets. *Xenotransplantation* **2**, 133-138.
89. Soderlund, J., Wennberg, L., Castanos-Velez, E. et al., 1999, Fetal porcine islet-like cell clusters transplanted to cynomolgus monkeys: an immunohistochemical study. *Transplantation* **67**, 784.
90. Groth, C.G., Andersson, A., Björken, C., Gunnarsson, R., Hellerström, C., Lundgren, G., Petersson, B., Swenne, I., and Östman, J., 1980, Transplantation of fetal pancreatic microfragments via the portal vein to a diabetic patients. *Diabetes* **29**, 80-83.
91. Groth, C.G., Korsgren, O., Tibell, A. et al., 1994, Transplantation of porcine fetal pancreas to diabetic patients. *Lancet* **344**, 1402-1404.
92. Bach, F.H., Fishman, J.A., Daniels, N. et al., 1988, Uncertainty in xenotransplantation: individual benefit versus collective risk. *Nat. Med.* **4**, 141-144.
93. Patience, C., Takeuchi, Y., and Weiss, R.A., 1997, Infection of human cells by an endogenous retrovirus of pigs. *Nat. Med.* **3**, 275-276.
94. Martin, U., Kiessig, V., Blusch, J.H., Haverich, A., von der Helm, K., Herden, T., and Steinhoff, G., 1998, Expression of pig endogenous retrovirus by primary porcine endothelial cells and infection of human cells. *Lancet* **352**, 666-667.
95. Van der Laan, L.J., Lockey, C., Griffeth, B.C. et al., 2000, Infection by porcine endogenous retroviruses after islet xenotransplantation in SCID mice. *Nature* **407**, 90-94.
96. Deng, Y.M., Tuch, B.E., and Rawlinson, W.D., 2000, Transmission of porcine endogenous retroviruses in severe combined immunodeficient mice xenotransplanted with fetal porcine pancreatic cells. *Transplantation* **70**, 1010-1016.
97. Heneine, W., Tibell, A., Switzer, W.M. et al., 1998, No evidence of infection with porcine endogenous retrovirus in recipients of porcine islet-cell xenografts. *Lancet* **352**, 695-699.
98. Paradis, K., Langford, G., Long, Z. et al., 1999, Search for cross-species transmission of porcine endogenous retrovirus in patients treated with living pig tissue. *Science* **285**, 1236-1241.
99. Soria, B., Skoudy, A., and Martin, F., 2001, From stem cells to beta cells: new strategies in cell therapy of diabetes mellitus. *Diabetologia* **44**. 407-415.
100. Edlund, H., 1958, Transcribing the pancreas. *Diabetes* **47**, 1817-1823.
101. Stoffers, D.A., Zinkin, N.T., Stanojevic, V., Clarke, W.L., and Habener, J.F., 1997, Pancreatic agenesis attributable to a single nucleotide deletion in the human IPF1 gene coding sequence. *Nat. Genet.* **15**, 106-110.

102. Apelqvist, A., Li, H., Sommer, L., Beatus, P., Anderson, D.J., Honjo, T., de Angelis, M., Lendahl, U., and Edlund, H., 1999, Notch signalling controls pancreatic cell differentiation. *Nature* **400**, 877-881.
103. Gradwohl, G., Dierich, A., Le Meur, M., and Guillemot, F., 2000, Neurogenin 3 is required for the development of the four endocrine cell lineages of the pancreas. *Proc. Natl. Acad. Sci. USA* **97**, 1607-1611.
104. Sosa-Pineda, B., Chowdhury, K., Torres, M., Oliver, G., and Gruss, P., 1997, The Pax 4 gene is essential for differentiation of insulin-producing beta cells in the mammalian pancreas. *Nature* **386**, 399-402.
105. Soria, B., Roche, E., Berna, G., Leon-Quinto, T., Reig, J.A., and Martin, F., 2000, Insulin-secreting cells derived from embryonic stem cells normalize glycemia in streptozotocin-induced diabetic mice. *Diabetes* **49**, 157-162.
106. Lumelsky, N., Blondel, O., Laeng, P., Velasco, I., Ravin, R., and McKay, R., 2001, Differentiation of embryonic stem cells to insulin-secreting structures similar to pancreatic islets. *Science* **292**, 1389-1394.
107. Assady, S., Maor, G., Amit, M., Itskovitz-Eldor, J., Skorecki, K.L., and Tzuckerman, M., 2001, Insulin production by human embryonic stem cells. *Diabetes* **50**, 1691-1697.
108. Zulewski, H., Abraham, E.J., Gerlach, M.J., Daniel, P.B., Moritz, W., Muller, B., Vallejo, M., Thomas, M.K., and Habener, J.F., 2001, Multipotential nestin-positive stem cells isolated from adult pancreatic islets differentiate ex vivo into pancreatic endocrine, exocrine, and hepatic phenotypes. *Diabetes* **50**, 521-533.
109. Ramiya, V.K., Maraist, M., Arfors, K.E., Schatz, D.A., Peck, A.B., and Cornelius, J.G., 2000, Reversal of insulin-dependent diabetes using islets generated in vitro from pancreatic stem cells. *Nat. Med.* **6**, 278-282.
110. Bonner-Weir, S., Taneja, M., Weir, G.C., Tatarkiewicz, K., Song, K.H., Sharma, A., and O'Neill, J.J., 2000, In vitro cultivation of human islets from expanded ductal tissue. *Proc. Natl. Acad. Sci. USA* **97**, 7999-8004.
111. Soria, B., Andreu, E., Berna, G., Fuentes, E., Gil, A., Leon-Quinto, T., Martin, F., Montanya, E., Nadal, A., Reig, J.A., Ripoll, C., Roche, E., Sanchez-Andres, and J.V., Segura, J., 2000, Engineering pancreatic islets. *Eur. J. Physiol.* **440**, 1-18.
112. Cheung, A.T., Dayanandan, B., Lewis, J.T., Korbutt, G.S., Rajotte, R.V., Bryer-Ash, M., Boylan, M.O., Wolfe, M.M., and Kieffer, T.J., 2000, Glucose-dependent insulin release from genetically engineered K cells. *Science* **290**, 1959-1962.
113. Lee, H.C., Kim, S.J., Kim, K.S., Shin, H.C., and Yoon, J.W., 2000, Remission in models of type 1 diabetes by gene therapy using a single-chain insulin analogue. *Nature* **408**, 483-488.
114. Shaw, J.A.M., Delday, M.I., Hart, A.W., and Docherty, K., 2002, Secretion of bioactive human insulin following plasmid-mediated gene transfer to non-neuroendocrine cell lines, primary cultures and rat skeletal muscle in vivo. *J. Endocrinol.* **172**, 653-672.
115. Riu, E., Mas, A., Ferre, T., Pujol, A., Gros, L., Otaegui, P., Montoliu, L., and Bosch, F., 2002, Counteraction of type 1 diabetic alterations by engineering skeletal muscle to produce insulin: insights from transgenic mice. *Diabetes* **51**, 704-711.
116. Ferber, S., Halkin, A., Cohen, H., Ber, I., Einav, Y., Goldberg, I., Barshack, I., Seijfers, R., Kopolovic, J., Kaiser, N., and Karasik, A., 2000, Pancreatic and duodenal homeobox gene 1 induces expression of insulin genes in liver and ameliorates streptozotocin-induced hyperglycemia. *Nat. Med.* **6**, 568-572.
117. Kahn, A., 2000, Converting hepatocytes to E-cells - a new approach for diabetes? *Nat. Med.* **6**, 505-506.
118. Weir, G.C., and Bonner-Weir, S., 1997, Scientific and political impediment to successful islet transplantation. *Diabetes* **46**, 1247-1256.

CELL-BASED THERAPY OF CHRONIC DEGENERATIVE DISEASES OF THE CENTRAL NERVOUS SYSTEM

Ye.V. Pankratov [1], A.I. Ivanov [1], T.D. Kolokoltsova [2], Ye.A. Nechayeva [2], I.F. Radayeva [2], L.I. Korochkin [3], A.V. Revischin [1], S.A. Naumov [1], I.A. Khlusovi [1], and A.I. Autenshlus [1]

[1]*Scientific and Clinical Center of Oncology and Neurology "Biotherapy", Novosibirsk, Russia;* [2]*State Research Center of Virology and Biotechnology "Vector", Novosibirsk, Russia;* [3]*Research Institute of Gene Biology, Moscow, Russia*

ABSTRACT

The traditional methods of pharmacotherapy of the degenerative diseases of the central nervous system do not frequently allow one to achieve the desired clinical effect. The fundamentally new approach for the treatment of severe neurological diseases is provided by the methods of biological medicine, in particular, transplantation of a complex of fetal tissues. Cell-based therapy was used to treat patients with multiple sclerosis; ante-, intra- and postnatal lesions; consequences of hemorrhagic and ischemic apoplexies; neuritis of facial nerve; sclerosis; Parkinson's disease; Alzheimer's disease; epilepsy and other types of pathologic process. The source material for obtaining a suspension of cells was the fetuses of allogenic origin. The suspension of brain cells in amounts of up to $1,5\cdot10^8$ cells and vitality not less than 40% was administered to the patients into liquor spaces using the method of endolumbar puncture. The total number of transplantations was 1900. Practically in all the cases FT was tolerated well. Positive clinical and immunologic changes were observed in the majority of the patients, thus, remission induction (in the patients with the progressive course of multiple sclerosis) for a period over 12 months was registered in 87.5% of the cases. Noteworthy that considerable changes were observed in immunograms: depression of antibody levels to brain-specific proteins, native and denatured DNA; quantitative and qualitative improvement of lymphocyte subpopulation indices, positive changes in the immunoregulatory index. Clinically, in 69% of the cases there was an improvement in more than one neurological defect and a change in the values of the Kurtzke scale towards a decrease by 2-3 points. The conduct of cell therapy with the MS patients under the acute process conditions after liquorosorption allowed the arresting of clinical manifestations and the creation of preconditions for further restoration. The retrobulbar transplantations provided a quick arrest of the retrobulbar neuritis clinical symptoms and in one case an almost complete restoration of vision in the patient with amaurosis (blindness). The remission duration has a marked direct dependence on the number of courses of endolumbar transplantations. Thus, the method of cell therapy with the use of human tissue transplantations is safe and can be used for different neurodegenerative lesions of the central nervous system. The high efficacy of the method suggests the possibility and necessity of using this method as an alternative of classical pharmacological therapy. An important element of cell therapy is the control after the state of the patient's immunity system.

1. INTRODUCTION

The traditional methods of pharmacotherapy of the degenerative diseases of the central nervous system do not frequently allow one to achieve the desired clinical effect. The fundamentally new approach for the treatment of severe neurological diseases is provided by the methods of biological medicine, in particular, transplantation of a complex of fetal tissues[1-3]. The therapeutic effects of fetal cell transplantation are connected with embryo-specific growth factors, cytokines, and other signal molecules capable of activating the regeneration and survival of cells in the recipient's body. It has been shown that donor cells getting embedded in the organism, partially or completely restore the disrupted molecular or cellular homeostasis and create stable foci of new healthy tissue in diseased organs[4]. Over the recent years, the use of cell transplantation for treating various pathological processes has become a remarkable phenomenon in clinical practice. The main efforts of scientists have been centered on the problem of treatment of degenerative diseases of the central nervous system and disorders of neurohumoral regulation.

In this connection, the goal of the present work was to develop technologies of cell-based therapy for organic lesions of the central nervous system and methods of preparation and certification of cell cultures used for transplantation.

2. MATERIALS AND METHODS

Fetuses of allogenic origin of 16-20-week gestation collected during medical abortions were used as the source material for obtaining a cell suspension. The donor's blood serum was examined for the presence of antibodies to the human immunodeficiency virus, herpes of types I and II, hepatitis B and C, HBs-antigen, syphilis, cytomegalia, rubella, toxoplasmosis, and chlamydia. The investigations were performed using the immunoenzyme method and the method of polymerase chain reaction.

The suspension of primary brain cell culture was obtained following the rules of asepsis. The material extracted was reduced to pieces with a diameter not exceeding 1 mm; the number of viable cells was counted. The concentration was $(0.5-1.0) \times 10^8$ cells per 1 ml; the doses of 1 ml each were poured into ampoules. The cryoprotector was used in order to protect the cells in the process of preservation. The ampoules with the cell suspension were frozen and stored at 196°C below zero. Before use the material was defrozen, the concentration and vitality of the cells were determined. The suspension of primary brain cell culture was certified in conformity with the standards[5].

The transplantation of cells was performed in an operating room or a medical treatment room. The suspension of brain cells in amounts of up to 1.5×10^8 cells and vitality not less than 40% was administered to the patients into liquor spaces using the method of endolumbar puncture. The course of treatment consisted of 2-3 endolumbar administrations of the cell suspension with an interval of 2-3 weeks. The patients received 3 to 8 transplantations during 1 to 3 courses of treatment at an interval of 6 months or 1 year.

Cell-based therapy was used in multiple sclerosis patients of 53 to 15 years of age with cerebrospinal form and steadily progressive course (n=129). Cell-based therapy was used to treat children of 6 months to 14 years of age with ante-, intra- and postnatal lesions of central nervous system (n=60). It was also used in patients with the consequences of hemorrhagic and ischemic apoplexies (n=62); the consequences of neuritis of facial nerve without contractures in paretic muscles (n=4); lateral amyotrophic sclerosis (n=6); Parkinson's disease (n=24); olivopontocerebellar degenerations (n=4); Alzheimer's disease (n=2); grand mal epilepsy and other types of pathological process.

The patients' states were evaluated proceeding from the dynamics of the indices of neurological, neuropsychological and immunological status. Complex examination of all the patients was performed in the course of treatment. The modified Kurtzke disability scale was used to calculate the summary neurological deficit[6]. The enzymoimmune method was employed to evaluate the humoral immune response to brain-specific proteins. The percentage of lymphocyte populations and subpopulations was determined with immunofluorescence method using monoclonal antibodies. The markers of T-lymphocytes, T-helpers/inductors, T-suppressors/cytotoxic and B-lymphocytes as well as those of natural killers were used in the work.

The statistical processing of the results was performed using standard programs.

3. RESULTS AND DISCUSSION

It is known that the Special International Convention on Human Rights in Biomedicine gave an official permission to use fetal organs and tissues for transplantation. None of the publications have reported any serious negative side effects of fetal cell transplantation with the exception for cases of microorganism or viral contamination[4]. As the initial donor's material can be infected, we paid a special attention to the contamination control of the donor and the cell material used for transplantation. Examinations of women's sera and cell suspensions did not detect antibodies to the human immunodeficiency virus, herpes of types I and II, hepatitis B and C, HBs-antigen, syphilis, cytomegalia, rubella, toxoplasmosis, and chlamydia. The results of microbiological tests showed the absence of mycoplasma, bacteria, fungi and yeast in the cell suspension.

As far as obtaining a cell suspension is concerned, it should be noted that the cells' viability directly depends on the time of taking the donor material. Our results are fully consistent with literature data[7]. The optimal period for the biological material delivery can be 2 to 3 hours, as within that period the cells' viability remained at the level of 80-85%; in 6 hours the viability decreased to 40%. Cryoconservation practically did not influence the percentage of viable cells.

Analyzing the cell suspension with immunofluorescent method revealed the presence of stem cells. (Figure 1).

It is known that donor fetal cells are successfully transported to different tissues of the recipient, however, at pathological processes in brain and spinal cord tissues, less traumatic endolumbar introduction into liquor spaces is preferable.

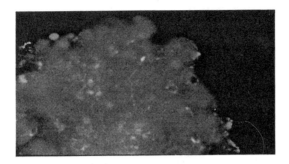

Figure 1. Brain stem cells.

It is known that donor fetal cells are successfully transported to different tissues of the recipient, however, at pathological processes in brain and spinal cord tissues, less traumatic endolumbar introduction into liquor spaces is preferable.

More than 1900 neurotransplantations were performed at central nervous system diseases. Good tolerance of cell-based therapy was observed in most cases. Only in 0.6% of cases transitory meningism, moderate headaches and subfebrility took place 2 – 3 hours after endolumbar transplantation. These lasted for a few hours and did not need any medical aid other than a single administration of analgesics.

Figures 2 and 3 present the data on the distribution of the patients according to the Kurtzke disability scale before and after the conducted treatment. It is seen that before the treatment the majority of the patients were persons with pronounced neurological deficit in the range from 4 to 7 points. The group with a deficit of 1 to 4 points (mark) by the Kurtzke scale is less representative. After the therapy, as is clearly seen in the histogram, a fairly representative group appears with absent or insignificantly manifested neurological deficit (1 point), which is mainly formed from the patients who had an index by the Kurtzke scale from 1 to 4 points before the treatment.

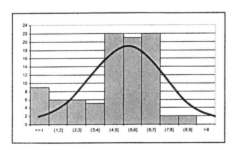

Figure 2. Distribution of the patients according to the Kurtzke disability scale before the treatment.

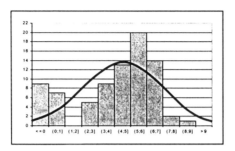

Figure 3. Distribution of the patients according to the Kurtzke disability scale after the treatment.

By the use of the cell-based therapy method, either stabilization or substantial regression of pathological symptomatology in multiple sclerosis patients has been achieved in the vast majority of cases (Figure 4).

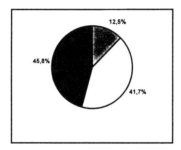

Figure 4. Structural distribution of the patients by the effect of the cell therapy (general group)/ Note: 12,5% - progressing process; 45,8% - stabilization; 41,7% -pronounced effect.

At complex inspection of the patients by multiple sclerosis before the treatment was revealed, that a considerable number of patients (26,9%) were infected with viruses (Table 1); herpes virus, cytomegalovirus, Epstein-Barr virus and associations of these viruses were isolated from the majority of patients. On this basis, antimicrobial therapy was an important element of therapy preceding endolumbar transplantation.

Table 1. Types of Infection in Multiple Sclerosis Patients

Type of infection	Incidence
Herpes simplex	28,6
Cytomegalovirus	28,6
Epstein-Barr	14,3
Chlamydiosis	7,1
Cytomegalovirus and herpes simplex	14,3
Cytomegalovirus and chlamydiosis	3,6
Cytomegalovirus and Epstein-Barr	3,6

Positive clinical and immunological changes were observed in the majority of the patients, thus, remission induction (in the patients with the progressive course of multiple sclerosis) for a period over 12 months was registered in 87.5% of the cases. Noteworthy that considerable changes were observed in immunograms: depression of antibody levels to brain-specific proteins, native and denatured DNA; quantitative and qualitative improvement of lymphocyte subpopulation indices, and positive changes were obtained in the immunoregulatory index. Clinically, in 69% of the cases there was an improvement in more than one neurological defect and a change in the values of the Kurtzke scale towards a decrease by 2-3 points, which is considered a good result of the treatment. It should be noted that the regression of pyramidal disorders (especially in the arms) and subcortical dysfunctions was the most pronounced, whereas sensor and coordination disorders proved to be resistant to the therapy. MRI in dynamics revealed in 12% of the patients with multiple sclerosis a quantitative decrease in demyelinization patches, their morphological organization manifest in a decrease in the dimensions and the structuring of the borders, which is a favorable morphological sign. The conduct of cell-based therapy with the multiple sclerosis patients under the acute process conditions after liquorosorption allowed the arresting of clinical manifestations and the creation of preconditions for further restoration. The retrobulbar transplantations provided a quick arrest of the retrobulbar neuritis clinical symptoms and in one case an almost complete restoration of vision in the patient with amaurosis (blindness).

Besides standard statistical data processing, a correlation analysis was performed the results of which provide evidence that the remission duration has a marked direct dependence on the number of courses of endolumbar transplantations R= + 0,95 (P< 0,05).

It should be also noted that we performed discriminant analysis with the purpose of cell-based therapy outcome prognosis. Statistical processing of the results with the use of this method allows one to build classifying functions using which one can give prognosis of the conducted treatment.

As a result of the calculations discriminant functions were obtained which in their characteristics can satisfy clinical requirements and be used with the purpose of treatment prognosis for the method of cell-based therapy. The classification problem of prognosis was solved at the level between the persons in whom the stabilization of the pathological process was observed after the conducted treatment and the patients in whom a pronounced clinical effect was noted. These linear functions had the following form (Table 2).

Table 2. Statistic Characteristics of Discriminant Diagnostic Functions

Function parameter	Function for Group 1	Function for Group 2
Disease continuance, years	0,0229	0,164
Kurtzke disability scale before treatment, conventional units	2,084	1,795
Immunoregulatory index with brain-specific protein before treatment, conventional units	35,35	38,38
CD8 lymphocytes with brain-specific protein before treatment, conventional units	1,715	1,831
Number of endolumbar injections of cells, conventional units	2,899	4,395
Constant	55,21	65,98

As can be seen, the suggested function includes a number of clinical and immunological parameters, which we used to evaluate the severity of the pathological process. Like correlation analysis, this kind of mathematical processing indicates that one of the most effective parameters is the number of transplantations, which essentially enables us to control the course of cell-based therapy.

The number of correct responses during the classification by the first function is 89%, by the second function 70%; the overall diagnostic efficacy is 80%. Checking on the control selection of 30 people not included in the statistical array during the build of the functions showed their sufficient diagnostic efficacy that is close to the calculated one.

4. CONCLUSION

Thus, the method of cell-based therapy with the use of human tissue transplantations is safe and can be used for different neurodegenerative lesions of the central nervous system. The high efficacy of the method suggests the possibility and necessity of using this method as an alternative of classic pharmacological therapy. An important element of cell-based therapy is control after the state of the patient's immunity system.

ACKNOWLEDGEMENTS

Corresponding member of RAMS, Professor Shmyrev V.I. — RF Presidential Administration Medical Center (Moscow); Dr. Khanykov A.I., MRC Biotherapy (Novosibirsk).

REFERENCES

1. Savelyev, S.V., and Lebedev, V.V., 1994, Transplantation of fetal and xenogenic nervous tissue at Parkinson's disease. *Bull. Exp. Biol. Med.* **4**, 369-372 (in Russian).
2. Pankratov, Ye.V., Autenshlus, A.I., and Mironov, N.V., 1997, Therapy of multiple sclerosis with human embryonic tissues; immunological control after treatment efficacy. *Int. J. Immunorehabil.* **4**, 113.
3. Mironov, N.V., Pankratov, Ye.V., and Autenshlus, A.I., 2001, Application of neurotransplantations of fetal and embryonic tissues of the human central nervous system in neurology. *J. Kremlin Med.* **2**, 23-25.
4. Repin, V.S., and Sukhikh, G.T., 1998, Medical cell biology, Moscow, 200 p.
5. *WHO Technical Report Series*, N 878, 1998, pp. 20-56 (in Russian).
6. Kurtzke, J.F., 1989, The disability scale for multiple sclerosis: apologia pro DSS. *Sua. J. Neurol.* **39**, 291-302.
7. Akimova, I.M., Gurchin, F.A., Shubin, N.A., and Gurchin, A.F., 1998, Viability of the cells of human embryo brain before and after cryoconcervation at homotransplantations. *Bull. Exp. Biol. Med.* **126**, 86-87 (in Russian).

CD34+ CELLS IN HEMATOPOIETIC STEM CELL TRANSPLANTATION

Taner Demirer
Department of Hematology/Oncology and Bone Marrow Transplant Unit, Ankara University Medical School, Ibn-i Sina Hospital, Sıhhıye, 06100 Ankara, Turkey

1. INTRODUCTION

Infusion of CD34+ cells, either autologous or allogeneic are being utilized with increasing frequency following the administration of myeloablative chemoradiotherapy for the treatment of hematologic malignancies or solid tumors. CD34+ cell collection does not require hospital admission or exposure to general anesthesia. Furthermore, many studies clearly documented rapid engraftment of both neutrophils and platelets with mobilized CD34+ cells compared to BM [1-3]. In this article, we will review issues concerning the optimization of yield, impact of the number of collected CD34+ cells and factors influencing the engraftment after hematopoietic stem cell transplantation (HSCT).

2. WHAT DOES AN ADEQUATE CD34+ CELL NUMBER MEAN?

A number of parameters, including nucleated and mononuclear cell number, quantity of granulocyte macrophage colony forming cells (CFU-GM), and the number of CD34+ cells (CD34 is an antigen expressed on stem and progenitor cells) present in the PBSC collection, have been used to assess the quality of a graft prior to its infusion [1-13]. Fernandez et al reported that neither the number of MNC/kg infused nor the number of CFU-GM/kg infused correlated with time to safe levels of granulocytes or self-sustaining levels of platelets, but did note a correlation between CD34+ cells infused and the speed of hematologic recovery[10]. In other studies, both CD34+ cell dose and CFU-GM graft content have been shown to predict the time to engraftment [9,14,15]. Bender et al have reported that rapid engraftment occurs when PBSC infusion contains 20×10^4 CFU-GM/kg or 2×10^6 CD34+ cells/kg [9]. Schwartzberg observed in 52 patients receiving chemotherapy-mobilized PBSCs that a threshold dose of 2.5×10^6 CD34+ cells/kg and 20×10^4 CFU-GM/kg correlated with rapid engraftment of neutrophils and platelets [15]. In another study which included 243 patients from Fred Hutchinson Cancer Research Center (FHCRC), patients receiving $> 2.5 \times 10^6$ CD34+ cells/kg had more rapid neutrophil ($p = .001$) and platelet recovery ($p = .0001$) than patients who received $< 2.5 \times 10^6$ CD34+ cells/kg. In patients receiving 2.5-5 or $> 5 \times 10^6$ CD34+ cells/kg there was no discernable difference in neutrophil kinetics but there was more rapid recovery of platelets ($p = .01$) in patients receiving the higher cell doses [8]. However, the threshold of 5×10^6 CD34+ cells/kg is not absolute and about 50% of patients who receive $2.5-5 \times 10^6$ CD34+ cells/kg will still have rapid recovery. Tricot reported on a series of 225 patients with myeloma who received CD34+ cells mobilized by cyclophosphamide (CY) and GM-CSF and used alone or with marrow. A threshold dose of 2.5×10^6 CD34+ cells/kg was found for patients receiving < 6 months of melphalan but $> 5 \times 10^6$ CD34+ cells/kg was required for rapid platelet recovery in patients who received > 12 months of melphalan [16]. This threshold effect for CD34+ cells has also been described using CFU-GM [9,15].

Rybka et al, in 94 patients, found that the CD34+ cell content of the graft serves as a reliable indicator of engraftment for granulocyte and platelets [11]. In that study, CD34+ cell content correlated significantly with the CFU-GM, BFU-E and CFU-GEMM content ($p < 0.0005$) and stepwise linear regression showed significant correlations between CD34+ cell content and days to granulocyte and platelet recovery ($p = 0.004$ and 0.03, respectively) [11]. Schiller determined that threshold dose to achieve hematopoietic recovery using PBSCs was 2×10^6 CD34+ cells/kg, below which engraftment was prolonged and incomplete [17]. Weaver et al found that the infusion of $\geq 5 \times 10^6$ CD34+ cells/kg was associated with an approximate 95% probability of achieving neutrophil and platelet recovery by 21 days after high dose chemotherapy [13]. Haas et al. reported a successful hematologic recovery within 2 weeks in patients receiving a CD34+ cells of $> 2.5 \times 10^6$/kg [18]. The minimum quantity of PBSCs required for successful engraftment is unknown but is probably between $2-3 \times 10^6$ CD34+ cells/kg. Although there may be some patients who have relatively rapid engraftment below this level, very prolonged platelet recovery has been observed in some patients who received $< 2 \times 10^6$ CD34+ cells/kg[7]. At low CD34+ cell doses there is probably, little if any, advantage of PBSCs over marrow due to the slow engraftment tempo.

3. FACTORS INFLUENCING AN OPTIMAL MOBILIZATION YIELD

Several reports have indicated that there is a significant inter-patient variation in the ability to mobilize CD34+ cells[7,8,16,18]. While many patients mobilize enough CD34+ cell in 1 or 2 collections for more than one transplant, a significant number of patients do not achieve acceptable CD34+ or CFU-GM numbers in PBSC products. Some investigators have reported that the time to recovery from the neutropenic nadir or thrombocytopenia separates patients who will have good CD34 collections and those who will not[16,19-22]. For example, patients with early hematologic recovery (< 9 days) have higher numbers of progenitor cells collected than patients with prolonged aplasia after the same therapy[7,13,23-25]. This observation likely reflects an indirect measurement of stem cell reserve. Two studies from FHCRC using analysis by linear regression of the logarithm of CD34+ cells collected found that lower age, marrow free of disease, lack of prior radiation, and lower number of prior chemotherapy regimens, were important factors influencing greater numbers of CD34+ cells in collections[7,8]. Demirer et al. reported that the percentage of marrow involvement, prior RT and number of prior chemotherapy regimens were important predictors of CD34+ cell yield in patients with multiple myeloma[26]. Seong et al. reported that previous pelvic radiotherapy, hypocellular marrow, and refractory disease were associated with poor harvests of CD34+ cells[27]. Similarly, Haas et al. reported that previous cytotoxic chemotherapy and radiation adversely affected the yield of CD34+ cells with each cycle of chemotherapy associated with an average decrease of 0.2×10^6 CD34+ cells/kg per pheresis in non-irradiated patients and large field radiotherapy reducing the collection yields by an average of 1.8×10^6 CD34+ cells/kg [18]. Tricot et al. reported a correlation between duration of exposure to previous chemotherapy, especially of alkylating agents, and mobilization yield in patients with multiple myeloma[16]. In that study, 91% of patients with exposure of < 6 months reached $> 5 \times 10^6$ CD34+ cells/kg as compared to only 28% of patients with exposure > 24 months. Recently, Glaspy et al. reported that frequency of previous chemotherapy, even with regimens which are not considered stem cell toxins can decrease the number of CD34+ cells harvested in patients with breast cancer. The median total number of CD34+ cells obtained was significantly greater in the group receiving ≤ 4 cycles (11.7 x 10^6/kg) than in the group receiving ≥ 5 cycles (4.68 x 10^6/kg) (p = .01)[28] However, these factors account for only about 1/2 of the inter-patient variability and do not fully explain differences. Even in normal donors who are presumed to have normal marrow function and have not received any chemotherapy, the administration of G-CSF 5-16 *ug*/kg results in wide intersubject CD34 yields and poor yields in 5-15% of donors[29-31].

4. WHEN IS THE BEST TIME FOR COLLECTION OF CD34+ CELLS?

The timing of PBSC collection is important in order to maximize the number of CD34+ cells harvested. The most reliable time for harvesting CD34+ cells is still under investigation. Apheresis usually is initiated 10 to 18 days after the administration of low to moderate dose chemotherapy. Following a chemotherapy-induced nadir, collections are usually initiated when the white blood cell (WBC) count recovers to > 1 x 10^9/L [14,32]. However, in one study investigators delayed collections until the WBC count was > 3 x 10^9/L [23]. Using this approach, sufficient number of CD34+ cells were collected in all patients with only a single leukapheresis. Ho *et al* observed that maximum mobilization following cyclophosphamide (CY), epirubicin and 5-fluorouracil with GM-CSF started consistently 2 days after the WBCs recovered to > 2 x 10^9/L after nadir, and remained elevated for 4 to 5 days[24]. Another study has suggested that a delay until the WBC exceeds 10 x 10^9/L may be more optimum[33]. Demirer and Bensinger observed poor CD34+ cell yields in patients who recover WBC to > 1 x 10^9/L but remain platelet transfusion dependent[34].

Several studies reported that monitoring daily CD34+ cell content in peripheral blood may also be useful to predict the best time to begin leukapheresis[25,33-36]. Siena *et al* recommended that apheresis begin when CD34+ cells first appear in the circulation during recovery from intensive chemotherapy-induced pancytopenia[25]. Haas *et al.* reported that, a CD34+ cell count of at least 50/*ul* in peripheral blood was highly predictive for a yield greater than 2.5 x 10^6 CD34+ cells/kg in a single apheresis [18]. Passos-Coelho *et al.* reported that percentage of peripheral blood CD34+ cells ≥ 0.5% and marrow CD34+ cells ≥ 2.5% following cyclophosphamide and GM-CSF were highly predictive of successful mobilization yield[37]. In that study, > 2.9 x 10^6 CD34+ cells/kg were collected after CY and GM-CSF mobilization in patients with greater than 2.5% CD34+ cells in the bone marrow harvest before PBSC mobilization. All patients with a large number of collected CD34+ cells had a peripheral blood CD34+ cell percentage greater than 0.5% just prior to apheresis[37]. Demirer et al. reported a significant correlation between WBC counts on the first day of collection and CD34+ cell yield[38]. In that study, as the WBC counts on the first day of collection increased, CD34+ cell yield on the first day increased[38].

Demirer et al. investigated the correlation of preleukapheresis circulating CD34+ cells/*ul,* WBC and platelet counts on the first day of apheresis with the yield of collected CD34+ cell counts[39]. A strong correlation was found between the early morning number of circulating CD34+ cells/*ul* in peripheral blood on the day of leukapheresis and the total amount of CD34+ cells obtained per leukapheresis ($r = 0.962$, $P < 0.001$). In that study, threshold numbers of circulating CD34+ cells required to obtain a particular number of CD34+ cells/kg with a single apheresis were calculated. The threshold numbers of peripheral blood CD34+ cell/*ul* in order to obtain $\geq 0.5 \times 10^6$/kg, $\geq 1 \times 10^6$/kg and $\geq 2.5 \times 10^6$/kg CD34+ cell in one collection were 5/*ul*, 12/*ul* and 34/*ul*, respectively. Threshold number of 34/*ul* of CD34+ cells was reached in 42.5% of patients and 88% of these patients reached the level of $\geq 2.5 \times 10^6$/kg in a single apheresis [39]. Despite low r values, WBC and platelet counts on the first day of apheresis were also correlated with the yield of collected CD34+ cells per kilogram ($r = 0.482$, $P < 0.01$ and $r = 0.496$ $P < 0.01$, respectively). That study showed that preleukapheresis circulating CD34+ cells/*ul* significantly better correlated with the yield of collected CD34+ cells than WBC and platelet counts on the first day of apheresis. The presence of ≥ 34 CD34+ cells/*ul* in the peripheral blood predicted the achievement of $\geq 2.5 \times 10^6$/kg CD34+ cells in a single apheresis. Based on this and previous studies mentioned above, this correlation constitutes the basis for the accepted clinical practice of guiding leukapheresis according to the daily peripheral blood CD34+ cell counts. The use of this threshold in the clinical practice may prevent unnecessary collections and decrease the procedure related cost [39].

Yu et al. from FHCRC found that a subpopulation of lysis-resistant cells in the peripheral blood, identified by Sysmex SE9500 and designated as HPC, can serve as surrogate marker predictive of the yield of CD34+ cells[40]. The results indicated that WBC and MNC in the peripheral blood were poor predictors of CD34 content, while HPC gave a correlation coefficient of 0.62. Another word, the HPC level in the peripheral blood had a stronger correlation with CD34+ cell yield than did WBC and MNC counts, but was weaker than the correlation between CD34+ cell count in the peripheral blood and CD34+ cell yield[40]. Although HPC enumeration does not predict the apheresis yield, there is still a correlation between preleukapheresis peripheral blood HPC and CD34+ cell counts by using Sysmex SE-9500 hematology analyzer which is a simple method. Flow cytometry is an expensive and time consuming method just to determine preleukapheresis peripheral blood CD34+ cell counts in order to determine the appropriate time for apheresis, therefore Sysmex SXE-9500 as a part of the automated blood differential can be a practical and cheap method which may prevent unnecessary attempts of flow measurement of preleukapheresis peripheral blood CD34+ cell counts.

5. DOES THE NUMBER OF INFUSED CD34+ CELLS HAS ANY IMPACT ON PERI-TRANSPLANT MORBIDITY ?

In one study, Demirer et al. investigated the effect of different doses of rhG-CSF following mobilization chemotherapy on yields of CD34+ cells and peri-transplant morbidities in patients with hematologic malignancies and solid tumors[41]. In that study, 50 patients were randomized to receive rhG-CSF 8 (n = 25) versus 16 (n = 25) *ug*/kg/day following mobilization chemotherapy regimens[41]. Median time between mobilization chemotherapy and the first apheresis in the low and high dose arms of rhG-CSF were 12 days (10-17) and 10 days (range 9-16) (P < 0.001). Twenty of 25 (80%) patients in the high dose rhG-CSF arm had bone pain as compared to 10 of 25 (40%) in the low dose arm (P = 0.004). The median number of CD34+ cells collected after 8 *ug*/kg/day of rhG-CSF was 2.36×10^6/kg (range 0.21-7.80) as compared to 7.99 (range 2.76-14.89) after 16 ug/kg/day (P < 0.001) [41]. Among patients randomized to 8 v 16 *ug*/kg, all (100%) achieved $\geq 4.0 \times 10^6$ CD34+ cells/kg and less aphereses were required to achieve $\geq 2.5 \times 10^6$ CD34+ cells/kg after the higher dose (P < 0.001). Twenty of 25 (80%) patients in the low dose and 23 of 25 (92%) in the high dose rhG-CSF arm underwent high dose chemotherapy (HDC) and autologous stem cell transplantation (ASCT). Median days of WBC engraftment in patients mobilized with 8 *ug*/kg and 16 *ug*/kg of rhG-CSF were 12 (range 10-20) and 9 (8-11), respectively (P < 0.001). But there was no difference between 2 groups regarding the other parameters of peritransplant morbidity such as days of platelet engraftment (P = 0.10), RBC (P = 0.56) and platelet transfusions (P = 0.22), days of TPN (Total parenteral nutrition) requirement (P = 0.84), days of fever (P = 0.93), days of antibiotics (P = 0.77), and number of different antibiotics which was used (P = 0.58)[41]. This small study showed that higher doses of rhG-CSF following a submyeloablative mobilization chemotherapy were associated with a clear dose response effect based on the collected CD34+ cell yields. Based on the parameters of peritransplant morbidity, 8 ug/kg/day is as effective as 16 ug/kg/day except a rapid neutrophil engraftment in the high dose arm. Therefore, in the routine clinical practice, higher doses of rhG-CSF may not be used for CD34+ cell collections following chemotherapy based mobilization regimens in this cost-conscious era[41].

6. IS THERE ANY BENEFIT OF POST-TRANSPLANT GROWTH FACTOR ADMINISTRATION ON PERI-TRANSPLANT MORBIDITY?

In one study, Demirer et al. evaluated the effect of post-transplant rhG-CSF administration on the parameters of peritransplant morbidity [42]. In that study, three sequential and consecutive cohorts of 20 patients each with hematologic malignancies and solid tumors received either post-transplant rhG-CSF at a dose of 5 ug/kg/day IV in the morning started on day 0, day 5, or no rhG-CSF. RhG-CSF was given until the absolute neutrophil count was greater than $5 \times 10^9/L$. Number of infused CD34+ cell counts were comparable among these 3 groups. Engraftment kinetics and other parameters of peritransplant morbidity such as transfusion and TPN requirements, fever, antibiotic administration as well as hospital stay were evaluated with univariate and multivariate analysis [42]. Patients receiving post-transplant rhG-CSF starting on day 0 and 5 recovered granulocytes more rapidly than those not receiving post-transplant rhG-CSF ($P < 0.001$ for ANC ≥ 0.5 and $1 \times 10^9/L$). Post-transplant rhG-CSF administration was not significantly associated with more rapid platelet engraftment in the univariate and multivariate analysis. Post-transplant rhG-CSF administration starting on day 0 and 5 were significantly associated with a decreased duration of fever ($P = 0.002$ and 0.001, respectively) and antibiotic administration ($P < 0.001$ and 0.006, respectively) compared to reference group of without rhG-CSF. Post-transplant rhG-CSF were also significantly associated with a short hospital stay compared to reference group of without rhG-CSF administration ($P < 0.001$ and 0.001, respectively). There was no difference among three arms regarding TPN and transfusion requirements. There was also no difference between day 0 and day 5 arms regarding the parameters of peritransplant morbidity [42]. In conclusion, post-transplant rhG-CSF administration is associated with a faster granulocyte recovery and shortened duration of hospitalization, fever as well as nonprophylactic antibiotic administration in patients who receive autologous stem cell transplantation. This study also showed that post-transplant rhG-CSF administration on day 5 may be as effective as day 0 administration on the clinical outcome. Day 5 administration instead of day 0 may be an economical approach in the routine clinical practice in this cost-conscious era.

7. CONTAMINATION OF PBSC COLLECTIONS WITH TUMOR CELLS

Recently, several reports have shown that CD34+ cell infusions frequently are contaminated with tumor cells [43-46]. Circulating neoplastic cells may be present in patients with certain malignancies regardless of tumor involvement by the marrow. The possibility of infusing cancer cells into patients at the time of stem-cell transplantation is known to occur in breast cancer, lymphomas, multiple myeloma and leukemias [44,45,47]. Brugger et al have shown that mobilization of CD34+ cells can in some circumstances result in tumor cell recruitment into the peripheral blood in patients with small cell lung cancer or stage IV breast cancer [43]. Several studies have demonstrated that 50-67% of patients with multiple myeloma have malignant cells in circulation at the time of CD34+ cell harvest [46, 48, 49]. The presence of these cells in circulation appears to correlate with disease activity and stage [48].

Despite the demonstration that leukemic cells infused with remission marrow can contribute to relapse, the overall significance of infused residual malignant cells to clinical relapse remains unknown [50]. It is, however, reasonable to assume that peripheral blood CD34+ cells may contain occult malignant cells and strategies should be developed to cope with this problem. Efforts to purge grafts of tumor cells have been carried out by incubation of grafts with chemotherapeutic drugs and tumor-specific monoclonal antibodies, and by positive selection for CD34+ stem cells [51]. Vescio et al reported that highly purified collection of CD34+ cells in patients with multiple myeloma showed no myeloma specific antigen despite an assay sensitivity of 1 tumor cell in 2,500 to 44,000 normal cells [52]. While such efforts have led to reductions in tumor cell numbers present in PBSC grafts, the impact of such approaches on relapse or patient survival has not yet been determined[51]. It is also important to realize that any purging strategies results in some loss of stem cells. CD34+ cell enrichment procedures have an average yield of only 50% [51]. The loss of such a large number of CD34+ cells after selection could compromise the speed of engraftment. It is likely that novel purging methods are needed which are able to preserve the majority of CD34+ cells.

8. FUTURE PROSPECTS

Although strategies for CD34+ cell mobilization are almost well described, there are still an ongoing effort in order to explore novel methods for mobilization of stem cells. Burns *et al.* reported the mobilization of a PBSC with anti-tumor activity using IL-2 plus G-CSF in patients with advanced breast cancer [53]. It has been shown that G-CSF administration to normal donors results in suppression of NK cell function in PBSC products. Since NK cell function can be markedly augmented by IL-2, authors hypothesized that in vivo mobilization with IL-2 and G-CSF for collection of PBSCs used for hematopoietic rescue may reverse NK suppressive effects of G-CSF and lead to an in vivo enhanced graft-versus-tumor effect in the immediate post-transplant period. Burns *et al.* concluded that the addition of IL-2 to G-CSF is safe, reverses NK dysfunction observed with G-CSF alone and increases cytotoxic effectors in the graft and in the patient early post-transplant. This infusion of an IL-2 activated graft may enhance the efficacy of early post-transplant immuno-therapy [53].

Although in this article we have only mentioned the role of CD34+ cells in hematopoietic stem cell transplantation, there are new and rapidly progressing aspects of the use of stem cells in different area of medicine [54]. Some studies suggested that hematopoietic stem cells can serve as an alternative to embryonic stem cells for tissue replacement after injury or disease such as stroke and heart infarct, Parkinson disease, cystic fibrosis, muscular dystrophy, and congenital liver diseases [54]. Because of the vast amount of knowledge accumulated in their handling for the purpose of transplantation and their relatively easy isolation, they would indeed be an ideal source of organ repair and reconstitution. The clinical prospects for the use of hematopoietic stem cells for these purposes largely depends on whether it will be possible to develop methods that increase the tissue conversion frequencies and noninvasive mobilization of progenitor cells.

REFERENCES

1. Demirer, T., Buckner, C.D., Appelbaum, F.R. *et al.*, 1995, Rapid engraftment after autologous transplantation utilizing marrow and recombinant granulocyte colony-stimulating factor-mobilized peripheral blood stem cells in patients with acute myelogenous leukemia. *Bone Marrow Transplantation* **15**, 915-922.
2. Demirer, T., Petersen, F.B., Bensinger, W.I., *et al.*, 1996, Autologous transplantation with peripheral blood stem cells collected after granulocyte colony-stimulating factor in patients with acute myelogenous leukemia. *Bone Marrow Transplantation* **18**, 29-34.
3. Demirer, T., Bensinger, W.I., and Buckner, C.D., 1999, Peripheral blood stem cell mobilization for high dose chemotherapy. *J. Hematotherapy* **8**, 103-113.

4. Rowley, S.D., Zuehlsdorf, M., Braine, H.G., *et al.*, 1987, CFU-GM content of bone marrow graft correlates with time to hematologic reconstitution following autologous bone marrow transplantation with 4-hydroperoxycyclophosphamide-purged bone marrow. *Blood* **70**, 271-275.
5. Demirer, T., and Bensinger, W.I., 1995, Optimization of peripheral blood stem cell collection. *Current Opinion in Hematology* **2**, 219-226.
6. Emminger, W., Emminger-Schmidmeier, W., Hocker, P., *et al.*, 1989, Myeloid progenitor cells (CFU-GM) predict engraftment kinetics in autologous transplantation in children. *Bone Marrow Transplantation* **4**, 415-420.
7. Bensinger, W.I., Longin, K., Appelbaum, F., *et al.*, 1994, Peripheral blood stem cells (PBSCs) collected after recombinant granulocyte colony stimulating factor (rhG-CSF): an analysis of factors correlating with the tempo of engraftment after transplantation. *Br J Haematol.* **87**, 825-831.
8. Bensinger, W.I., Appelbaum, F.R., Rowley, S., *et al.*, 1995, Factors that influence collection and engraftment of autologous peripheral blood stem cells. *J. Clin. Oncol.* **13**(10), 2547-2555.
9. Bender, J.G., To, L.B., Williams, S., *et al.*, 1992, Defining a therapeutic dose of peripheral blood stem cells. *J. Hematotherapy* **1**, 329-341.
10. Fernandez, H.F., Noto, T.A., Morrell, L., *et al.*, 1994, Early engraftment of mobilized autologous peripheral blood progenitor cells collected by large volume leukapheresis. *Blood* **84**, (Suppl. 1, Abstract 365).
11. Rybka, W.B., Kiss, J.E., Lister, J., *et al.*, 1994, Graft CD34+ cell content predicts engraftment following allogeneic and autologous hematopoietic stem cell transplantation. *Blood* **84**, (Suppl. 1, Abstract 338).
12. Pecora, A.L., Brochstein, J.A., Jennis, A., *et al.*, 1994, Total CD34+ cell content and CD34+CD33 subset predict time to neutrophil and platelet engraftment and hospital discharge in patients following high-dose chemotherapy with primed peripheral blood progenitor cells. *Blood* **84**, (Suppl. 1, Abstract 342).
13. Weaver, C.H., Birch, R., Schwartzberg, L., *et al.*, 1994, CD34 content of peripheral blood progenitor cells (PBPC) is the single most powerful predictor of recovery kinetics in patients receiving myeloablative high-dose chemotherapy and PBPC infusion. *Blood* **84**, (Suppl. 1, Abstract 388).
14. Smith, R., Sweetenham, J.W., 1994, A mononuclear cell dose of 3×10^8/kg is sufficient to predict early multilineage engraftment in patients undergoing high dose therapy and transplantation with cryopreserved peripheral blood progenitor cells for malignant lymphoma. *Blood* **84**, (Suppl.1, Abstract 364).
15. Schwartzberg, L., Birch, R., Blanco, R., *et al.*, 1993, Rapid and sustained hematopoietic reconstitution by peripheral blood stem cell infusion alone following high-dose chemotherapy. *Bone Marrow Transplant.* **11**, 369-374.
16. Tricot, G., Jagannath, S., Vesole, D., *et al.*, 1995, Peripheral blood stem cell transplants for multiple myeloma: Identification of favorable variables for rapid engraftment in 225 patients. *Blood* **85**, 588-596.
17. Schiller, G., Rosen, L., Vescio, R., *et al.*, 1994, Threshold dose of autologous CD34 positive peripheral blood progenitor cells required for engraftment after myeloablative treatment for multiple myeloma. *Blood* **84**, (Suppl. 1, Abstract 813).
18. Haas, R., Mohle, R., Fruhauf, S., *et al.*, 1994, Patient characteristics associated with successful mobilizing and autografting of peripheral blood progenitor cells in malignant lymphoma. *Blood* **83**, 3787-3794.
19. Spencer, V., Smith, J., Kulkarni, S., *et al.*, 1992, Does transplantation of a high number of CD34 cells predict more rapid engraftment following high-dose chemotherapy. *Proc ASCO* **11**, 131 (Abstract).
20. Mortimer, J., Hendricks, D., Goodnough, L.T., *et al.*, 1993, Pheresis of peripheral blood progenitor cells directed by CD34 counts. *Proc. ASCO* **12**, 467 (Abstract).

21. Reid, C.D.L., Kirk, A., Muir, J., et al., 1989, The recovery of circulating progenit or cells after chemotherapy in AML and ALL and its relation to the rate of bone marrow regeneration after aplasia. Br. J. Haematol. 72, 21-27.
22. Cantin, G., Marchand-Laroche, D., Bouchard, M.M., et al., 1989, Blood-derived stem cell collection in acute nonlymphoblastic leukemia: Predictive factors for a good yield. Exp. Hematol. 17, 991-996.
23. Pettengell, R., Morgenstern, G.R., Woll, P.J., et al., 1993, Peripheral blood progenitor cell transplantation in lymphoma and leukemia using a single apheresis. Blood 82, 3770-3777.
24. Ho, A.D., Gluck, S., Germond, C., et al., 1993, Optimal timing for collections of blood progenitor cells following induction chemotherapy and granulocyte-macrophage colony-stimulating factor for autologous tx in advanced breast cancer. Leukemia 7, 1738-1744.
25. Siena, S., Bregni, M., Brando, B., et al., 1991, Flow cytometry for clinical estimation of circulating hematopoietic progenitors for autologous transplantation in cancer patients. Blood 77, 400-409.
26. Demirer, T., Buckner, C.D., Gooley, T., et al., 1996, Factors influencing collection of peripheral blood stem cells in patients with multiple myeloma. Bone Marrow Transplantation 17, 937-941.
27. Seong, D., Anderson, B., Korbling, M., et al.,1995, Predicting parameters of successful peripheral blood stem cell (PBSC) collection after chemo/cytokine primed mobilization in relapsed hodgkin's disease. ASCO 14, 321 (Abstract 951).
28. Glaspy, J., Chap, L., Menchaca, D., et al., 1995, Effect of prior chemotherapy on peripheral blood progenitor cell (PBPC) harvests in patients with breast cancer. ASCO 14, 319 (Abstract 943).
29. Dreger, P., Haferlach, T., Eckstein, V., et al., 1994, G-CSF mobilized peripheral blood progenitor cells for allogeneic transplantation: safety, kinetics of mobilization, and composition of the graft. Br. J. Haematol. 87, 609-613.
30. Bensinger, W.I., Weaver, C.H., Appelbaum, F.R., et al., 1995, Transplantation of allogeneic peripheral blood stem cells mobilized by recombinant human granulocyte colony stimulating factor. Blood 85, 1655-1658.
31. Schmitz, N., Dreger, P., Suttorp, M., et al., 1995, Primary transplantation of allogeneic peripheral blood progenitor cells mobilized by filgrastim (Granulocyte colony-stimulating factor). Blood 85, 1666-1672.
32. Elias, A.D., Ayash, L., Anderson, K.C. et al., 1992, Mobilization of peripheral blood progenitor cells by chemotherapy and granulocyte-macrophage CSF for hematologic support after high-dose intensification for breast cancer. Blood 79, 3036-3044.
33. Dreger, P., Marquardt, P., Haferlach, T., et al., 1993, Effective mobilization of peripheral blood progenitor cells with Dexa-BEAM and G-CSF-timing of harvesting and composition of the leukapheresis product. Br. J. Cancer 68, 950-957.
34. Demirer, T., Buckner, C.D., Bensinger, W.I., et al., 1996, Optimization of peripheral blood stem cell mobilization. Stem Cells 14,106-116.
35. Bender, J.G., Williams, S.F., Myers, S., et al., 1992, Characterization of chemotherapy mobilized peripheral blood progenitor cells for use in autologous stem cell transplantation. Bone Marrow Transplant. 10, 281-285.
36. Hohaus, S., Goldschmidt, H., Ehrhardt, R., et al.,1993, Successful autografting following myeloablative conditioning therapy with blood stem cells mobilized by chemotherapy plus RHG-CSF. Exp. Hematol. 21(4), 508-514.
37. Passos-Coelho, J.L., Braine, H.G., Davis, J.M., et al., 1995, Predictive factors for peripheral- blood progenitor-cell collections using a single large-volume leukapheresis after cyclophosphamide and GM- CSF mobilization. J. Clin. Oncol. 13, 705-714.
38. Demirer, T., Buckner, C.D., Storer, B., et al., 1997, Effect of different chemotherapy regimens on peripheral-blood stem-cell collections in patients with breast cancer receiving granulocyte colony stimulating factor. J. Clin. Oncol. 15(2), 684-690.

39. Demirer, T., İlhan, O., Aylı, M., et al., Monitoring of peripheral blood CD34+ cell counts on the first day of apheresis is highly predictive for efficient CD34+ cell yield. *Therapeutic Apheresis* (in press).
40. Yu, J., Leisenring, W., Fritschle, W., et al., 2000, Enumeration of HPC in mobilized peripheral blood with the Sysmex SE9500 predicts final CD34+ cell yield in the apheresis collection. *Bone Marrow Transplant*, **25**, 1157-1164.
41. Demirer, T., Aylı, M., Ozcan, M., et al., 2002, Mobilization of peripheral blood stem cells with chemotherapy and recombinant human granulocyte-CSF (Rh-GCSF): A randomized evaluation of different doses of Rh-GSCF. *Br.J. Haematol.* **116**, 468-474.
42. Demirer, T., Aylı, M., Daglı, M., et al., Influence of post-transplant recombinant human granulocyte-colony stimulating factor (RhG-CSF) administration on peritransplant morbidity in patients undergoing autologous stem cell transplantation. *Br. J. Haematol.* (in press).
43. Brugger, W., Bross, K.J., Glatt, M., et al., 1994, Mobilization of tumor cells and hematopoietic progenitor cells into peripheral blood of patients with solid tumors. *Blood* **83**, 636-640.
44. Ross, A.M., Cooper, B.W., Lazarus, H.M., et al., 1993, Detection and viability of tumor cells in peripheral blood stem cell collections from breast cancer patients using immunocytochemical and clonogenic assay techniques. *Blood* **82**, 2605-2610.
45. Vora, A.J., Toh, C.H., Peel, J., et al., 1994, Use of granulocyte colony-stimulating factor (G-CSF) for mobilizing peripheral blood stem cells: risk of mobilizing clonal myeloma cells in patients with bone marrow infiltration. *Br. J. Haematol.* **86**, 180-182.
46. Gibson, J., Pope, B., Petersen, A., et al.,1994, G-CSF stimulated PBSC harvests in myeloma contain immature malignant plasma cells. *Blood* **84**, (Suppl. 1, Abstract 422).
47. Brockstein, B., Ross, A., Hollingsworth, K., et al., 1995, Tumor cell contamination of bone marrow harvest products: clinical consequences in a cohort of advanced breast cancer patients undergoing high-dose chemotherapy. *ASCO* **14**, 327 (Abstract 975).
48. Owen, R.G., Child, J.A., Rawson, A., et al., 1994, Detection of contaminating cells in PBPC harvests and the efficacy of CD34 selection in patients with multiple myeloma. *Blood* **84**, (Suppl. 1, Abstract 1392).
49. Witzig, T.E., Gertz, M.A., Pineda, A.A., et al., 1994, Detection of monoclonal plasma cells in the peripheral blood stem cell harvests of patients with multiple myeloma. *Blood* 84 (Suppl. 1, Abstract 882).
50. Rill, D.R., Moen, R.C., Buschle, M., et al., 1992, An approach for the analysis of relapse and marrow reconstitution after autologous marrow transplantation using retrovirus-mediated gene transfer. *Blood* **79**, 2694-2700.
51. Shpall, E.J., Jones, R.B., Bearman, S.I., et al., 1994, Transplantation of enriched CD34-positive autologous marrow into breast cancer patients following high-dose chemotherapy: influence of CD34-positive peripheral -blood progenitors and growth factors on engraftment. *J. Clin. Oncol.* **12**, 28-36.
52. Vescio, R.A., Hong, C., Cao, J., et al., 1994, The hematopoietic stem cell antigen, CD34, is not expressed on the malignant cells in multiple myeloma. *Blood* **84**, 3283-3290.
53. Burns, L., Weisdorf, D., Ogle, K., et al., 1997, Mobilization of a PBPC graft with anti-tumor activity using interleukin-2 plus G-CSF in patients with advanced breast cancer. *Blood* **90**(10), (Suppl. 1, Abstract 2634).
54. Graf, T., 2002, Differentiation plasticity of hematopoietic cells. *Blood* **99**, 3089-3101.

THE EFFECTS OF DIFFERENT GROWTH FACTORS ON HUMAN BONE MARROW STROMAL CELLS DIFFERENTIATING INTO HEPATOCYTE-LIKE CELLS

Yu-Shih Weng, Hsien-Yi Lin, Yi-Jung Hsiang, Cheng-Ta Hsieh, and Wen-Tyng Li

Department of Cell-Tissue Engineering, Biomedical Engineering Center, Industrial Technology Research Institute, Hsinchu, 310 Taiwan.

1. INTRODUCTION

Stem cells are self-renewable and are thought to be the pluripotent cells that can differentiate into a variety of cells or tissue types. For many years, adult stem cells harvested from bone marrow have been used therapeutically. In 1999, Pittenger et al.[1] published the methods to induce differentiation of human mesenchymal stem cells into different cell types of mesodermal lineages. Theise et al.[2,3] have demonstrated that hepatocytes, from endodermal lineage, can be derived from bone marrow in human and mice. Hepatocyte engraftment from bone marrow cells have been confirmed by double FISH (fluorescence in situ hybridization) after bone marrow transplantation. Lagasse et al.[4] further demonstrated that purified hematopoietic stem cells from adult mouse bone marrow rescued fumarylacetoacetate hydrolase (FAH) deficient mice and restored the biochemical function of their liver. Alison et al.[5] showed that the human adult hematopoietic stem cell population is capable of yielding an epithelial lineage in chronically damaged liver. $\beta_2 m^-/Thy-1^+$ cells from rat and human bone marrow were integrated with hepatic cell plates and were differentiated into mature hepatocytes after intraportal infusion into rat livers studied by Avital et al.[6] β_2m^-/Thy-1$^+$ cells also differentiated into mature hepatocytes in a culture system simulating liver regeneration and containing cholestatic serum. Oh et al.[7] and Schwartz et al.[8] have succeeded in differentiating rat bone marrow cells and multipotent adult progenitor cells from bone marrow into hepatocyte-like cells by addition of growth factors in the culture medium. Hamazaki et al.[9] induced hepatic maturation in mouse embryonic stem cells *in vitro*. Other studies[10] suggest that the microenvironment of embryonic liver, including growth factors and cell-cell interactions, is critical for regulating liver development. Acidic FGF and HGF were known to play important roles in the early- and mid-developmental stages of liver development. So far, none have succeeded to induce human bone marrow stromal cells (BMSC) differentiation into hepatocytes in culture.

To induce hepatic differentiation of human BMSCs, the microenvironment of embryonic liver development was mimicked. The effects of different growth factors, including aFGF, HGF, SCF, or IL-6, on human BMSCs were investigated in this study. As a result, a combination of aFGF, HGF and Dex was found to be an optimal condition for inducing differentiation of human BMSCs into hepatocyte-like cells. The other growth factors, including IL-6 and SCF, showed no effect on differentiation of BMSCs.

2. MATERIALS AND METHODS

2.1 Chemicals and Cytokines

IL-6 and stem cell factor (SCF) were purchased from Serotec (UK). Hepatocyte growth factor (HGF) and acidic fibroblast growth factor (aFGF) were from BD Biosciences (USA). Modified Eagle Medium α Medium (α-MEM), non-essential amino acids (NEAA) solution, and antibiotic-antimycotic solution were from Invitrogen (Grand Island, New York, USA). Fetal bovine serum (FBS) was from Hyclone (Logan, Utah, USA). Human bone marrow stromal cells (BMSC, passage 2) were from Cesco™ (Hsinchu, Taiwan, ROC). Antibodies against CD29 and CD34 were from Serotec (UK), and those against CD44, CD45 and human albumin were from DAKO (Denmark). Chamber slides and cultureware were from Nunc (Denmark). DAPI (4',6'-diamidino-2-phenylindole), dexamethasone (Dex) and other chemicals were from Sigma-Aldrich (St. Louis, Missouri, USA).

2.2 Cell Culture

Human BMSCs were propagated in .-MEM medium containing 10% FBS (lot selected for rapid growth of human BMSCs), 1x antibiotic-antimycotic, NEAA and incubated at 37°C with 5% humidified CO_2. The culture medium was changed every 2-3 days. The cells were trypsinized at 90% confluence and passaged at 1:3. Human BMSCs were routinely characterized by their expression of cell surface antigens by flow cytometeric analysis (Beckman Coulter flow cytometer, Miami, Florida, USA) and differentiation down specific cell lineages by cell staining[1]. To test osteogenic potential of human BMSCs, the cells were induced in osteogenic medium for 2 weeks, and calcium deposition was observed by Alizarin red-S stain. To test adipogenic potential of BMSCs, the cells were induced in adipogenic medium for 2 weeks, and neutral lipid was observed by Oil Red stain. To test chondrogenic potential of BMSCs, the cells were induced in chondrogenic medium for 2 weeks, and glycosaminoglycan was stained by Safranin-O stain. Human BMSCs at passage 4 were used for hepatocyte differentiation experiments.

2.3 Differentiation of Human BMSCs into Hepatocyte-like Cells

To induce hepatocyte differentiation, human BMSCs were seeded in Δ MEM medium containing 10% FBS and cultured on 16-well chamber slides coated with 0.1% collagen type I at a density of 10^2 to 10^3 cells/well. After one day, human BMSC propagation medium was removed and serum-free media supplemented with various cytokines or combinations of cytokines was added. Cytokines used included 100 ng/ml aFGF, 100 ng/ml HGF, 100 ng/ml SCF, 100 ng/ml IL-6, and 10^{-8}M dexamethasone. Cultures were evaluated daily by inverted microscope. The expression of albumin was examined over time by immunofluorescence and reverse transcriptase-polymerase chain reaction (RT-PCR).

2.4 Immunofluorescence

Undifferentiated and differentiated human BMSCs were fixed in 2% formaldehyde at room temperature for 10 min, and washed twice with PBS. In between each wash, cells were allowed to sit at room temperature for 5 min. Slides were incubated in PBS/10% FBS solution for 10 to 20 min to prevent non-specific binding of antibodies. Slides were incubated sequentially in FITC-conjugated antibody specifically against human albumin (1:250 dilutions in 0.1% saponin/PBS/10% FBS solution) at room temperature for 20 min. Slides were washed twice with PBS/10% FBS. The nuclei of the cells were stained with DAPI. Cells were examined by fluorescence microscopy (Leica DM LB Microscope & Digital imaging analysis system, Germany).

2.5 RT-PCR

Total RNAs were extracted from BMSCs treated with different growth factors for 14 days by using Trizol reagent (Invitrogen, USA). Complementary DNA was synthesized from total RNAs by using SuperScript II first-strand synthesis system with oligo (dT) (Invitrogen, USA). PCR was performed by using rTaq DNA polymerase (Takara Biochemicals, Japan). β-actin gene expression was used as an endogenous control. The sequences of PCR primer pairs were as following:
 albumin (sense): 5'-AAACCTCTTGTGGAAGAGCC-3'
 albumin (antisense): 5'-CAAAGCAGGTCTCCTTATCG-3'
 β-actin (sense): 5'-GTAGGGCGCCCCAGGCACCA-3'
 β-actin (antisense): 5'-CTCCTTAATGTCACGCACGAT-3'

3. RESULTS

3.1 Characterization of Human BMSCs

Human BMSCs at passage 4 were characterized by flow cytometric and differentiation analysis. Figure 1 shows the result of flow cytometric analysis. These cells were positive for CD44 and CD29 and negative for CD34 and CD45 markers. This phenotype is consistent with what was reported for human mesenchymal stem cells previously.[1] Differentiation analysis with osteogenic, adipogenic, and chondrogenic induction showed that these cells could differentiate into these cell lineages in two weeks of induction (Figure 2). It indicated that these cells did have multi-lineage differentiation potential.

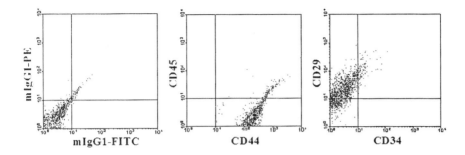

Figure 1. Flow cytometric analysis of human BMSCs. BMSCs were co-stained with either CD44-FITC and CD45-PE or CD34-FITC and CD29-PE.

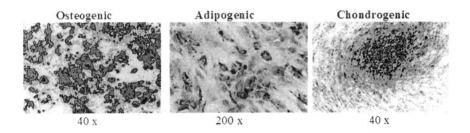

Figure 2. Human BMSCs differentiate to mesenchymal lineages. Osteogenesis was indicated by calcium deposition that stained with Alizarin red-S. Adipogenesis was indicated by the accumulation of neutral lipid that stained with Oil Red. Chondrogenesis was shown by glycosaminoglycan secretion stained by Safranin-O.

3.2 Morphological Characterization of Human BMSCs Differentiation

During embryonic development of mice, the initial event of liver ontogeny occurs on embryonic day 9 (E9). In this early stage, FGFs, derived from adjacent cardiac mesoderm, commit the foregut endoderm to form the liver primodium. The liver bud proliferates and migrates into surrounding septum transversum, which consists of loose connective tissue containing collagen. Here, hepatic precursors contact with connective tissue matrix. During and after the mid-stage of hepatogenesis, surrounding mesenchymal cells secrete HGF and support fetal hepatocytes. At late stage, from E12 through E16, the fetal liver becomes the major site for hematopoiesis. In this stage, hematopoietic cells produce oncostatin M that induces maturation of murine fetal hepatocytes[9]. IL-6 was demonstrated for its particular role in murine liver regeneration[11]. Fujio et al.[12] indicated that SCF/c-kit might, possibly in combination with other growth factors/receptors, be involved in the early activation of hepatic stem cells as well as the expansion and differentiation of oval cells.

Based on the previous reports for embryonic development and liver regeneration, we applied growth factors and extracellular matrix to induce hepatic differentiation of human BMSCs *in vitro*. Cytokines including HGF, aFGF, IL-6, and SCF were tested individually or in combinations to observe their effects on human BMSCs under inverted microscopy. As shown in figure 3, we found HGF and aFGF plus HGF induced morphological changes of human BMSCs from fibroblast-like to polygonal- or round-shape. When the cells were treated with HGF, their cytoplasm spread after 5 days, then shrank gradually, and the cell morphology ended up in polygonal shape with granules inside which were hepatocyte-like. As the cells were cultured for 24 days in HGF, the percentage of differentiated cells increased to 25% (data not shown). Interestingly, the combination of aFGF and HGF stimulated a higher percentage of cells to change their morphology than HGF alone did. When human BMSCs were cultured in medium containing aFGF, HGF and Dex, the percentage of differentiated cells increased up to 40% (data not shown).

3.3 Immunofluorescence of Human BMSCs Differentiation into Hepatocyte-like Cells

We further evaluated hepatocyte differentiation by immunofluorescence for albumin expression, a late marker for hepatocyte differentiation. Human BMSCs were cultured on 0.1% collagen I coated slides in serum free medium with different cytokines for 24 days. The nuclei of human BMSCs were stained with DAPI and albumin expression was confirmed over time by FITC-conjugated human albumin specific antibody stain. Cells treated with HGF, aFGF or aFGF plus HGF expressed high levels of albumin at day 16. Cells treated with IL-6 and SCF showed no albumin expression (Figure 4).

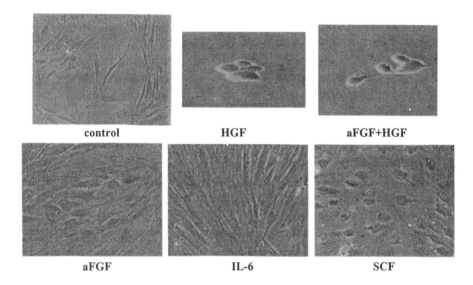

Figure 3. Phenotypic characterization of human BMSCs differentiation to hepatocyte-like cells (200 x). Phenotypic changes of human BMSCs were observed daily under inverted microscope. When the cells were treated with HGF, aFGF or aFGF plus HGF, the morphology of human BMSCs changed from fibroblast-like to polygonal or round shape after 9 days.

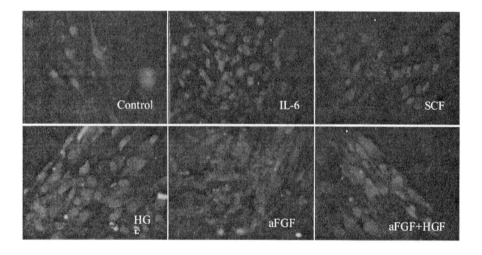

Figure 4. Immunochemical characterization of human BMSCs differentiation to hepatocyte-like cells. The nuclei of human BMSCs were stained by DAPI (blue) and albumin expression (green) was confirmed by FITC-conjugated human specific albumin antibody stain. Cells treated with HGF, aFGF or aFGF plus HGF expressed albumin at day 16. No albumin expression was observed in IL-6 or SCF treated cells.

3.4 Demonstration of aFGF and HGF Induced Albumin Gene Expression by RT-PCR

We further confirmed hepatocyte differentiation by RT-PCR as shown in figure 5. Albumin mRNA expression was not detected in human BMSCs without cytokine treatment or with IL-6, SCF, FGF-4 treatment. Cells received aFGF, HGF or aFGF plus HGF treatment exhibited albumin mRNA expression. The result is consistent with immunofluorescence analysis shown in Figure 4.

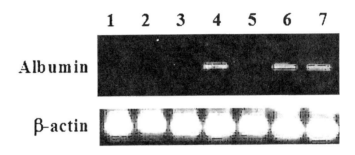

Figure 5. RT-PCR confirmed that hepatocyte-like phenotype. E-actin was used as an endogenous control. Lane 1: negative control, no cytokine treatment; lane 2: IL-6; lane 3: SCF; lane 4: aFGF; lane 5: FGF-4; lane 6: HGF; lane 7: HGF plus aFGF. Cells treated with aFGF, HGF or aFGF plus HGF expressed albumin at day 14. No albumin expression was observed in IL-6, SCF or FGF-4 treated cells.

4. DISCUSSION

To understand hepatic potential of human BMSCs, cytokines involved in liver development or regeneration including IL-6, SCF, aFGF, HGF, and FGF-4 were tested. We have evaluated phenotypic changes, albumin production, and albumin mRNA expression of undifferentiated and differentiated human BMSCs. Different effects were observed. Neither IL-6 nor SCF induced the expression of albumin at gene or protein expression level. Instead, aFGF, HGF and combination of the two showed hepatic differentiation potential.

Although we found human BMSCs morphologically changed 9 days after HGF or HGF plus aFGF treatment, not all the cells with polygonal or round shape were stained by antibody against human albumin. Interestingly, some fibroblast-like cells were stained by antibody against human albumin. The observation might be due to the heterogeneity of cell population in BMSCs. These fibroblast-like cells might be the precursor of liver cells or billiary duct cells, which also express albumin. In addition to the effects by the supplement of growth factors, the differentiated cells might provide some cues for their surrounding cells to differentiate and cell-cell interaction might play a role in the induction of differentiation.

HGF, a potent mitogen for hepatocytes, is a ubiquitous growth factor which reacts with its receptor, c-met, in many cells types. In our study, 60% to 75% of cells in the human BMSC cultures were not induced to differentiate to albumin positive cells by HGF. Previous studies showed that human BMSCs expressed HGF receptor, c-met. C-met positive cells in BMSCs might act as the target for HGF to induce differentiation of BMSCs into hepatocyte-like cells. To further address this question, BMSCs expressed c-met can be selected and tested for their ability to differentiate into hepatocytes.

IL-6 was shown to involve in liver regeneration, which mainly acts on hepatocytes. SCF was elucidated to participate in the activation of hepatic stem cells as well as expansion and differentiation of oval cells. However, we showed that IL-6 and SCF had no effects on human BMSC differentiation. It seems reasonable to explain the difference by assuming that the hepatic stem cells in liver and bone marrow are different populations of cells. Our results suggest that the combination of HGF and aFGF is capable of inducing hepatic differentiation of human BMSCs *in vitro*. It will be interesting to know what the intrinsic properties of hepatic stem cells within human BMSC populations are and whether these stem cells share any characteristics of embryonic stem cell derived hepatic stem cells.

BMSCs, also termed mesenchymal stem cells, are thought to give rise to tissues of mesodermal origin. However, liver is an organ derived from endoderm. Our results suggest that human BMSCs have the potential to transdifferentiate into cells of endodermal origin. The mechanism of transdifferentiation will be another issue to be investigated.

Further experiments to characterize the hepatocyte-like cells are required. At molecular level, expression of hepatocyte-specific genes, such as α-fetoprotein and CK18 will be determined by RT-PCR. Immunostaining with antibodies against hepatocyte-specific proteins and surface marker identification in these cells are also important. Furthermore, liver-specific function such as albumin secretion, urea production, and cytochrome P450 activity will be analyzed. The success of our study may facilitate application of human BMSCs in cell therapy for chronic liver diseases.

ACKNOWLEDGEMENTS

This work was supported by grants 90-EC-2-A-17-0337 (903XS4D31) and 91-EC-2-A-17-0337 (A311XS4180) from Ministry of Economic Affair, ROC. We are grateful to Prof. Jung-Sang Huang's (St. Louis University, USA) technical advice.

REFERENCES

1. Pittenger, M.F., Mackay, A.M., Beck, S.C., Jaiswal, R.K., Douglas, R., Mosca, J.D., Moorman, M.A., Simonetti, D.W., Craig, S., and Marshak, D.R., 1999, Multilineage potential of adult human mesenchymal stem cells. *Science* **284**, 143-147.
2. Theise, N.D., Badve, S., Saxena, R., Henegariu, O., Sell, S., Crawford, J.M. and Krause, D.S., 2000, Derivation of hepatocytes from bone marrow cells in mice after radiation-induced myeloablation. *Hepatology* **31**, 235-240.
3. Theise, N.D., Nimmakayalu, M., Gardner, R., Illei, P.B., Morgan, G., Teperman, L., Henegariu, O., and Krause, D.S., 2000, Liver from bone marrow in humans. *Hepatology* **32**, 11-16.
4. Lagasse, E., Connors, H., Al-Dhalimy, M., Reitsma, M., Dohse, M., Osborne, L., Wang, X., Finegold, M., Weissman, I.L., and Grompe, M., 2000, Purified hematopoietic stem cells can differentiate into hepatocytes *in vivo. Nature Med.* **6**, 1229-1234.
5. Alison, M.R., Poulson, R., Jeffery, R., Dhillon, A.P., Quaglia, A., Jacob, J., Novelli, M., Prentice, G., Williamson, J., and Wright, N.A., 2000, Hepatocytes from non-hepatic adult stem cells. *Nature* **406**, 257.
6. Avital, I., Inderbitzin, D., Aoki. T., Tyan, D.B., Cohen, A.H., Ferraresso, C., Rozga, J., Arnaout, W.S., and Demetriou, A.A., 2001, Isolation, characterization, and transplantation of bone marrow-derived hepatocyte stem cells. *Biochem. Biophys. Res. Commun.* **288**, 156-164.
7. Oh, S.H., Miyazaki, M., Kouchi, H., Inoue, Y., Sakaguchi, M., Tsuji, T., Shima, N., Higashio, K., and Namba, M., 2000, Hepatocyte growth factor induces differentiation of adult rat bone marrow cells into a hepatocyte lineage in vitro. *Biochem. Biophys. Res. Commun.* **279**:500-504.
8. Schwartz, R.E., Reyes, M., Koodie, L., Jiang, Y., Blackstad, M., Lund, T., Lenvik, T., Johnson, S., Hu, W.-S., and Verfaillie, C.M., 2002, Multipotent adult progenitor cells from bone marrow differentiate into functional hepatocyte-like cells. *J. Clin. Invest.* **109**, 1291-1302.
9. Hamazaki, T., Iiboshi, Y., Oka, M., Papst, P.J., Meacham, A.M., Zon, L.I., and Terada, N., 2001, Hepatic maturation in differentiating embryonic stem cells *in vitro. FEBS Lett.* **497**, 15-19.
10. Zaret, K.S., 2001, Hepatocyte differentiation: from the endoderm and beyond. *Curr. Opin. Genet. Develop.* **11**, 568-574.
11. Aldeguer, X., Debonera, F., Shaked, A., Krasinkas, A.M., Gelman, A.E., Que, X., Zamir, G.A., Hiroyasu, S., Kovalovich, K.K., Taub, R., and Olthoff, K.M., 2002, Interleukin-6 from intrahepatic cells of bone marrow origin is required for normal murine liver regeneration. *Hepatology* **35**, 40-48.
12. Fujio, K., Evarts, R.P., Hu, Z., Marsden, E.R., and Thorgeirsson, S.S., 1994, Expression of stem cell factor and its receptor, c-kit, during liver regeneration from putative stem cells in adult rat. *Lab. Invest.* **70**, 511-516.

OXIDATIVE DNA DAMAGE BIOMARKERS USED IN TISSUE ENGINEERED SKIN

Henry Rodriguez[1], Pawel Jaruga[1], Mustafa Birincioğlu[2], Peter E. Barker[1], Catherine O'Connell[1], and Miral Dizdaroğlu[1]
[1]*DNA Technologies Group, Chemical Science and Technology Laboratory, National Institute of Standards and Technology, 100 Bureau Drive, Mail Stop 831, Gaithersburg, MD 20899-8311, U.S.A.;* [2]*Department of Pharmacology, Medical School, Inönü University, Malatya, Turkey*

1. INTRODUCTION

The process of tissue engineering often involves the mixing of cells with polymers that may cause inflammation to the tissue and thus elevate the level of endogenous free radical production. In order to assure that such composite materials are free of genetic changes that might occur from inflammation during the development phase of the product, our laboratory is responding to the need for test methods used to assess the safety and performance of tissue-engineered materials. Specifically, we are identifying cellular biomarkers that could be used during the *in vitro* development phase of tissue-engineered materials to ensure that cells have not undergone any inflammatory response during the development or shipment of the product. Using GC/MS technology, we have screened for a total of five genomic modified base DNA biomarkers in tissue-engineered skin and compared the levels to control cells, neonatal fibroblasts and neonatal keratinocytes. No significant level of damage was detected compared to control cells. LC/MS technology was used in the validation of one of the oxidatively modified DNA lesions. Nearly identical results were obtained when measuring the nucleoside with LC/MS. Biomarker programs such as this can provide the basis for an international reference standard of cellular biomarkers that can aid in the development and safety of tissue engineered medical products.

1.1 Initial Comments

Tissue engineering is an emerging area of biotechnology that will provide replacement tissues for patients, as well as complex, functional biological systems for research and testing in the pharmaceutical industry. There are two forms of tissue engineering: one in which cells are grown in culture and seeded onto a material, and in the other where an implanted material induces a specific response such as tissue regeneration *in vivo*. The former approach is used to create skin substitutes, while the latter is used to accelerate nerve regeneration as an example.

The need for alternative, immediate and permanent wound closure materials has created a multi-million dollar industry to manufacture skin substitutes for wound coverage and wound healing. Estimates for the number of hospitalizations from burns range from 60,000-80,000 annually, and costs for recovery from acute injuries range from US$36,000-117,000 per patient[1-2]. The knowledge gained from cultured epidermal autografts, in which a small skin biopsy is cultured to produce extended epidermal sheets, led to the development of skin equivalents in which donor tissue with limited immunogenicity are used.

A new research area of tissue engineering involves the investigation of how living cells interact and respond to synthetic biomaterial surfaces. The clinical development underlying such scientific research includes a number of novel tissue-engineered products that include replacement skin as a synthetic dermal matrix for burn patients and chronic ulcer patients. The first tissue-engineered organ, which has progressed from lab bench to accepted patient care, has been skin. Skin being the largest and most highly complex organ in the human body, is the most affected organ in traumatic injuries. Research and development in the field of wound dressing has resulted in the fabrication and production of a wide variety of synthetic and biological dressings. There are now several commercially available products that fall into two categories: dermal skin substitutes and combined epidermal and dermal skin substitutes. Dermal skin substitutes include AlloDerm® (LifeCell, Inc., Branchburg, NJ) a dermal matrix lacking immunogenic cells, and Integra® (Integra LifeSciences Holdings Corp., Plainsboro, NJ), a combination of dermal fibroblasts and bovine collagen. Dermagraft® (Applied Tissue Sciences, La Jolla, CA) consists of non-immunogenic neonatal fibroblasts cultured on a polyglactin mesh and has been used to treat burns[3] and diabetic foot ulcers[4]. Combined epidermal and dermal skin substitutes include Apligraf® (Organogenesis, Inc, Canton, MA), the first mass-produced skin product comprised of fibroblasts and keratinocytes (derived from human neonatal foreskin) in a type I bovine collagen extracellular matrix. This product has been approved by the Food and Drug Administration (FDA) for treatment of partial thickness and full thickness skin loss due to venous stasis ulcers[5-6]. Apligraf is a bilayered living skin analog with appearance and handling characteristics that are similar to normal human skin[7]. TestSkin II® (Organogenesis, Inc, Canton, MA) is equivalent to Apligraf and is sold for the purposes of *in vitro* research.

The aim of this program was to help identify cellular biomarkers and measurement technologies that could be used to assure that tissue-engineered skin products are free of genetic changes that could occur during the development phase. These biomarkers could help better understand the cellular mechanisms of how cells react to inflammatory stimuli from different matrices. Specifically, we looked at oxidative damage to DNA by free radicals.

Free radicals are produced in living cells by normal metabolism and by exogenous sources such as carcinogenic compounds and ionizing radiations[8]. Of the free radicals, the highly reactive hydroxyl radical (•OH) causes damage to DNA and other biological molecules[8-10]. Scientific studies have shown that free radicals are implicated in many diseases of the older population, such as cancer, arthritis, cataracts, Alzheimer's disease and Parkinson's disease[8]. It was therefore important to determine if significant levels of free radical-induced damage to DNA (a biomarker of cellular inflammation) had occurred to the tissue-engineered product.

In this study, tissue-engineered skin (TestSkin II®; Organogenesis, Inc, Canton, MA) was obtained and separated into its two cellular layers (Epidermal component consisting of neonatal human keratinocytes and the Dermal component consisting of neonatal human fibroblasts) (Figure 1).

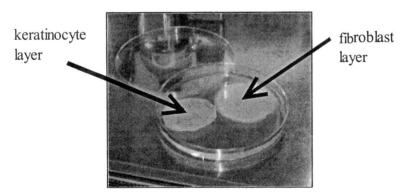

Figure 1. TestSkin II® from Organogenesis separated into individual cell layers.

DNA was isolated and compared to the DNA from neonatal control cells (neonatal human dermal fibroblasts and neonatal human epidermal keratinocytes) and HeLa cells that have not undergone the tissue engineering process. It was also compared to calf thymus DNA (ctDNA).

2. EXPERIMENTAL PROCEDURES

Certain commercial equipment or materials are identified in this paper in order to specify adequately the experimental procedures. Such identification does not imply recommendation or endorsement by the National Institute of Standards and Technology, nor does it imply that the materials or equipment identified are necessarily the best available for the purpose.

2.1 Cell Culture and DNA Isolation

HeLa cells were placed in antibiotic-free Dulbecco's Modified Eagle Medium containing 10% (v/v) fetal bovine serum and grown in 175 cm^2 flasks at 37 °C in a humidified cell culture incubator with 5% CO_2/95% air. Medium was aspirated off and cells were rinsed with 20 mL of 1X Phosphate Buffered Saline (PBS). Cells were detached by adding 3 mL trypsin/EDTA solution. Human dermal neonatal fibroblast cells (HDFn; Cascade Biologics, Portland, Oregon) were cultured in Medium 106 supplemented with Low Serum Growth Supplement (LGGS) in the absence of antibiotics and antimycotics (Cascade Biologics, Portland, Oregon). Medium was aspirated off, and cells were rinsed and detached as above. Trypsin/EDTA solution was immediately removed and an aliquot of 3 ml of Trypsin neutralizer solution (Cascade Biologics, Portland, Oregon) was added to each flask. Human epidermal neonatal keratinocyte cells (HEKn; Cascade Biologics, Portland, Oregon) were cultured in EpiLife medium supplemented with Human Keratinocyte Growth Supplement (HKGS) in the absence of antibiotics and antimycotics (Cascade Biologics, Portland, Oregon) and then treated as above. Calf thymus DNA was purchased from the Sigma Chemical Corporation.

DNA was isolated from cells using a blood and cell culture DNA kit (Qiagen, Valencia, CA). DNA was recovered by spooling, washed once in 70% ethanol, and then air-dried. DNA was dissolved in 10 mM sodium phosphate buffer at a concentration of 0.3 mg/mL and dialyzed against water for 18 h at 4°C. Water outside the dialysis bags was changed three times during the course of the dialysis. Subsequently, DNA concentration was determined by UV spectroscopy. Aliquots of this solution containing 100 µg of DNA were dried under vacuum in a SpeedVac.

2.2 TestSkin II: Fibroblast/Keratinocyte Separation and DNA Isolation

<u>Separating Cell Layers</u>. A TestSkin II® disk (Organogenesis, Inc., Canton, MA) was placed in a 150 mm^2 sterile petri dish containing 35 mL 1x PBS and incubated at room temperature for 30 min in a cell culture hood. PBS was removed and replaced with 40 mL protease type X solution (0.5 mg/mL 1x PBS) and incubated at 37 °C for 2 h in a humidified cell culture incubator with 5% CO_2/95% air. Epidermal layer (keratinocytes; gray top layer) was gently separated from the dermal layer (fibroblasts; white bottom layer) using sterile forceps.

<u>Separating Individual cells and DNA Isolation</u>. Epidermal layer was placed in a 50-mL polypropylene conical tube containing 40 mL trypsin-versene and incubated in a 37 °C water bath for 2 h. The dermal layer was placed in a 175-cm^2 T-flask containing 180 mL collagenase solution [60 mL collagenase (4.17 mg/mL H_2O) and 120 mL collagenase pre-mix (120 ml 1x PBS, 14 mL of 2.5% trypsin solution, 1 mL filtered 0.45% glucose solution)] and incubated at 37 °C in a humidified cell culture incubator with 5% CO_2/95% air for 2 h. Independently, each respective tube was agitated every 15 min. Cells were pelleted by centrifugation (1300 x g/4 °C for 5 min) and rinsed twice with 20 mL 1x PBS with centrifugation (1300 x g/4 °C for 5 min) between each rinse step. Cells were eventually suspended in 4-mL 1x PBS and counted using a cell culture hemocytometer. DNA was isolated from the cells using a blood and cell culture DNA kit (Qiagen, Valencia, CA).

2.3 Analyses of Oxidatively-Modified DNA Bases by LC/MS and GC/MS

This work has been previously discussed in detail[11].

3. CONCLUSION

Oxidative damage to DNA can be measured by a variety of analytical techniques, which each has its own advantages and drawbacks[12-13]. Most of these techniques measure only a single product with no spectroscopic evidence for identification. Techniques that use mass spectrometry provide unequivocal identification and quantification of DNA damage[13]. For over a decade, gas chromatography/mass spectrometry (GC/MS) has been used for the measurement of DNA base and sugar lesions, and DNA-protein crosslinks in cells and *in vitro*[13]. Recently, liquid chromatography/tandem mass spectrometry (LC/MS/MS) and liquid chromatography/mass spectrometry (LC/MS) emerged as new techniques for the measurement of modified nucleosides in DNA. For this reason, we employed the use of GC/MS and LC/MS in the validation of one of the oxidatively modified DNA lesions.

Using GC/MS technology, we have screened for a total of 5 genomic DNA biomarkers in tissue-engineered skin (TestSkin II®) and compared the levels to control cells: neonatal fibroblasts and neonatal keratinocytes, including cultured HeLa cells and commercially available ctDNA. The biomarkers consisted of FapyAdenine, FapyGuanine, 8-OH-Guanine, 5-OH-Uracil, and 5-OH-Cytosine. For 8-OH-Guanine (a free base), its nucleoside form (8-OH-dGuanosine) was also monitored suing LC/MS (Figure 2; data only shown for 8-OH-Guanine).

Results showed that the level of oxidative DNA damage was found to be at background/endogenous levels (approximately 1-10 modified molecules/10^6 DNA bases). Nearly identical results were obtained when measuring the nucleosides with LC/MS. Therefore, no significant level of damage was detected compared to control cells.

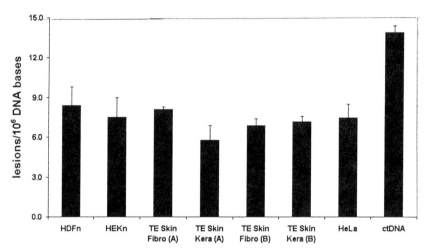

Figure 2. Level of 8-OH-Guanine in various samples using GC/MS technology. HDFn: Human Dermal Fibroblasts neonatal; HEKn: Human Epidermal Keratinocytes neonatal; TE Skin Fibro (A & B): Fibroblast cells isolated from TestSkin II products – "A & B" each represent three independent TestSkin fibroblast layers combined into one; TE Skin Kera (A & B); Keratinocyte cells isolated from TestSkin II products – "A & B" each represent three independent TestSkin keratinocyte layers combined into one; HeLa: HeLa DNA isolated from cultured cells; ctDNA: calf thymus DNA commercially obtained. S.D. error bars are based on triplicate measurement analysis.

The National Institute of Standards and Technology is making a concerted effort to identify cellular biomarkers for the field of tissue-engineered medical products. These studies can provide the basis for an international reference standard of cellular biomarkers that can aid in the development and safety of tissue-engineered medical products.

REFERENCES

1. Saffle, J.R., Davis, B., and Williams, P., 1995, Recent outcomes in the treatment of burn injury in the United States: a report from the American Burn Association Patient Registry. *J.Burn Care Rehabil.* **16**, 219-232.
2. Brigham, P.A. and McLoughlin, E., 1996, Burn incidence and medical care use in the United States: estimates, trends, and data sources. *J.Burn Care Rehabil.* **17**, 95-107.
3. Hansbrough, J.F., 1997, Dermagraft-TC for partial-thickness burns: a clinical evaluation. *J.Burn Care Rehabil.* **18**, S25-S28.
4. Gentzkow, G.D., Iwasaki, S.D., Hershon, K.S., Mengel, M., Prendergast, J.J., Ricotta, J.J., Steed, D.P., and Lipkin, S., 1996, Use of dermagraft, a cultured human dermis, to treat diabetic foot ulcers. *Diabetes Care* **19**, 350-354.
5. Falanga, V., Margolis, D., Alvarez, O., Auletta, M., Maggiacomo, F., Altman, M., Jensen, J., Sabolinski, M., and Hardin-Young, J., 1998, Rapid healing of venous ulcers and lack of clinical rejection with an allogeneic cultured human skin equivalent. Human Skin Equivalent Investigators Group. *Arch. Dermatol.* **134**, 293-300.
6. Sabolinski, M.L., Alvarez, O., Auletta, M., Mulder, G., and Parenteau, N.L., 1996, Cultured skin as a 'smart material' for healing wounds: experience in venous ulcers. *Biomaterials* **17**, 311-320.
7. Wilkins, L.M., Watson, S.R., Prosky, S.J., Meunier, S.F., and Parenteau, N.L., 1994, Development of a bilayered living skin construct for clinical applications. *Biotechnol.Bioeng.* **43**, 747-756.
8. Halliwell, B. and Gutteridge, J.M.C., 1999, *Free Radicals in Biology and Medicine*, Third Edition, Oxford Science Publ., Oxford.
9. Dizdaroglu, M., 1992, Oxidative damage to DNA in mammalian chromatin. *Mutat.Res.* **275**, 331-342.
10. Breen, A.P., and Murphy, J.A., 1995, Reactions of oxyl radicals with DNA. *Free Radic. Biol. Med.* **18**:, 1033-1077.
11. Jaruga, P., Birincioglu, M., Rodriguez, H., and Dizdaroglu, M., 2002, Mass spectrometric assays for the tandem lesion 8,5'-cyclo-2'-deoxyguanosine in mammalian DNA. *Biochemistry* **41**, 3703-3711
12. Collins, A., Cadet, J., Epe, B., and Gedik, C., 1997, Problems in the measurement of 8-oxoguanine in human DNA. Report of a workshop, DNA oxidation, held in Aberdeen, UK, 19-21 January, 1997. *Carcinogenesis* **18**, 1833-1836.
13. Dizdaroglu, M., 1998, Mechanisms of free radical damage to DNA. In Aruoma, O. I. and Halliwell, B., eds., *DNA & Free Radicals: Techniques, Mechanisms & Applications*, pp. 3-26. OICA International, Saint Lucia.

BIOMARKERS USED TO DETECT GENETIC DAMAGE IN TISSUE ENGINEERED SKIN

Catherine O'Connell[1], Peter E. Barker[1], Michael Marino[2], Patricia McAndrew[2], Donald H. Atha[1], Pawel Jaruga[1], Mustafa Birincioğlu[3], Miral Dizdaroğlu[1], and Henry Rodriguez[1]
[1]*DNA Technologies Group, Chemical Science and Technology, Laboratory, National Institute of Standards and Technology, 100 Bureau Drive, Mail Stop 831, Gaithersburg, MD 20899-8311, U.S.A.;* [2]*Transgenomic, Inc., Gaithersburg, MD,U.S.A.;* [3]*Department of Pharmacology, Medical School, İnönü University, Malatya, Turkey*

1. INTRODUCTION

In this study, tissue-engineered skin (TestSkin II) was obtained, separated into its two cellular layers (epidermis and dermis) and DNA was extracted. The first biomarker tested consisted of screening for DNA point mutations in the p53 gene, the most commonly mutated gene in skin cancer. To ensure the accuracy of the results, two measurement technologies that incorporate internal calibration standards were used. It was shown that tissue-engineered skin did not contain mutations in this gene at the level of sensitivity of capillary electrophoresis-SSCP and Denaturing High Performance Liquid Chromatography. Results were compared to control cells (neonatal fibroblasts and neonatal keratinocytes) and fibroblasts that were obtained from a 55 year-old and 96 year-old human donor. The second set of biomarkers tested looked at the loss of the Y-chromosome. Using Fluorescent In Situ Hybridization technology, Y chromosome loss was examined in the tissue-engineered skin, normal control lymphocytes, and neonatal and aged (55 and 96 year-old) donor control cells. Y-chromosome loss was only detected in the fibroblasts from the 96 year-old donor. Biomarkers such as p53 mutations and chromosome loss can provide the basis for an international reference standard of cellular biomarkers to aid in the development and safety of tissue engineered medical products.

1.1 Initial Comments

Tissue engineering is an emerging area of biotechnology that will provide replacement tissues for patients, as well as complex, functional biological systems for research and testing in the pharmaceutical industry. There are two forms of tissue engineering: one whereby cells are grown in culture and seeded onto a material, and in the other in which an implanted material induces a specific response such as tissue regeneration *in vivo*. The former approach is used to create skin substitutes, while the latter is used to accelerate nerve regeneration, for example.

The aim of the DNA Technologies Group tissue engineering program at the National Institute of Standards and Technology (NIST) is to identify cellular biomarkers and measurement technologies that could be used to assure that tissue-engineered skin products are free of genetic changes that could occur during the development phase. In this study, we looked at two potential biomarkers: (1) DNA point mutations in the p53 gene, the most commonly mutated gene in skin cancer[1-2] and (2) loss of the Y-chromosome, a common occurrence in aging[3]. In the accompanying study presented at this meeting, oxidative damage to DNA by free radicals was also studied.

DNA mutation can be measured by a variety of analytical techniques, which have their own advantages and drawbacks[4]. Most of these techniques scan for mutations within a region of the gene of interest. If mutations are found, the specific region involved can be sequenced. Alternatively, if hotspot regions for mutations are known and are not overly large, direct DNA sequencing may be used. A drawback for direct sequence analysis is its lack of sensitivity in detecting mixtures of wild type and mutant DNA (~20% for automated fluorescent sequencing) and the presence of mutations spanning large regions of a gene. To examine the tissue engineered products for p53 mutations, two measurement technologies that incorporate NIST internal calibration standards[5-6] were used. It was shown that tissue engineered skin did not contain mutations in this gene at the level of sensitivity of single strand conformation polymorphism-capillary electrophoresis (CE-SSCP) and Denaturing High Performance Liquid Chromatography (DHPLC) analysis. Results were compared to control cells (neonatal fibroblasts and neonatal keratinocytes) and fibroblasts that have not gone through the tissue engineering process. These were obtained from a 55 year-old (YO) and 96 YO human donor. To examine these products for Y-chromosome loss, Fluorescent In Situ Hybridization (FISH) technology was used. No detectable loss of Y-chromosome was found in the tissue-engineered skin and neonatal controls cells. Y-chromosome loss was found in the fibroblasts from the 96 YO donor as expected. Biomarkers such as p53 mutations and chromosome loss can provide the basis for an international reference standard of cellular biomarkers that can aid in the development and safety of tissue-engineered medical products.

2. EXPERIMENTAL PROCEDURES

Certain commercial equipment or materials are identified in this paper in order to specify adequately the experimental procedures. Such identification does not imply recommendation or endorsement by the National Institute of Standards and Technology, nor does it imply that the materials or equipment identified are necessarily the best available for the purpose.

2.1 Cell Culture and DNA Isolation

Human dermal neonatal fibroblast cells (HDFn; Cascade Biologics, Portland, Oregon, Catalog Number C-004-25P) and fibroblasts obtained from a 55 YO & 96 YO donor (Coriell Cell Repositories, Camden, New Jersey, Catalog Numbers AG06287 and AG04059B, respectively) were cultured in Medium 106 supplemented with Low Serum Growth Supplement (LGGS) in the absence of antibiotics and antimycotics (Cascade Biologics, Portland, Oregon). Medium was aspirated off, and cells were rinsed with 20 mL of 1X PBS. Cells were detached by adding 3 mL trypsin/EDTA solution. The trypsin/EDTA solution was immediately removed and an aliquot of 3 ml of Trypsin neutralizer solution (Cascade Biologics, Portland, Oregon) was added to each flask. Human epidermal neonatal keratinocyte cells (HEKn; Cascade Biologics, Portland, Oregon, Catalog Number C-001-25P) were cultured in EpiLife medium supplemented with Human Keratinocyte Growth Supplement (HKGS) in the absence of antibiotics and antimycotics (Cascade Biologics, Portland, Oregon) and then treated as above. Normal male lymphocytes were donated by a volunteer. These were cultured for 72 hr in RPMI 1640 (80% v/v), 20% v/v fetal calf serum, 2 mM/L glutamine with penicillin-streptomycin (100 U; 100 µg/ml) at 37 °C with 5% CO_2.

DNA was isolated from cells using a blood and cell culture DNA kit (Qiagen, Valencia, CA). DNA was recovered by spooling, washed once in 70% ethanol, and then air-dried. DNA was dissolved in 10 mM sodium phosphate buffer at a concentration of 0.3 mg/mL and dialyzed against water for 18 h at 4 °C. Water outside the dialysis bags was changed three times during the course of the dialysis. Subsequently, DNA concentration was determined by UV spectroscopy. Aliquots of this solution containing 100 µg of DNA were dried under vacuum in a SpeedVac.

2.2 Y Chromosome Analysis

Cells were treated with hypotonic solutions, fixed, air dried, and slides were prepared using standard procedures[7]. Briefly, lymphocytes were treated with 75 mM KCl for 10 min at 37 °C, and keratinocytes and fibroblasts were treated with 24 mM Na_3Citrate for 20 min at 37 °C prior to fixation. Cells were collected from these hypotonic solutions by mild centrifugation, fixed (methanolic acetic acid 3:1 v/v) and spun out of fresh, ice cold fixative three times before air dried slides were prepared. FISH methods for the whole chromosome painting (WCP®) Y SpectrumGreen™ probe were followed according to manufacturer's instructions (Vysis item #32 122024, Downers Grove, IL). Visualization and image capture systems have been previously described[8].

2.3 TestSkin II®: Fibroblast/Keratinocyte Cell Layer Separation Followed by DNA Isolation

Separating Cell Layers. A TestSkin II® disk (Organogenesis, Inc., Canton, MA) was placed in a 150 mm^2 sterile petri dish containing 35 mL 1x PBS and incubated at room temperature for 30 min in a cell culture hood. PBS was removed and replaced with 40 mL protease type X solution (0.5 mg/mL 1x PBS) and incubated at 37 °C for 2 h in a humidified cell culture incubator with 5% CO_2/95% air. Epidermal layer (keratinocytes; gray top layer) was gently separated from the dermal layer (fibroblasts; white bottom layer) using sterile forceps.

Separating Individual cells and DNA Isolation. Epidermal layer was placed in a 50-mL polypropylene conical tube containing 40 mL trypsin-versene and incubated in a 37 °C water bath for 2 h. The dermal layer was placed in a 175-cm^2 T-flask containing 180 mL collagenase solution [60 mL collagenase (4.17 mg/mL H_2O) and 120 mL collagenase pre-mix (120 ml 1x PBS, 14 mL of 2.5% trypsin solution, 1 mL filtered 0.45% glucose solution)] and incubated at 37 °C in a humidified cell culture incubator with 5% CO_2/95% air for 2 h. Independently, each respective tube was agitated every 15 min. Cells were pelleted by centrifugation (1300 x g/4 °C for 5 min) and rinsed twice with 20 mL 1x PBS with centrifugation (1300 x g/4 °C for 5 min) between each rinse step. Cells were eventually suspended in 4-mL 1x PBS and counted using a cell culture hemocytometer. DNA was isolated from the cells using a blood and cell culture DNA kit (Qiagen, Valencia, CA).

2.4 Analyses of p53 Status

Amplification of p53 exons 5-9. PCR primers to amplify a 2 kilobase region of the p53 gene containing exon 5-9 have been previously described[5]. The 2 kb fragment was amplified in a 20 µL reaction volume containing the following: 250 ng genomic DNA, 1X PCR buffer H (Invitrogen, Carlsbad, CA), 500 nMol/L each primer, 2.0 mmol/L $MgCl_2$, 2.5 U *AmpliTaq Gold®* DNA Polymerase, and 200 umol/L each dNTP. Thermal cycling conditions were as follows: pre-amplification denaturation: (1 cycle), 94 °C for 5 min; amplification (35 cycles): denaturation, 94 °C for 30 s; annealing, 66 °C for 30 s; elongation, 72 °C for 40 s; final elongation: (1 cycle), 72 °C for 7 min. A Perkin Elmer 9700 thermal cycler and was used for amplification.

Exon-specific Amplification. For mutation detection, 1 µL of the 2 kilobase amplification products was reamplified with exon-specific fluorescent labeled PCR primers. NIST standard clones were used for both positive and negative exon specific controls at 50 ng per PCR reaction. 1 µL of a 1:10 dilution of these amplification products was analyzed by CE-SSCP. The exon-specific primers (cat. # 6398-1) were purchased from Clontech Laboratories (Palo Alto, CA). The fluorescent labeled primers labeled with FAM (5-carboxyfluorescein), 5' primer, and JOE (2', 7'-dimethoxy-4',5'-dichloro-6-carboxyfluorescein), 3' primer were provided by PE, Applied Biosystems Division. A Perkin Elmer 9700 thermal cycler and *GeneAmp®* PCR core reagents (Perkin Elmer, Part No. N808-0009) were used for all amplifications. PCR reactions contained: 1X PCR buffer II, 500 nMol/L fluorescently labeled primers, 1.5 mMol/L $MgCl_2$, 2.5 units *AmpliTaq®* DNA Polymerase, and 200 µMol/L each of dATP, dCTP, dGTP and dTTP. Thermal cycling conditions were as follows: pre-amplification denaturation: (1 cycle), 94 °C for 3 min; amplification (35 cycles): denaturation, 94 °C for 30 s; annealing, 66 °C for 30 s; elongation, 72 °C for 40 s; final elongation: (1 cycle) 72 °C for 7 min.

2.5 CE-SSCP Analysis

Fluorescent-labeled PCR samples were prepared for electrophoresis by combining 10.5 µL deionized formamide with 0.5 µL 0.3 N NaOH, 1 µL water, 1 µL of PCR sample (diluted 1:10) and 0.5 µL of GENESCAN-500 TAMRA (6-carboxy-tetramethyl - rhodamine) - labeled internal size standard. The mixture was heated for 2 min at 95 °C and chilled on ice. SSCP separations were performed using the Perkin Elmer/Applied

Biosystems PRISM™ Model 310 Genetic Analyzer. All separations were performed using the Perkin Elmer, Applied Biosystems GENESCAN™ capillary and polymer system (41 cm X 50 μm capillary, 3% GENESCAN™ polymer containing 10% glycerol in 1X TBE). This capillary and polymer system was chosen because previous studies demonstrated its high resolution and reproducibility for the detection of sequence-induced mobility differences in double-stranded DNA fragments[6]. Samples were electrokinetically injected (10 s, 7 KV) and separated at 30 °C, 13 KV. Data were collected and analyzed using Perkin Elmer/Applied Biosystems PRISM™ and GENESCAN™ software, version 2.0.2.

2.6 DHPLC Analysis

The samples were analyzed on the WAVE® 3500HT DNA Fragment Analysis System (Transgenomic, Inc. Omaha, Nebraska). The stationary phase consists of alkylated nonporous polystyrene-divinlybenzene particles, and the mobile phase consists of buffer (A) 0.1M triethylammonium acetate (TEAA), and (B) 0.1M TEAA; 25% acetonitrile (v/v). The PCR products were denatured for 4 minutes at 94 °C and cooled to room temperature at a rate of 1 °C/min. Ten to 20 μL of PCR products were applied to the DNASep preheated reverse phase column (Transgenomic Inc.) As previously, described, the temperature for optimal resolution of heteroduplex and homoduplex DNA detection was determined by analyzing the melting of a PCR fragment of each exon while the temperature was increased by 1 °C increments from 50° C until the fragment was completely melted[9]. The analysis temperature for each fragment was chosen as the temperature at which about ~75% of the DNA was present as an alpha helix[9]. The experimental DNA melting data was analyzed using Wavemaker software (Transgenomic, Inc.) included with the DHPLC analysis system.

3. CONCLUSION

The first potential biomarker examined was the presence of p53 mutations in the tissue-engineered skin products. Two commonly used scanning techniques were used to search for DNA mutations within the hot spot regions of the p53 gene: CE-SSCP and DHPLC analysis. NIST internal calibration standards were used to confirm analytical validity of the two systems. Figure 1 displays the results for mutational analysis of the p53 exon 7. In panels A and B, CE-SSCP and DHPLC results indicate that mutations were not detected in this region. Mutations were also not detected in the DNAs from the normal neonatal keratinocyte and fibroblast primary cells, including that obtained from the 55 YO and 96 YO human donors. A control containing a single point mutation in exon 7 (M5) is shown for CE-SSCP, and demonstrates that this technology produces a shift in the migration of one of the two DNA strands. Comparable changes in the chromatographic profile of this control have been observed for DHPLC[10].

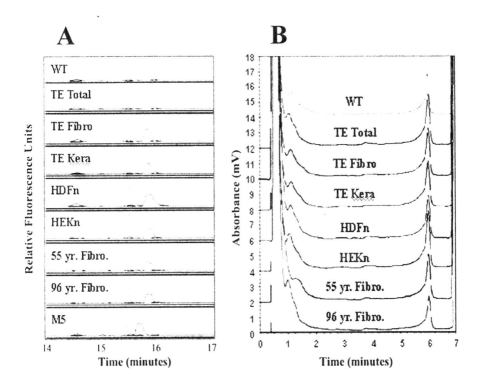

Figure 1. Mutational analysis of the p53 exon 7. Panel A: CE-SSCP analysis, Panel B: DHPLC analysis. For both panels, WT is wild type p53, exon 7 control from NIST p53 Standard Reference Material (in development); TE Total is TestSkin II® keratinocyte DNA and fibroblast DNA combined into one sample material; TE Fibro is TestSkin II® fibroblast DNA; TE Kera is TestSkin II® keratinocyte DNA; HDFn is human dermal fibroblast neonatal control DNA; HEKn is human epidermal keratinocyte neonatal DNA; 55 YO is fibroblast DNA from fibroblast cells obtained from a 55 YO donor; 96 YO is fibroblast DNA obtained from a 96 YO donor; M5 is mutant p53, exon 7 control DNA at aa 249 (AGG to AGT) from NIST p53 Standard Reference Material (in development).

The second biomarker examined was the loss of the Y chromosome. To determine background levels for these experiments, the rates of Y chromosome loss were estimated in control and aged fibroblasts (Table 1). After short-term culture, no instances of Y chromosome loss were seen in normal lymphocytes (PBLs), neonatal fibroblast cells, neonatal keratinocytes, and fibroblasts from a 55 YO subject. Y chromosome loss was also undetectable in the tissue-engineered skin product after separation into fibroblast and keratinocytes components. Fibroblasts from a 96 YO control subject showed Y chromosome loss at a rate of 8%.

Table 1. Y Chromosome in Peripheral Blood Cultures, Fibroblasts and TE Samples*

	% Cells with Y chromosome detected by FISH	Cells Scored
Age-Dependent Exp.		
Control PBL	100%	158
55 YO fibroblasts	100%	164
96 YO fibroblasts	92%	245
Tissue Culture Exp.		
Control PBL	100%	216
HDFn	100%	176
HEKn	100%	128
Tissue Engineered Skin Exp.		
Control PBL	99%	150
TE Skin fibroblasts	99%	214
TE Skin keratinocytes	99%	160

* Control PBL is peripheral blood lymphocyte cells; 55 YO fibroblasts is fibroblast cells obtained from a 55 YO donor; 96 YO fibroblasts is fibroblast cells obtained from a 96 YO donor; HDFn is human dermal fibroblast neonatal control cells; HEKn is human epidermal keratinocyte neonatal control cells; TE Skin fibroblasts is fibroblast cells obtained from TestSkin II®; TE Skin keratinocytes is keratinocyte cells obtained from TestSkin II®.

The National Institute of Standards and Technology is making a concerted effort to identify cellular biomarkers for the field of tissue-engineered medical products. These studies can provide the basis for an international reference standard of cellular biomarkers that can aid in the development and safety of tissue-engineered medical products.

REFERENCES

1. Hussain, S.P., Hofseth, L.J., and Harris, C.C., 2001, Tumor suppressor genes: at the crossroads of molecular carcinogenesis, molecular epidemiology and human risk assessment. *Lung Cancer* **34**, S7-15.

2. Whittaker, S., 2001, Molecular genetics of cutaneous lymphomas. *Ann. N. Y. Acad. Sci.* **941**, 39-45.
3. Stone, J.F., and Sandberg, A.A., 1995, Sex chromosome aneuploidy and aging. *Mutat. Res.* **338**, 107-113.
4. Cotton, R.G., 2000, Methods in clinical molecular genetics. *Eur. J. Pediatr.* **159**, S179-S182.
5. O'Connell, C.D., Tian, J., Juhasz, A., Wenz, H.M., and Atha, D.H., 1998, Development of standard reference materials for diagnosis of p53 mutations: analysis by slab gel single strand conformation polymorphism. *Electrophoresis* **19**, 164-171.
6. Atha, D.H., Wenz, H.M., Morehead, H., Tian, J., and O'Connell, C.D., 1998, Detection of p53 point mutations by single strand conformation polymorphism: analysis by capillary electrophoresis. *Electrophoresis* **19**, 172-179.
7. Barch, M., Knutsen, T., and Spurbeck, J., 1997, *The AGT Cytogenetics Laboratory Manual*, 3rd ed., Lippincott-Raven Publishing, New York.
8. Barker, P.E., and Schwab, M., 1993, Junction mapping of translocation chromosomes by fluorescence *in situ* hybridization (FISH) and computer image analysis in human solid tumors. *Methods in Molecular Genetics* **2**, 129-154.
9. Keller, G., Hartmann, A., Mueller, J., and Hofler, H., 2001, Denaturing high pressure liquid chromatography (DHPLC) for the analysis of somatic p53 mutations. *Lab. Invest.* **81**, 1735-1737.
10. O'Connell, C.D., Tully, L., Devaney, J., Marino, M., Jakupciak, J.P., and Atha, D.H. A standard reference material for the detection of p53 mutations. Manuscript in preparation.

DESIGN PEPTIDE SCAFFOLDS FOR REGENERATIVE MEDICINE

Shuguang Zhang and Carlos E. Semino
Center for Biomedical Engineering, Massachusetts Institute of Technology, Cambridge, MA 02139-4307, U.S.A.

1. INTRODUCTION

Regenerative and reparative medicine require two key complementary ingredients: the biological scaffolds and stem cells, both embryonic and adult stem cells. Designs of new scaffolds at the molecular level have become increasingly important for such an endeavor. New technology through molecular self-assembly as a fabrication tool will become integral part of new medicine in the coming years. We are inspired from nature through understanding the molecular self-assembly phenomena. Self-assembly phenomena are ubiquitous in nature. The two basic elements in molecular self-assembly are chemical complementarity and structural compatibility, through weak and noncovalent interactions. We have defined the path to understand these principles. Several self-assembling peptide systems have been developed for regenerative medicine including "molecular Lego" forming a nanofiber scaffold hydrogel. "molecular carpet" for surface biological engineering; and peptide nanotubes and nanovesicles, or "molecular capsule" for protein and gene deliveries. These self-assembling peptide systems are simple, versatile and easy to produce for large scale. These self-assembly peptide systems represent a significant advance in the molecular engineering of scaffolds for regenerative medicine.

1.1 Programmed Assembly and Molecular Self-Assembly

When construction of a house, one can first prefabricate various construction units, the wall, doors, windows, lighting system, kitchen cabinets, etc. These units can then be programmably assembled together according to their design and functions.

The conventional process engineering approach to produce the nanoscale materials requires expensive and sophisticated instrument and machinery, often requires large-scale materials. On the other hand, molecular engineering of nanoscale biological materials requires unconventional approaches. One of approaches is to design individual construction units and to facilitate them to self-assemble into well ordered structures.

Self-assembly is ubiquitous in nature at all scales, from macroscopic to microscopic scales, from meters to nanometers. Assemblies of schools of fish in the ocean, flocks of birds in the sky, herds of wild animals on the vast plain are examples of such self-assembling phenomena. At the microscopic scale, oil droplets self-assemble in water, assembly of DNA into double helix, of four individual polypeptide chains and heme/iron into functional hemoglobin, and of RNA and ribosomal proteins into ribosome that manufacture proteins in the cell, are all great examples of molecular self-assembly. Self-assembly describes the spontaneous association of numerous individual entities into a coherent organization and well-defined structures to maximize the benefit of the individual without external instructions.

Molecular self-assembly is the spontaneous organization of molecules under thermodynamic equilibrium conditions into structurally well-defined and stable arrangements through numerous weak and noncovalent interactions. These molecules undergo self-association forming hierarchical structures. The key engineering principle for molecular self-assembly is to artfully design the molecular building blocks that are able to undergo spontaneously stepwise interactions and assemblies through the formations of numerous noncovalent weak chemical bonds. These typically include hydrogen bonds, ionic bonds, electrostatic interaction, van der Waals interaction, water-mediated interaction to assemble these molecules into some well-defined and stable hierarchical molecular and macroscopic structures. Although each of the bonds and interactions is rather week, the collective interactions can result in very stable structures and materials. The key elements in molecular self-assembly are chemical complementarity and structural compatibility.

2. DESIGNED SELF-ASSEMBLING PEPTIDE SYSTEMS

A new class of peptide based-biological scaffolds was serendipitously discovered from the self-assembly of ionic self-complementary peptides[1,2]. The building motif was first found as a motif in a yeast protein, zuotin that was characterized to bind left-handed Z-DNA[3]. A number of peptide molecular self-assembly systems have since been designed and developed. This systematic analysis of a variety of peptide motifs provided insight into the chemical and structural principles of peptide self-assembly. These peptides are short, simple to molecular-design, extremely versatile, easy to synthesize and to be purified by HPLC to homogeneity. Several types of self-assembling peptides have been systematically studied. It is believed additional different types will be discovered and developed in the coming years. This class of biological peptide scaffold has a considerable potential for a number of applications, including scaffolding for reparative and regenerative medicine, drug delivery of molecular medicine, as well as biological surface engineering.

2.1 Peptide Scaffold Construction Units

The construction motif for the peptide scaffold, like "molecular Lego", form beta-sheet structures in aqueous solution because they contain two distinct surfaces, one hydrophilic, the other hydrophobic (Table 1). Like Lego bricks that have pegs and holes and can only be assembled into particular structures, these peptides can do so at the molecular level. The hydrophobic side can be designed with increasing hydrophobicity so that the mechanic strength of the scaffold can also be enhanced. The unique structural feature of these peptides is that they form complementary ionic bonds with regular repeats on the hydrophilic surface (Fig. 1). The complementary ionic sides have been classified into several moduli, *i.e.* modulus I, II, III, IV, etc., and mixed moduli. This classification is based on the hydrophilic surface of the molecules that have alternating + and - charged amino acid residues, either alternating by 1, 2, 3, 4 and so on. For example, molecules of modulus I have - + - + - + - +, modulus II, - - + + - - + +, modulus, IV - - - - + + + +. These well-defined sequences allow them to undergo ordered self-assembly, resemblance of some situation found in well-studied polymer assemblies.

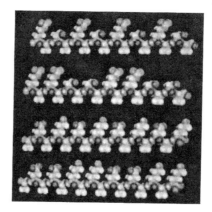

Figure 1. Molecular models of the extended beta-strand structures of individual molecules are shown for (A) RAD16-I, (B) RAD16-II, (C) EAK16-I, (D) EAK16-II. The distance between the charged side chains along the backbone is approximately 6.8 Å; the methyl groups of alanines are found on one side of the sheet and the charged residues are on the other side. Conventional beta-sheet hydrogen bond formation between the oxygen and hydrogen on the nitrogen of the peptide backbones is perpendicular to the page.

Table 1. Designed Self-Assembling Peptides

Name	Sequence (N->C)	Ionic Modulus	Structure
RADA16-I	+ - + - + - + - n-RADARADARADARADA-c	I	E
RGDA16-I	+ - + - + - + - n-RADARGDARADARGDA-c	I	r.c.
RADA8-I	+ - + - n-RADARADA-c	I	r.c.
RAD16-II	+ + - - + + - - n-RARADADARARADADA-c	II	E
RAD8-II	+ + - - n-RARADADA-c	II	r.c.
EAKA16-I	- + - + - + - + n-AEAKAEAKAEAKAEAK-c	I	E
EAKA8-I	- + - + n-AEAKAEAK-c	I	r.c.
RAEA16-I	+ - + - + - + - n-RAEARAEARAEARAEA-c	I	E
RAEA8-I	+ - + - n-RAEARAEA-c	I	r.c.
KADA16-I	+ - + - + - + - n-KADAKADAKADAKADA-c	I	E
KADA8-I	+ - + - n-KADAKADA-c	I	r.c.

Name	Sequence	Charge pattern	Class	Structure
EAH16-II	n-AEAEAHAHAEAEAHAH-c	- - + + - - + +	II	E
EAH8-II	n-AEAEAHAH-c	- - + +	II	r.c.
EFK16-II	n-FEFEFKFKFEFEFKFK-c	- - + + - - + +	II	E
EFK12-I	n-FEFKFEFKFEFK-c	- + - + - +	I	E
EFK8-II	n-FEFKFEFK-c	- + - +	I	E
ELK16-II	n-LELELKLKLELELKLK-c	- - + + - - + +	II	E
ELK8-II	n-LELELKLK-c	- - + +	II	E
EAK16-II	n-AEAEAKAKAEAEAKAK-c	- - + + - - + +	II	E
EAK12	n-AEAEAEAEAKAK-c	- - - - + +	IV/II	E/Δ
EAK8-II	n-AEAEAKAK-c	- - + +	II	r.c.
KAE16-IV	n-KAKAKAKAEAEAEAEA-c	+ + + + - - - -	IV	E
EAK16-IV	n-AEAEAEAEAKAKAKAK-c	- - - - + + + +	IV	E
KLD12-I	n-KLDLKLDLKLDL-c	+ - + - + -	I	E
KLE12-I	n-KLELKLELKLEL-c	+ - + - + -	I	E
RAD16-IV	n-RARARARADADADADA-c	+ + + + - - - -	IV	E
DAR16-IV	n-ADADADADARARARAR-c	- - - - + + + +	IV	E/Δ
DAR16-IV*	n-DADADADARARARARA-c	- - - - + + + +	IV	E/Δ
DAR32-IV	n-(ADADADADARARARAR)-c	- - - - + + + +	IV	E/Δ
EHK16	n-HEHEHKHKHEHEHKHK-c	+-+-++++-+-++++	N/A	r.c.
EHK8-I	n-HEHEHKHK-c	+-+-++++	N/A	r.c.

Notations: E, beta-sheet; Δ, alpha-helix; r.c., random coil. The numbers follow the name denote the length of the peptides or amino acids.

Upon the addition of monovalent alkaline cations or the introduction of the peptide solutions into physiological media, these peptides spontaneously assemble to form macroscopic structures. Because they have extremely high water content, greater than 99% water, often used at 1-10mg/ml solution (w/v), so they can be readily fabricated into various geometric shapes (Fig. 2) [4-7]. Scanning EM and AFM reveals that the matrices are made of interwoven nanofibers having 10-20 nm in diameter and pores about 50-200 nm in diameter [1, 4-9].

The molecular structure and proposed complementary ionic pairings of the peptides between positively charged lysines and negatively charged glutamates in an overlap arrangement are modeled in Fig. 1. This structure represents an example of this class of self-assembling beta-sheet peptides that undergo spontaneously association under physiological conditions. If the charged residues are substituted, *i.e.*, the positive charged lysines are replaced by positively charged arginines and the negatively charged glutamates are replaced by negatively charged aspartates, there are essentially no drastic effects on the self-assembly process. However, if the positively charged resides, Lys and Arg are replaced by negatively charged residues, Asp and Glu, the peptide can no longer undergo self-assembly to form macroscopic materials although they can still form beta-sheet structures in the presence of salt. If the alanines are changed to more hydrophobic residues, such as Leu, Ile, Phe or Tyr, the molecules have a greater tendency to self-assemble and form peptide matrices with enhanced strength [5, 9-11].

A number of mammalian cells have been tested and all have been found to be able to form stable attachments with the peptide scaffolds (Table 3)[4]. Several peptide scaffolds have been used to test for their ability to support cell proliferation and differentiation. These results suggested that the peptide scaffolds can not only support various types of cell attachments, but can also allow the attached cells to proliferate and differentiate. For example, rat PC12 cells on peptide matrices were exposed to NGF, they underwent differentiation and exhibited extensive neurite outgrowth. In addition, when primary mouse neuron cells were allowed to attach the peptide scaffolds, the neuron cells projected lengthy axons that followed the specific contours of the self-assembled peptide surface and made active and functional connections [6].

The fundamental design principles of such self-assembling peptide systems can be readily extended to polymers and polymer composites, where co-polymers can be designed and produced. We have learned a great deal from nature, has gone many steps further and will continue to create new biological scaffolds for regenerative medicine[12-16].

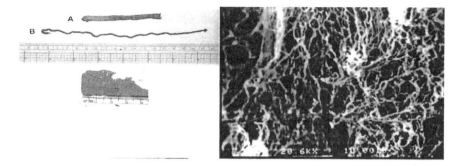

Figure 2. Peptide scaffold hydrogel form 3-dimensional biological materials from self-assembly of the peptide motifs (A-C). Several geometric forms have been fabricated as a tape, a rope and a sheet. Additional forms can be easily produced since the peptide scaffolds contain >99% water in a hydrogel texture. D) SEM image of RDA16-I peptide nanofiber scaffold. The scaffold is self-assembled from individual interwoven nanofibers (1, 4, 6). The diameter of the fiber is about 10-20 nm and the enclosures are about 50-200 nm. Under high resolution by atomic force microscopy, the nanofibers are revealed to be a left-handed double helix with regular repeats in the initial stage of the self-assembly [9].

2.2 Surfactant Peptides

Nature also produced diverse biological building motifs. One of which is the ubiquitous lipid molecule that has a hydrophilic head and a hydrophobic tail. It is well known that in water lipid molecules, either nature occurring or synthetic, undergo self-assembly to form well-order vesicles, microtubules and others structures[17]. Since lipid molecules belong to surfactant materials, we also designed lipid-like, or surfactant-like peptides that share similar properties except at a nanoscale.

We design another class of peptide scaffold. In this case, this class of peptides have distinct 2 ends, one hydrophobic and the other hydrophilic with charged residues, either negatively asparate and glutamate or positively charged lysine, histidine or arginine (Table 2)[18-21].

These surfactant peptides form both nanotubes and nanovesicles in water. The process is rather dynamic and they can undergo self-assembly and disassembly because the individual surfactant peptides are small and can disassociate and associate into the assemblies. This is much like the situation of people get in and out of a theater or a sport stadium. The overall structure remains largely intact but the individual moments suggest the dynamic phenomenon. The Brownian motion of the peptides in water permits similar dynamic event.

Table 2. Surfactant Peptides*

	−		− −
A6D	AAAAAAD	A6D2	AAAAAADD
	−		− −
V6D	VVVVVVD	V6D2	VVVVVVDD
	− −		− −
L6D2	LLLLLLDD	I6D2	IIIIIIDD
	− −		− −
G4D2	GGGGDD	G6D2	GGGGGGDD
	− −		− −
G8D2	GGGGGGGGDD	G10D2	GGGGGGGGGGDD
	+		+ +
KA6	KAAAAAA	K2A6	KKAAAAAA
	+		+ +
KV6	KVVVVVV	K2V6	KKVVVVVV
	+ +		+ +
K2L6	KKLLLLLL	H2V6	HHVVVVVV

*The surfactant peptides. They have distinct ends, a hydrophilic head and hydrophobic tail. The heads can be either negative, as in the case of biological lipids, or positive, like some synthetic cationic lipids. The hydrophobic tails can vary according to the various degree of hydrophobicity. The + and − refer to the positive and negative charges, respectively.

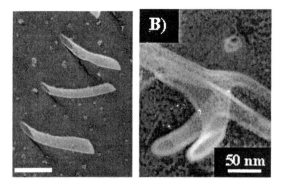

Figure 3. Quick-freeze/deep-etch TEM image of V_6D (A) and G6D2 (B) dissolved in water at high-resolution. The images show the dimensions, 30-50 nm in diameters with openings of nanotube ends clearly visible. The strong contrast shadow of the platinum coat also suggests the hollow tubular structure. The bar in A is 100 nm.

A few molecular models were built to explain the observations. These models are presented in figure 4. The tube structure is carried out with V6D peptide, which has a negatively charged aspartic acid as the head; and the vesicle structure is carried out with KV6 where the positively charged lysine is the head. Both peptides have valine, which has 3 carbon of isopropyl group on the side chain, as the hydrophobic tails.

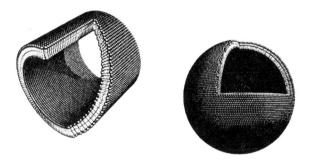

Figure 4. Potential packing pathway of V_6D peptide nanotube formation. Each peptide monomer is 2 nm, and the diameter of the modeled bilayer nanotube is 50 nm. Each peptide may interact with one another to form a closed ring which in turn stack on top of one another, ultimately yielding a nanotube. Both molecular models of nanotube with − charged V6D (A) and nanovesicles with + charged KV6 (B) are presented.

These designed surfactant peptides will likely find applications for encapsulation of molecular drugs, DNA and RNA genes, RNAi, miRNA and siRNA that can silence particular genes effectively. These encapsulated molecules can be delivered into cells.

3. BIOLOGICAL SURFACE ENGINEERING

To produce medical devices from non-biologically compatible materials, it is often required to coat the surface to produce a suitable environment for cells, resemblance of extracellular environment. We have previously demonstrated that design of particular peptide with the specific ligands to modify the surface is feasible [15, 22]. Unlike coating surfaces with modified polymers and other non-orientated ligands, that often result in low density of ligands with a less ideal surface, the designed peptides contain the ligands directly link to the peptide coating with all ligands exposed. Furthermore, the peptide coating is often a only a few nanometers (Fig. 5). The cells on the surface can also be arranged in a specific manner when combining with micro-contact printing or ink-jet printing (Fig. 6).

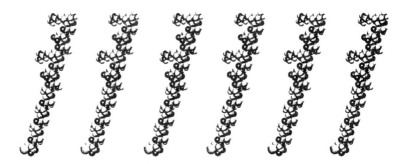

Figure 5. The surface engineering peptide. Each peptide has 3 distinct parts: 1) the ligand that can interact with cells, 2) the linker that serves as the spacer between the cells and the surface. The spacer can be designed to be flexible, when using glycines, or stiff, when using leucine or isoleucine. 3) The anchor that covalently link the peptide to the surface. In this particular case, it is cysteine that binds to gold atoms. Other anchor residues can also be used, such as asparate or glutamate that can be activated to covalently bind to amino surface. Or, lysine that can be activated to couple to the aldehyde surface.

Each peptide has 3 distinct parts: 1) the ligand that can interact with cells, 2) the linker that serves as the spacer between the cells and the surface. The spacer can be designed to be flexible, when using glycines, or stiff, when using leucine or isoleucine. 3) The anchor that covalently link the peptide to the surface. In this particular case, it is cysteine that binds to gold atoms. Other anchor residues can also be used, such as asparate or glutamate that can be activated to covalently bind to amino surface. Or, lysine that can be activated to couple to the aldehyde or ester surface.

Molecular engineering cell-friendly surfaces at the nanometer scale using fabricated patterns in combination with the designed surface active peptide with ligands will likely find uses in modify medical devices for implantation. Likewise, these active peptides will likely to induce smoothly interface grafting of the tissue with the newly introduced devices and reduce the undesired rejection. This peptide will likely reduce the need of some polymers that are not optimized for tissue repair and tissue engineering. Like weave a Turkish rug, we call the surface engineering technology "molecular carpeting".

 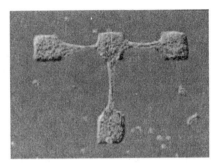

Figure 6. Biological surface engineering using microcontact printing and surface coating peptides. The panel on the left shows the cells are organized as parallel arrays. The right panel shows the fabricated letter **T** with cells confined in it. The scale bars are 100 microns.

Cells on the biological engineered surface can be precisely organized and confined in the predetermined surface coated with designed peptides. The peptides coated surfaces are only a few nanometer thick, it uses much less materials, thus may likely reduce undesirable side effect such as corrosion. Such a surface engineering technology will likely be broadly applicable to study cell-cell communications and coat medical devices requiring implantation in the body.

4. THE CELLS

Cells are the other half of the ingredients for reparative and regenerative medicine. There have been concerted efforts to develop new embryonic stem (ES) and progenitor cells for such purpose. A great deal of information is available for many types of cells including mouse and human ES and progenitor cells. However, new methods are still needed and a suitable technology for expansion of these cells with controlled and desired differentiation still remains tremendous challenge.

4.1 Stem and Progenitor Cells

Considerable progress has been made towards controlling differentiation of embryonic stem cells in cell cultures based on the use of cellular factors that promote maturation of specific cell lineages, including muscular cells, hematopoietic cells, neurons, pancreatic E-cells, etc. Advances is slower with adult stem and progenitor cells because of their more complex cell division kinetics and differentiation programs' as well as their expanding difficulty in culture. It is known that stem cells can divide asymmetrically to produce a new stem cell and a progenitor cell. The progenitor cell subsequently undergoes differentiation and maturation to form functional tissues. In the case of adult "stem cell differentiation" it is the microenvironment of the progenitor cell residence that is likely to be most important in dictating the type of mature functional cells that they develop. The molecular-engineered microenvironments designed to produce differentiated cells from adult stem cells need to support both adult stem cell proliferation and progeny differentiation [23].

A major goal in reparative and regenerative medicine is the molecular engineering of biological materials capable of supporting growth and functional differentiation of cells and tissues in a controlled manner. Much progress has been made in the last decade in developing biopolymeric materials, such as poly-lactic acid (PLA), polyglycolic acid (PGA), hyaluronic acid, alginates and other biocompatible scaffolds. In general, these polymers are composed by fibers in the micro-scale ~10-100 ɼm in diameter.

We have described, in the previous section, a peptide scaffold, that is made by the interweaving of self-assembling peptide nanofibers of 10-20 nm in diameter. The peptide scaffolds consist of greater than 99% water content (1-10 mg/ml, w/v) [1, 4-7]. These nanofibers are 3 orders of magnitude thinner than other biopolymer microfibers. Thus they truly embody cells in a 3-dimensional environment. Several peptide scaffolds have been shown to support a variety of mature differentiated cell functions [5-7]. However, these designed peptide scaffolds have not been previously evaluated for their ability to support stem cell differentiation and function.

Given the ability of self-assembling peptide scaffold to support mature cell function, we investigated whether they could also promote differentiation of adult stem cells. For these studies, we used an adult rat hepatocyte putative stem cell line that was clonally derived.

The results indicate that the peptide scaffold provides a microenvironment that promotes normal stem cell division kinetics and enhanced progenitor cell differentiation. The differentiated progeny display several characteristics of mature hepatocytes, including expression of inducible cytochrome p450 enzymes (such as CYP1A1, CYP1A2, and CYP2E1) that have the ability to produce complex metabolic products (Figure 7)[24]. Because the stem cell-progeny cell structure is a general feature of adult mammalian tissues, the stem cell-peptide scaffold culture established here have broad application to a variety of tissues of interest in biomedical research and regenerative medicine.

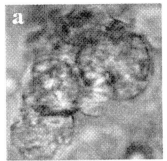 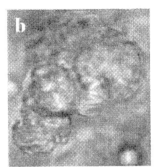

Figure 7. Putative adult liver stem cells were cultured in peptide peptide scaffolds for two weeks. Cellular spheroids showing releasing of resofurin after 30 minutes of *in vivo* incubation in presence of the substrate 7-ethoxyresofurin (CYP1A1 activity). Cells were photographed on bright field and fluorescence. Both images were combined. **a**, before incubation; **b**, after incubation. Bar = 50 μm.

4.2 Other Cells

A variety of cells have been studied using the peptide scaffold as a culture source. These include cell lines in the early studies and primary derived cells from animals in recent studies. It appears that all cells studied to date have shown that the several peptide scaffolds are excellent matrices for cell attachment, induced differentiation, controlled expansion as well as gene expression perform biological functions. Furthermore, many colleagues have independently found that a variety of cells would be suitable to be cultured on the scaffold in 3-D (personal communications). Some of the cells are listed in Table 3.

Table 3. Cells Studied in the Peptide Scaffold Hydrogel

Cell Type	Cell Line	Primary cells
Mouse fibroblast	NIH-3T3	Mouse cerebellum granule cells*•
Chicken embryo fibroblast	CEF	Mouse & rat hippocampal cells*•
Chinese hamster ovary	CHO	Rat adult neural stem cells*•
Monkey kidney cells	Cos7	Rat adult stem cells
Human cervical carcinoma	Hela	Rabbit & mouse cardiac myocytes*
Human osteosarcoma	MG63	Bovine aortic endothelial cells*
Human hepatocellular carcinoma	HepG2	Human endothelial cells*
Hamster pancreas	HIT-T15	Human foreskin fibroblast*
Human embryonic kidney	HEK293	Bovine chondrocytes* (calf & adult)
Human neuroblastoma•	SH-SY5Y	Human epidermal keratinocytes*
Rat pheochromocytoma•	PC12	Rat neural tissues*•

Various cell type attachment or encapsulated to the peptide scaffold. Visual assessment of cell attachment was performed using phase contrast microscopy for over a period of two weeks. * refers to cells derived from primary cultures. • refers to neuronal cells.

It is likely that the list will grow over time when more and more people use the peptide scaffold in a broad range of studies. It is anticipated that new observations will be made, new applications will be found and new therapies will be developed in the coming years.

5. ENCAPSULATION

The combination of the peptide scaffold and the cells encapsulated in it may likely produce novel and unexpected results. Since the peptide scaffold is entirely made of amino acids with the nanoscale cells are familiar with, the cells will likely exhibit behaviors quite different from the conventional petri dish conditions. Cells themselves can produce and secrete growth factors, cytokines, hormone and other messenger molecules into the local environment, a molecular gradient will likely to be established. This is crucial for further cell interactions and tissue development when multiple cell types are co-encapsulated. Likewise, when encapsulate embryonic stem cells and/or progenitor cells, it is possible to preferentially induce these cells into a particular cell or tissue lineage using a combination of growth factors, inhibitors and other signaling molecules.

The scaffolds injected in to animals have been so far not to elicit measurable immune responses, informatory reactions in several types of animals including rats, mice, rabbits, hamster and goats. These preliminary test and observations suggest that the peptide scaffold is inert in animals. Thus, it paves the way for further development of cell based therapies for humans.

6. CONCLUSIONS

Designed new scaffolds are needed to foster the cell expansion and controlled differentiation for reparative and regenerative medicine. These peptide scaffolds described here are built at the single molecular level from bottom up. They can be systematically designed for special biochemical and mechanical properties, tailored for specific cell types, modified to incorporate biological cues. These construction motifs can be used as the building blocks and the fabrication of the scaffolds is through molecular self-assembly. It is likely that the nanoscale nature of the building materials for the scaffolds is one of the key factors. The peptide scaffolds are not only made of nanofibers, but also with extremely high water content, often greater than 99% (99.5-99.8% water, or 2-5 mg/ml, w/v). There, the cells are not only truly encapsulated in 3-D environment, but they also can move freely in all dimensions. Such a system is likely closer to the in vivo environment. Furthermore, the nanofiber scaffold with the nanopores may allow the establishment of the molecular gradient locally so that a tissue-like environment may be achieved.

The designed surfactant peptides may used to encapsulate small molecular drugs, DNA/RNA genes, RNAi, siRNA, miRNA to specifically regulate the gene expression patterns, cell cycle events, cell differentiation, tissue and organ development.

In combination with stem cells (embryonic and adult) and progenitor cells, we can encapsulate these cells in the peptide scaffold, inducing them to differentiate into desired cell types and to form tissues with specific growth factors and cytokines, and then apply the cell-scaffold systems into needed tissues. These designed peptide scaffolds fabricated through molecular self-assembly will likely play an increasingly important role for broad range of applications in reparative and regenerative medicine.

We have also engaged other activities to further understand and to develop the peptide-based materials for reparative and regenerative medicine. We designed the scaffolds for neural injury repair[25-26] and for gene delivery[27]. We also try to understand the physical and molecular basis of how the single peptide molecules, only a few nanometers in dimension, can self-assemble into well- ordered macrostructures[28]. Moreover, we also wish to push the emerging field of nature- inspired and designed biological materials further along with other investigators to foster nano-biotechnology[29].

ACKNOWLEDGEMENTS

We thank Steve Santoso, Geoffrey von Maltzahn, Wonmuk Hwang and other members of our lab for carrying out experiments. We gratefully acknowledge the supports over the years by grants from the US Army Research Office, Office of Naval Research, Defense Advanced Research Project Agency/Naval Research Laboratories, NSF CCR-0122419 to MIT Media Lab's Center for Bits & Atoms, NSF/MIT BPEC, National Institute of Health. We also gratefully acknowledge the generous educational donation of computer cluster from the Intel Corporation.

REFERENCES

1. Zhang, S., Holmes, T., Lockshin, C., and Rich, A., 1993, Spontaneous assembly of a self-complementary oligopeptide to form a stable macroscopic membrane. *Proc. Natl. Acad. Sci. USA* **90**, 3334-3338.
2. Zhang, S., Lockshin, C., Herbert, A., Winter, E., and Rich, A., 1992, Zuotin, a putative Z-DNA binding protein in *Saccharomyces cerevisiae*. *EMBO. J*, **11**, 3787-3796.
3. Zhang, S., Lockshin, C., Cook, R., and Rich, A., 1994, Unusually stable beta-sheet formation of an ionic self-complementary oligopeptide. *Biopolymers* **34**, 663-672.
4. Zhang, S., Holmes, T., DiPersio, M., Hynes, R.O., Su, X., and Rich, A., 1995, Self-complementary oligopeptide matrices support mammalian cell attachment. *Biomaterials* **16**, 1385-1393.
5. León, E.J, Verma, N., Zhang, S., Lauffenburger, D.A., and Kamm, R.D., 1998, Mechanical properties of a self-assembling oligopeptide matrix. *J. Biomaterials Science: Polymer Edition* **9**, 297-312.
6. Holmes, T. , Delacalle, S., Su, X., Rich, A., and Zhang, S., 2000, Extensive neurite outgrowth and active neuronal synapses on peptide scaffolds. *Proc. Natl. Acad. Sci. USA* **97**, 6728-6733.
7. Kisiday, J., Jin, M., Kurz, B., Hung, H., Semino, C., Zhang, S., and Grodzinsky, A.J., 2002, Self-assembling peptide hydrogel fosters chondrocyte extracellular matrix production and cell division: implications for cartilage tissue repair. *Proc. Natl. Acad. Sci. USA* **99**, 9996-10001.
8. Caplan, M. Moore, P., Zhang, S., Kamm, R.D., and Lauffenburger, D.A., 2000, Self-assembly of a beta-sheet oligopeptide is governed by electrostatic repulsion. *Biomacromolecules* **1**, 627-631.
9. Marini, D., Hwang, W., Lauffenburger, D.A, Zhang, S., and Kamm, R.D., 2002, Left-handed helical ribbon intermediates in the self-assembly of a beta-sheet peptide. *NanoLetters* **2**, 295-299.
10. Caplan, M., Schwartzfarb, E., Zhang, S., Kamm, R., and Lauffenburger, D.A., 2002, Control of self-assembling oligopeptide matrix formation through systematic variation of amino acid sequence. *Biomaterials* **23**, 219-227.
11. Caplan, M.R., Schwartzfarb, E.M., Zhang, S., Kamm, R.D., and Lauffenburger, D.A., 2002, Effects of systematic variation of amino acid sequence on the mechanical properties of a self-assembling, oligopeptide biomaterial. *J. Biomaterials Science Polymer Edition* **13**, 225-236.
12. Zhang, S., and Altman, M., 1999, Peptide self-assembly in functional polymer science and engineering. *Reactive and Functional Polymers* **41**, 91-102.
13. Zhang, S., 2001, Molecular self-assembly. *Encyclopedia of Materials: Science & Technology*, Elsevier Science, Oxford, UK, pp.5822-5829.
14. Zhang, S., and Altman, M., 2001, Self-assembling peptide systems in biology, engineering and medicine. *Crete Meeting Proceedings* (Ed. Aggeli, A., Boden, N. & Zhang, S.) Kluwer Academic Publishers, Dordrent, The Netherlands pp. 343-360.
15. Zhang, S., 2002, Emerging biological materials through molecular self-assembly *Biotechnology Advances* **20**, 321-339.
16. Zhang, S., Marini, D., Hwang, W., and Santoso, S., 2002, Design nano biological materials through self-assembly of peptide & proteins. *Current opinion in Chemical Biology* **6**, 865-871.
17. Schnur, J.M., 1993, Lipid Tubules: A Paradigm for Molecularly Engineering Structures. *Science,* **262**, 1669-1676.
18. Vauthey, S., Santoso, S., Gong, H., Watson, N., and Zhang, S., 2002, Molecular self-assembly of surfactant-like peptides to form nanotubes and nanovesicles. *Proc. Natl. Acad. Sci. USA* **99**, 5355-5360.

19. Santoso, S., Hwang, W., Hartman, H., and Zhang, S., 2002, Self-assembly of surfactant-like peptides with variable glycine tails to form nanotubes and nanovesicles. *NanoLetters* **2**, 687-691.
20. Santoso, S., Vauthey, S., and Zhang, S., 2002, Structures, functions, and applications of amphiphlic peptides. *Current Opinion in Colloid & Interface Science* **7**, 262-266.
21. von Maltzahn, G., Vauthey, S., Santoso, S., and Zhang, S., 2003, Positively charged surfactant-like peptides self-assemble into nanostructures. *Langmuir* **19**, (In press, May 27, Cover article).
22. Zhang, S., Yan, L., Altman, M., Lässle, M., Nugent, H., Frankel, F., Lauffenburger, D., Whitesides, G., and Rich, A., 1999, Biological surface engineering: A simple system for cell pattern formation. *Biomaterials* **20**, 1213-1220.
23. Semino, C., 2003, Can we build artificial stem cell compartments? *J. Biomedicine & Biotechnology* **3**, (In press).
24. Semino, C.E., Merok, J.R., Crane, G., Panagiotakos, G., Zhang, S., and Sherley, J.L., 2003, A three-dimensional peptide hydrogel culture system for enhanced hepatic putative progenitor cell differentiation. (Submitted).
25. Semino, C.E., Kasahara, J., Hayashi, Y., and Zhang, S., 2003, Entrapment of mitotically active hippocampal neural cells in self-assembling peptide hydrogel. (Submitted).
26. Ellis-Behnke, R., Semino, C.E., Zhang, S., and Schneider, G.E., 2003, Peptide nanofiber hydrogel scaffold for brain lesion repair (Submitted).
27. Schwartz, J. & Zhang, S., 2000, Peptide-mediate cellular delivery. *Current Opinion in Molecular Therapeutics* **2**, 162-167.
28. Hwang, W., Marini, D.M., Kamm, R.D., and Zhang, S., 2003, Supramolecular structure of helical ribbons self-assembled from a b-sheet peptide. *J. Chem. Physics* **118**, 389-397.
29. Santoso, S., and Zhang, S., 2003, Nanomaterials through molecular self-assembly. *Encyclopaedia of Nanotechnology* (In press).

PROGRESSES IN SYNTHETIC VASCULAR PROSTHESES: TOWARD THE ENDOTHELIALIZATION

Mathilde Crombez and Diego Mantovani
Bioengineering and Biotechnology Unit, St-François d'Assise Hospital Research Centre and Laval University, Department of Materials Engineering, Laboratory for Biomaterials and Bioengineering, Quebec City, G1K 7P4, Canada

1. INTRODUCTION

Since the 1970s, arterial prostheses made of PET (Poly-Ethylene-Teraphtalate, Dacron) and ePTFE (expanded Poly-Tetra-Fluoro-Ethylene, microporous Teflon) have been widely used to replace large (internal diameter more than 10 mm) and medium vessels (between 6 and 10 mm). It is estimated that more than a million prostheses are implanted world-wide annually.[1] About 550,000 of these implantations are performed in the USA. Over 65% of them, however, have to be removed during the 10 following years because of complications, such as thrombosis, infection, and pseudo-aneurysms.[2] In the past few decades, much has been done to investigate the origin of these unexpected complications, but a clear theory has yet to be worked out. Nonetheless, complete endothelialization, i.e., coverage of the luminal surface by a monolayer of endothelial cells (ECs), has never been observed in synthetic vascular prostheses implanted in humans. The lack of this neo-intima is considered to be the primary cause of complications. Because this natural hemocompatible boundary inhibits thrombosis development it would be an ideal covering layer for the internal surface of prostheses.

Tissue Engineering, Stem Cells and Gene Therapies
Edited by Y. Murat Elçin, Kluwer Academic / Plenum Publishers, 2003

Historically, several attempts have been made to improve the long-term survival of small-diameter prosthetic vascular grafts through the use of EC seeding.[3] Such a strategy soon proved to be ineffective for long-term implantation. Indeed, EC linings do not spontaneously attach strongly enough to prosthetic grafts, to withstand the shear stresses of blood flow to the cells.[4]

The importance of developing a pro-active surface, i.e., one that leads to EC adhesion and proliferation, became clear. Since 1985, biomaterial researchers have focused on immobilisation of suitable biomolecules to the luminal surface of prosthetic grafts as a means to promote interactions between the prosthesis and the surrounding tissue. Furthermore, by developing pro-active materials that provide signalling to cells, we may be able to improve tissue formation for applications in tissue engineering and wound healing. However, to determine which signals have to be generated for a specific application, we need a complete understanding of how the signals may affect cell behaviour. The current major difficulties lie in the partial knowledge we have about cell signalling in the vascular wall. An effective arterial prosthesis that can exhibit "endothelialization" will need to take advantage of advances in both materials science and cell physiology. In the following pages, we will schematically review the strategies for choosing the appropriate biomolecules, for making them adhere to the inert prosthesis, and for inducing them to express signals to surrounding cells and tissue. Finally, we will present our group's strategy to induce such signalling on the surfaces of synthetic arterial prostheses.

2. CELL SIGNALLING IN THE ARTERIAL INTIMA

2.1 Adhesion

Attachment of mammalian blood and tissue cells to other cells, extracellular matrices, and biomaterial surfaces is controlled by various families of adhesion receptors.[5] When the substratum is a cell surface, the term "receptor" is used for the molecules on the surface of the free cells and "ligand" for the complementary molecules on the substratum. The adhesion will be as strong, on a logarithmic curve, as the binding affinity between the receptor and the ligand. Among the super-families of adhesion receptors, the selectins and the integrins seem to play predominant and complementary roles in cell capture. Moreover, they mediate EC migration and new blood vessel formation by interacting with glyco-conjugates. Finally, direct interaction of integrins with proteoglycans has been reported to be involved in adhesion of ECs to the basement membrane.[6]

2.1.1 Selectins

The selectin family is composed of three members named after the cells in which they were originally discovered.[7] E-selectin is produced exclusively by ECs after cytokine activation. Its counter-receptors are on neutrophils, monocytes, eosinophils, lymphocyte subsets, and some tumour cells. L-selectin is expressed on leukocytes and its target cells are activated ECs. P-selectin is preformed and stored for rapid release in ECs activated by cytokines. Its target cells are the same as those for E-selectin. E and P-selectin are involved in angiogenesis. Moreover recombinant human soluble E-selectin stimulates chemotaxis of HUVEC and is preferentially synthesized by angiogenic or proliferating ECs. Prior work has shown that L- and P-selectin binding are similar in their ability to be inhibited by many compounds containing sulphate groups. L-selectin seems less promiscuous and may require a more specific sequence for recognition, since it requires calcium.[8] Many injuries (stroke, myocardial ischemia, etc.) for which P- and L-selectin inhibitory interactions are considered to be of potential value in restoring blood flow are already routinely treated with heparin, on the assumption that its anticoagulant properties will be of therapeutic value.[9] Significantly, the best effects of thrombolytic therapy for acute myocardial infarction are seen when heparin is included in the treatment regimen.[10] In such instances, it seems that heparin works primarily by providing protection from P- and L-selectin–mediated reperfusion injury, rather than by its anticoagulant action. Finally, it can be concluded that low doses of HE and HS on a synthetic prosthesis can also prevent thrombus development.

2.1.2 Integrins

Integrins are the principal receptors on animal cells for binding most extracellular matrix proteins.[11] They encompass a large family of heterodimeric glycoproteins. Central to the function of integrins is their ability to shift between active and inactive ligand binding states.[12] A striking feature of many integrins is their ability to bind multiple ligands.[13]

Under static conditions, the anchorage-dependent adhesion of ECs relies on the interaction of integrins with ECM. When cells are exposed to shear stress, such interaction must be reinforced if they are to withstand the shearing forces.[14] Integrins act as mechanical transducers that can translate the outside forces on a cell into biochemical signals leading to adhesion.[15] Adhesions undergo constant remodelling, an indication that there is an increase in the on-off rate between integrins and their cognate ECM substrates.[16]

Integrin-mediated cell adhesiveness, migration rate, and signalling messages can be modulated by growth factors.[17] Cell movement during tissue repair is also integrin-dependent. Activated or proliferative ECs express high levels of alphaVß3. Consistent with this notion, the integrin alphaVß3 is required for angiogenesis *in vivo*.[18] During cell adhesion mediated by interaction between the integrin alphaVß3 and its ECM substrates, mitogen-activated protein kinases (MAPKs) are activated by shear stress.[19] As the function of the integrin alphaVß3 appears to be critical to formation and maintenance of newly formed blood vessels,[20] it seems that either fibronectin or vitronectin could be immobilised onto a synthetic prosthesis, for the purpose of inducing cell adhesion.

2.2 Proliferation

Growth factors are mostly known for their ability to induce cell proliferation. Among them, basic fibroblast growth factor (bFGF, FGF-2) and vascular endothelial growth factor (VEGF) have received by far the most attention, the former because of its high level of effectiveness and the latter because of its apparently central regulatory role in angiogenesis. FGF seems to be secreted only when cells are damaged.[21] As a potent stimulator of angiogenesis, it can stimulate proliferation of both fibroblasts and vascular ECs by binding- with HS in the sub-endothelial ECM and in the basement membrane of various tissue and blood vessels. Thus to induce the formation of endothelium, VEGF is well suited because of its high specificity in only activating ECs.[22]

Among the five VEGF isoforms identified, the predominant one is the $VEGF_{165}$ homodimer, a 45 kDa protein that signals through two endothelial-cell transmembrane-receptor tyrosine kinases: VEGFR1 (Flt-1) and VEGFR2 (KDR/Flk-1).[23] The half-life of circulating VEGF is less than 3 min, probably because it binds readily, but with low affinity, to HSPGs on the luminal surface of the vascular endothelium. VEGF can be either stored in the ECM, through HS, or produced by cells. Heparin-binding domains mediate VEGF/GAG/receptor interactions, which are critical for effective signal transduction and stimulation of EC proliferation.[24] VEGF has been detected in autologous vessels following bypass and arterial injury and may partly account for improved patency in natural arteries.[25] At least three mechanisms could account for improvement in endothelium-dependent flow of collateral-dependent limbs after VEGF therapy. First, in calves, VEGF therapy significantly increases the blood pressure of the ischemic limb;[26] such improved perfusion pressure may lead to repair of dysfunctional endothelium. A second and intriguing possibility is a direct improvement in endothelial function by VEGF. *In vitro* studies have shown that endothelial function in coronary microcirculation perfused via collateral vessels is preserved by continuous administration of bFGF.[27] bFGF protects ECs from apoptosis and is known to modulate integrin expression by EC.[28] VEGF, through up-regulation of both the integrin alphaVß3 and adhesion proteins such as fibronectin or vitronectin, may similarly inhibit apoptosis by enhancing EC adhesion to matrix proteins.[29] VEGF may also enhance survival of ECs, and may directly repair presumed EC damage by protracted ischemia, thereby restoring normal endothelium-dependent flow.[30] Third, the possibility that the documented improvement in endothelium-dependent flow is due to newly formed VEGF-induced collateral vessels cannot be discounted. Indeed, among the various molecules known to affect EC physiology, VEGF is a major multifunction cytokine that regulates angiogenesis and vasculogenesis.[31] In addition to being potently and specifically mitogenic for ECs, VEGF also serves diverse functions such as modulating vascular permeability and stimulating EC migration.

Human umbilical-vein ECs (HUVEC) bind, internalise, and degrade VEGF.[32] Binding is time- and concentration-dependent and is saturable. Internalisation of bFGF has been reported to be slower than for VEGF.[33] In cells further away from the wound, VEGF is internalised via a classical receptor-mediated endocytosis pathway and accumulated in the endosomal compartment, whereas in the ECs at the wound site, VEGF (either released by activated macrophages or platelets) is rapidly taken up and translocated to the nucleus.[34] VEGF nuclear accumulation may thus play a role in stimulating coagulation and fibrinolysis pathways and in affecting vascular EC physiology in ways that are independent of VEGF growth-promoting effects and permeability properties.

Finally, Heparan Sulphate ProteoGlycan can potentiate the activity of VEGF and possibly that of bFGF when immobilised onto a surface by (1) promoting the accumulation of cytokines at high concentrations in an appropriate location for encounters with their target cells; (2) activating cytokines through conformational changes in the bound cytokine; (3) promoting conformation-dependent association or polymerisation of cytokines and their receptors and facilitating assembly of the appropriate molecular complex to initiate signal transduction; and (4) protecting cytokines from both chemical and physiological degradation.[35]

3. INCORPORATING CELL-SIGNALS INTO THE SURFACE OF A SYNTHETIC PROSTHESIS

In this section, we will review the processes for transforming an arterial prosthesis from a synthetic and inert device into a proactive one that looks more like a living natural vessel than an inert synthetic polymer. To accelerate vascular prosthesis endothelialization, one may try covalent grafting of selected molecule, thereby allowing ECs to find anchor points and form the desired endothelium. The cells can subsequently take part in the remodelling process, thus allowing permanent implantation of the materials and maintenance of the appropriate mechanical properties.

3.1 Grafting Adhesion Molecules

Fibrin coatings were first used to improve vascular-graft haemocompatibility.[36] After implantation, collagen IV, vitronectin, FN, and VEGF replaced the fibrin, an indication of the importance of the latter molecules.[37] Unfortunately, a fibrin mesh may also retain other molecules, various cell types, and lipids so that one must weigh the risk of requiring the eventual prosthesis explantation later on.

Since 1985, fibronectin has been used to enhance EC adherence to synthetic substrates.[38] Coating a bioglass with fibronectin reduces the time required for cell spreading and changes the morphology of the attached cells from an elongated shape to an extremely flattened one.[39] It has also been reported with regard to e-PTFE grafts and polyester elastomers that fibronectin does not significantly increase initial attachment but does increase the percentage of inoculum remaining after perfusion.[40] Fibronectin, collagen type-1, and gelatin-coated ammonia-plasma modified PTFE have been tested with seeded human ECs.[41] The areas in the vicinity of the RGD site are involved in the contact surface between ligands and integrins.[42]

Although platelets adhere to fibrinogen, vWF, IgG, or fibronectin immobilized on polystyrene, limited binding to either albumin or vitronectin has been detected.[43] Vitronectin, may thus be immobilized for the purpose of enhancing cell adhesion without inducing coagulation.[44] If we consider the subendothelial matrix as a standard, the level of platelet adhesion is high for HA and decreases respectively for HE, CS, DS, and KS, with ESHS-coated membranes being completely inert to platelets.[45] The number of platelets deposited on plasma-treated polystyrene PS-CO(2) coated with albumin-heparin conjugate is twice as high on PS-CO(2) coated with albumin.[46] ECs adhering to and proliferating on this coating significantly decrease the number of platelets that adhere to the surface. The immobilisation of cell adhesion peptides on the surface of implantable biomaterials may enhance the endothelialization.[47]

3.2 Covalent Linking of Growth Factors

Growth factor proteins are a possible way to give biomaterials the ability to regulate cell functions such as proliferation, differentiation, and apoptosis.[48] They can be covalently immobilised onto various matrices by different chemical methods. This type of stimulation by non-diffusing growth factors makes it possible to regulate tissue formation with artificial biomaterials. The biological activity of VEGF covalently linked to bovine serum albumin (BSA) has also been assessed.[49] BSA, which was used as a 'basecoat' layer in this surface binding study, is abundant in the blood, making it a good candidate for *in vivo* testing. The results show that cells cannot internalise covalent linkage of growth factor to the surface, as is the case *in vivo*. Permanent linkage probably leads to permanent stimulation of the cells. It was thus impossible to regulate the endothelium, limited here to a cell monolayer, and maintain homeostasis. This interpretation will have to be confirmed by long-term studies.

Although VEGF is a well-established initiator of angiogenesis, its presence is often insufficient for the formation of a complex, mature vascular network.[50] The endothelialization pathway requires adhesion, non-coagulation signals, and proliferation. Thus, growth-factor binding can be combined with grafting of adhesion and/or anticoagulant molecules to enhance the endothelialization process. Immobilisation of a single specific molecule is less efficient in prosthesis endothelialization than co-immobilization.[51]

3.3 Local Delivery of Growth Factors

Growth factors can also be delivered locally. A fibrin glue (FG) suspension for delivering a variety of angiogenic factors,[52] and an *in vitro* controlled release system for delivering VEGF via calcium alginate microspheres to promote vigorous angiogenesis[53] have already been investigated for applications in tissue engineering and wound healing.

A porous polymer scaffold that can deliver multiple growth factors has been made from poly(lactide-co-glycolide) (PLG).[54] This process allows for sustained protein delivery and maintains the biological activity of incorporated and released growth factors, even at low doses.[55] VEGF and bFGF have been incorporated into engineered tissues and have facilitated blood-vessel growth. Growth is facilitated more by VEGF than by bFGF.

Finally, impregnating the gelatinous layer of grafts with VEGF enhances trans-anastomotic tissue ingrowth and transmural capillary ingrowth.[56]

4. BIOACTIVE PROSTHESIS DESIGN

The idea of incorporating cell signalling onto the surface of a synthetic prosthesis, in order to develop a bioactive prosthesis, is very recent and has probably been made possible by advances in cell and molecular biology. For example, in 1992, Schneider et al. envisaged a uniform, naturally produced, subendothelial extracellular matrix as a coating for vascular grafts before implantation.[57] This substrate was found to provide an appropriate bilayer for EC adhesion, growth, and differentiation, in comparison to prostheses coated with fibronectin or basement membrane extracts. Such a substrate requires both adhesive glycoproteins (fibronectin, laminin, collagen) and proteoglycans (heparan sulphate) as well as potent EC growth factors (bFGF and VEGF). Starting from a study of cell-signalling mechanisms in the neointima, that study have shown that it is not only possible but even desirable to immobilise specific biomolecules in order to promote the endothelialization of the prosthesis.

We have recently developed a method to generate a covalent bound between the surface and the biomolecules.[58] By using an home-made radio-frequency glow discharge reactor,[59] VEGF was successfully grafted onto ePTFE vascular prostheses, as well as other biomolecules that are heavily involved in cell signalling, onto the surface of ePTFE synthetic vascular prostheses.[60] A cell migration test showed that the growth factor was still available for cells (Figure 1).

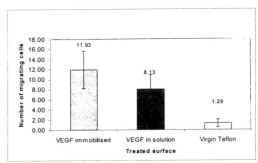

Figure 1. Cell migration as a function of the surface treatment. The number of migrating cells was high for cells migrating on the surface of a commercial Teflon prosthesis on which VEGF was previously immobilised than for those migrating on VEGF-added culture medium, and on commercial Teflon prostheses (Virgin Teflon).

These strategies have resulted in effective delivery of growth factors to ECs and also to circulating leukocytes that result from post-surgery inflammation. We have thus gained new insights not only into the process of endothelium and vascular regeneration but also into the regulation of inflammation. We now know that platelet adhesion is prevented by the presence of negatively charged HSPGs that are left exposed to cells after VEGF internalisation. Therefore, a prosthesis with grafted adhesive molecules and VEGFs immobilized onto HSPGs would probably be conducive to EC growth and result in total tissue reconstruction. In fact, the prosthesis would mimic the cellular membrane of a non-existent producer cell that secretes growth factors and adhesion molecules. Further efforts in biomaterials science should concentrate on developing this process *in vivo*. The functional biological properties of the prosthesis may be greatly enhanced through spatial regulation of signals to ECs.

ACKNOWLEDGEMENTS

The work from our laboratory was supported by grants from the National Science and Engineering Research Council (Canada) and the *Fonds Quebecois pour la Recherche sur la Nature et les Technologies* (Québec). Mathilde Crombez benefited of a Grant from the Research Center of St-François d'Assise Hospital for her M.Sc. studies.

REFERENCES

1. Szycher, M., 1991, Medical and Pharmaceutical Markets for Medical Plastics. In *High Performance Biomaterials*. Lancaster: Technomic Co, London, pp 1-25.
2. Guidoin, R., Chakfé, N., Maurel, S., How, T., Batt, M., Marois, M., and Gosselin, C., 1993, Expanded Polytetrafluoroethyene arterial prostheses in humans: Histopathological study of 298 surgically excised grafts. *Biomaterials* 14, 678-693.
3. Herring, M., Gardner, A., Peigh, P., Madison, D., Baughman, S., Brown, J., and Glover, J., 1984, Patency in canine inferior vena cava grafting: Effects of graft material, size, and endothelial seeding, *J. Vasc. Surg.* 1, 877-887.
4. Isner, J.M., and Takayuki, A., 1998, Therapeutic angiogenesis, *Front. Biosci.* 5, 49-69.
5. Jang, Y., Lincoff, A.M., Plow, E.F., and Topol, E.J., 1994, Cell adhesion molecules in coronary artery disease, *J. Am. Coll. Cardiol.* 24, 1591-1601.
6. Dejana, E., Languino, L.R., Colella, S., Corbascio, G.C., Plow, E., Ginsberg, M., and Marchisio, P.C., 1988, The localization of a platelet GpIIb-IIIa-related protein in endothelial cell adhesion structures, *Blood* 71, 566-572.
7. Lekatsas, J., and Koulouris, S., 2001, The role of selections in the development of coronary atherosclerosis, *Hellenic J. Cardiol. (Athens)* 42, 4-11.

8. Norgard-Sumnicht, K.E., Varki, N.M., and Varki, A., 1993, Calcium-dependent heparin-like ligands for L-selectin in nonlymphoid endothelial cells, *Science* **261**, 480-483.
9. Koenig, A., Norgard-Sumnicht, K., Linhardt, R., and Varki, A., 1998, Differential interactions of heparin and heparan sulfate glycosaminoglycans with the selectins. Implications for the use of unfractionated and low molecular weight heparins as therapeutic agents, *J. Clin. Invest.* **101**, 877-889.
10. White, H.D., 1997, Is heparin of value in the management of acute myocardial infarction?, *Cardiovasc. Drugs Ther.* **11**, 111-119.
11. Giancotti, F.G., and Ruoslahti, E., 1999, Integrin signaling, *Science* **285**, 1028-1032.
12. Beglova, N., Blacklow, S.C., Takagi, J., and Springer, T.A., 2002, Cysteine-rich module structure reveals a fulcrum for integrin rearrangement upon activation, *Nat. Struct. Biol.* **9**, 282-287.
13. Hafdi, Z., Lesavre, P., Tharaux, P.L., Bessou, G., Baruch, D., and Halbwachs-Mecarelli, L., 1997, Role of alpha v integrins in mesangial cell adhesion to vitronectin and von Willebrand factor, *Kidney Int.* **51**, 1900-1907.
14. Gimbrone, M.A. Jr., Nagel, T., and Topper, J.N., 1997, Biomechanical activation: An emerging paradigm in endothelial adhesion biology, *J. Clin. Invest.* **100**, 61-65.
15. Shyy, J.Y., and Chien, S., 1997, Role of integrins in cellular responses to mechanical stress and adhesion, *Curr. Opin. Cell. Biol.* **9**, 707-713.
16. Davies, P.F., Robotewskyj, A., and Griem, M.L., 1994, Quantitative studies of endothelial cell adhesion. Directional remodeling of focal adhesion sites in response to flow forces, *J. Clin. Invest.* **93**, 2031-2038.
17. Maheshwari, G., Brown, G., Lauffenburger, D.A., Wells, A., and Griffith, L.G., 2000, Cell adhesion and motility depend on nanoscale RGD clustering, *J. Cell. Sci.* **113**, 1677-1686.
18. Brooks, P.C., Clark, R.A., and Cheresh, D.A., 1994, Requirement of vascular integrin alpha v beta 3 for angiogenesis, *Science* **264**, 569-571.
19. Jo, H., Sipos, K., Go, Y.M., Law, R., Rong, J., and McDonald, J.M., 1997, Differential effect of shear stress on extracellular signal-regulated kinase and N-terminal Jun kinase in endothelial cells, *J. Biol. Chem.* **272**, 1395-1401.
20. Stromblad, S., and Cheresh, D.A., 1996, Integrins, angiogenesis and vascular cell survival, *Chem. Biol.* **3**, 881-885.
21. Steed, D.L., 1997, The role of growth factors in wound healing, *Surg. Clin. North Am.* **77**, 575-586.
22. Ishihara, M., Sato, M., Hattori, H., Saito, Y., Yura, H., Ono, K., Masuoka, K., Kikuchi, M., Fujikawa, K., and Kurita, A., 2001, Heparin-carrying polystyrene (HCPS)-bound collagen substratum to immobilize heparin-binding growth factors and to enhance cellular growth, *J. Biomed. Mater. Res.* **56**, 536-544.
23. Ferrara, N, and Keyt, B., 1997, Vascular endothelial growth factor: Basic biology and clinical implications, *Experimental Supplementum* **79**, 209-232.
24. Schlessinger, J., Lax, I., and Lemmon, M., 1995, Regulation of growth factor activation by proteoglycans: What is the role of the low affinity receptors? *Cell* **83**, 357-360.
25. Hamdan, A.D., Aiello, L.P., Misare, B.D., Contreras, M.A,. King, G.L., LoGerfo, F.W., and Quist, W.C., 1997, Vascular endothelial growth factor expression in canine peripheral vein bypass grafts, *J. Vasc. Surg.* **26**, 79-86.
26. Takeshita, S., Zheng, L.P., Brogi, E., Kearney, M., Pu, L.Q., Bunting, S., Ferrara, N., Symes, J.F., and Isner, J.M., 1994, Therapeutic angiogenesis: A single intra-arterial bolus of vascular endothelial growth factor augments revascularization in a rabbit ischemic hindlimb model, *J. Clin. Invest.* **93**, 662-670.

27. Sellke, F.W., Wang, S.Y., Friedman, M., Harada, K., Edelman, E.R., Grossman, W., and Simons, M., 1994, Basic FGF enhances endothelium-dependent relaxation of the collateral-perfused coronary microcirculation, *Am. J. Physiol.* **267**, 1303-1311.
28. Fuks, Z., Persaud, R.S., Alfieri, A., McLoughlin, M., Ehleiter, D., Schwartz, J.L., Seddon, A.P., Cordon-Cardo, C., and Haimovitz-Friedman, A., 1994, Basic fibroblast growth factor protects endothelial cells against radiation-induced programmed cell death *in vitro* and *in vivo*, *Canc. Res.* **54**, 2582-2590.
29. Spyridopoulos, I., Brogi, E., Kearney, M., Sullivan, A.B., Cetrulo, C., Isner, J.M., and Losordo, D.W., 1997, Vascular endothelial growth factor inhibits endothelial cell apoptosis induced by tumor necrosis factor-alpha: Balance between growth and death signals, *J. Mol. Cell Cardiol.* **29**, 1321-1330.
30. Brooks, P.C., Montgomery, A.M., Rosenfeld, M., Reisfeld, R.A., Hu, T., Klier, G., and Cheresh, D.A., 1994, Integrin alpha v beta 3 antagonists promote tumor regression by inducing apoptosis of angiogenic blood vessels, *Cell* **79**, 1157-1164.
31. Ferrara, N., and Davis-Smyth, T., 1997, The biology of vascular endothelial growth factor, *Endocr. Rev.* **18**, 4-25.
32. Bikfalvi, A., Sauzeau, C., Moukadiri, H., Maclouf, J., Busso, N., Bryckaert, M., Plouet, J., and Tobelem, G., 1991, Interaction of vasculotropin/vascular endothelial cell growth factor with human umbilical vein endothelial cells: Binding, internalization, degradation, and biological effects, *J. Cell. Physiol.* **149**, 50-59.
33. Bikfalvi, A., Dupuy, E., Inyang, A.L., Fayein, N., Leseche, G., Courtois, Y., and Tobelem, G., 1989, Binding, internalization, and degradation of basic fibroblast growth factor in human microvascular endothelial cells, *Exp. Cell. Res.* **181**, 75-84.
34. Li, W., and Keller, G., 2000, VEGF nuclear accumulation correlates with phenotypical changes in endothelial cells, *J. Cell. Sci.* **113**, 1525-1534.
35. Letourneur, D., Machy, D., Pelle, A., Marcon-Bachari, E., D'Angelo, G., Vogel, M., Chaubet, F., and Michel, J.B., 2002, Heparin and non-heparin-like dextrans differentially modulate endothelial cell proliferation: *In vitro* evaluation with soluble and crosslinked polysaccharide matrices, *J. Biomed. Mater. Res.* **60**, 94-100.
36. Nikolaychik, V.V., Samet, M.M., and Lelkes, P.I., 1994, A new, cryoprecipitate based coating for improved endothelial cell attachment and growth on medical grade artificial surfaces, *ASAIO J.* **40**, 846-852.
37. Lyman, D.J., Murray-Wijelath, J., Ambrad-Chalela, E., and Wijelath, E.S., 2001, Vascular graft healing. II. FTIR analysis of polyester graft samples from implanted bi-grafts, *J. Biomed. Mater. Res.* **58**, 221-237.
38. Williams, S.K., Jarrell, B.E., Friend, L., Radomski, J.S., Carabasi, R.A., Koolpe, E., Mueller, S.N., Thornton, S.C., Marinucci, T., and Levine, E., 1985, Adult human endothelial cell compatibility with prosthetic graft material, *J. Surg. Res.* **38**, 618-629.
39. Seitz, T.L., Noonan, K.D., Hench, L.L., and Noonan, N.E., 1982, Effect of fibronectin on the adhesion of an established cell line to a surface reactive biomaterial, *J. Biomed. Mater. Res.* **16**, 195-207.
40. Kesler, K.A., Herring, M.B., Arnold, M.P., Glover, J.L., Park, H.M., Helmus, M.N., and Bendick, P.J., 1986, Enhanced strength of endothelial attachment on polyester and polytetrafluoroethylene graft surfaces with fibronectin substrate, *J. Vasc. Surg.* **3**, 58-64.
41. Lu, A., and Sipehia R., 2001, Antithrombotic and fibrinolytic system of human endothelial cells seeded on PTFE: The effects of surface modification of PTFE by ammonia plasma treatment and ECM protein coatings, *Biomaterials* **22**, 1439-1446.

42. Tweden, K.S., Harasaki, H., Jones, M., Blevitt, J.M., Craig, W.S., Pierschbacher, M., and Helmus, M.N., 1995, Accelerated healing of cardiovascular textiles promoted by an RGD peptide, *J. Heart Valve Dis.* **4**, 90-97.
43. Marchand-Brynaert, J., Detrait, E., Noiset, O., Boxus, T., Schneider, Y.J., and Remacle, C., 1999, Biological evaluation of RGD peptidomimetics, designed for the covalent derivatization of cell culture substrata, as potential promotors of cellular adhesion, *Biomaterials* **20**, 1773-1782.
44. Pieper, J.S., Hafmans, T., Veerkamp, J.H., and van Kuppevelt, T.H., 2000, Development of tailor-made collagen-glycosaminoglycan matrices: EDC/NHS crosslinking, and ultrastructural aspects, *Biomaterials* **21**, 581-593.
45. Baumann, H., and Keller, R., 1997, Which glycosaminoglycans are suitable for antithrombogenic or athrombogenic coatings of biomaterials? Part II: Covalently immobilized endothelial cell surface heparan sulfate (ESHS) and heparin (HE) on synthetic polymers and results of animal experiments, *Semin. Thromb. Hemost.* **23**, 215-223.
46. Bos, G.W., Scharenborg, N.M., Poot, A.A., Engbers, G.H., Beugeling, T., van Aken, W.G., and Feijen J., 1999, Blood compatibility of surfaces with immobilized albumin-heparin conjugate and effect of endothelial cell seeding on platelet adhesion, *J. Biomed. Mater. Res.* **47**, 279-291.
47. Mann, B.K., and West, J.L., 2002, Cell adhesion peptides alter smooth muscle cell adhesion, proliferation, migration, and matrix protein synthesis on modified surfaces and in polymer scaffolds, *J. Biomed. Mater. Res.* **60**, 86-93.
48. Ito, Y., Chen, G., and Imanishi, Y., 1998, Artificial juxtacrine stimulation for tissue engineering, *J. Biomater. Sci. Polym. Ed.* **9**, 879-890.
49. Stone, D., Phaneuf, M., Sivamurthy, N., LoGerfo, F.W., and Quist, W.C., 2002, A biologically active VEGF construct *in vitro*: implications for bioengineering-improved prosthetic vascular grafts, *J. Biomed. Mater. Res.* **59**, 160-165.
50. Yancopoulos, G.D., Davis, S., Gale, N.W., Rudge, J.S., Wiegand, S.J., and Holash, J., 2000, Vascular-specific growth factors and blood vessel formation, *Nature* **407**, 242-248.
51. Doi, K., and Matsuda, T., 1997, Enhanced vascularization in a microporous polyurethane graft impregnated with basic fibroblast growth factor and heparin, *J. Biomed. Mater. Res.* **34**, 361-370.
52. Tassiopoulos, A.K., and Greisler, H.P., 2000, Angiogenic mechanisms of endothelialization of cardiovascular implants: A review of recent investigative strategies, *J. Biomater. Sci. Polym. Ed.* **11**, 1275-1284.
53. Elcin, Y.M., Dixit, V., and Gitnick, G., 2001, Extensive *in vivo* angiogenesis following controlled release of human vascular endothelial cell growth factor: Implications for tissue engineering and wound healing, *Artif. Organs* **25**, 558-565.
54. Richardson, T.P., Peters, M.C., Ennett, A.B., and Mooney, D.J., 2001, Polymeric system for dual growth factor delivery, *Nature Biotechnol.* **19**, 1029-1034.
55. Sheridan, M.H., Shea, L.D., Peters, M.C., and Mooney, D.J., 2000, Bioabsorbable polymer scaffolds for tissue engineering capable of sustained growth factor delivery, *J. Control Release* **64**, 91-102.
56. Masuda, S., Doi, K., Satoh, S., Oka, T., and Matsuda, T., 1997, Vascular endothelial growth factor enhances vascularization in microporous small caliber polyurethane grafts, *ASAIO J.* **43**, 530-534.
57. Schneider, A., Melmed, R.N., Schwalb, H., Karck, M., Vlodavsky, I., and Uretzky, G., 1992, An improved method for endothelial cell seeding on polytetrafluoroethylene small caliber vascular grafts, *J. Vasc. Surg.* **15**, 649-656.

58. Crombez, M., 2002, M.Sc. Thesis, *Progresses in synthetic vascular prostheses: Toward the endothelialization*. Laval University, Québec City, Canada.
59. Mantovani, D., Castonguay, M., Pageau, J.P., Fiset, M., and Laroche, G, 2000, Ammonia RF-Plasma Treatment of Tubular ePTFE Vascular Prostheses, *Plasmas and Polymers*, **4**, 207-228 ; Chevallier, P., Castonguay, M., Turgeon, S., Dubrulle, N., Mantovani, D., McBreen, P.H., Wittmann, J.C., and Laroche, G., 2001, Ammonia RF-plasma on PTFE surfaces: Chemical characterization of the species created on surface by vapor – phase chemical derivatization. *J. Phys. Chem.B* **105**, 12490-12497.
60. Crombez, M., Chevallier, P., C-Gaudreault, R., Laroche, G., and Mantovani, D., 2002, Grafting of heparan sulfate/vascular endothelial growth factor complex onto synthetic substrates to improve hemocompatibility, *Proceeding of the Symposium on Advanced Materials for Biomedical Applications*, D. Mantovani Ed., Canadian Institute of Mining, Metallurgy and Petroleum, pp. 49-66. (see also Badeau, M., *et al.* pp. 67-78 and Chevallier, P., *et al.* pp. 269-286).

ADHESION AND GROWTH OF RAT AORTIC SMOOTH MUSCLE CELLS ON LACTIDE-BASED POLYMERS

Lucie Bačáková[1], Monika Lapčíková[2], Dana Kubies[2,3], and František Rypáček[2]

[1]*Centre for Exp. Cardiovascular Research, Institute of Physiology, Acad. Sci. CR, Vídeňská 1083, 142 20 Prague;* [2]*Institute of Macromolecular Chemistry, Acad. Sci. CR, and* [3]*Centre for Cell Therapy and Tissue Repair, Heyrovsky Sq. 2, 162 06 Prague, Czech Republic*

ABSTRACT

Biodegradable materials based on polymers of hydroxy acids are studied for application in artificial vascular substitutes. Polymers with functional surfaces are being developed, carrying specific recognition structures to affect selectively the adhesion and proliferation of endothelial cells (EC) and vascular smooth muscle cells (VSMC). This preliminary study focuses on evaluation of adhesion and growth of VSMC on surfaces of polylactide polymers and those modified by amphiphilic polylactide/poly(ethylene oxide) copolymers. Poly(L-lactic acid), PLLA, and poly(DL-lactic acid), PDLLA, and a block copolymer of lactide with a carboxylated poly(ethylene oxide) segment, PLLA-b-PEO-COOH, were synthesized by controlled polymerization of L and D,L-lactide, respectively, and using Δ-hydroxy-Z-carboxymethyl-PEO as a macroinitiator for the copolymer. Films of polymers were deposited on glass coverslips by a spin-coating method. Uncoated glass coverslips and Falcon dishes were used as control substrates. VSMC were obtained from the thoracic aorta of young adult male Wistar rats by explantation method and seeded in Dulbecco-Modified Eagle MEM with 10% foetal bovine serum. The number of adhering cells, their shape, size of cell-material contact area and cell population doubling time were evaluated from day 1 to 7 after seeding. It was found that both PLLA and especially PDLLA relatively well supported adhesion and growth of VSMC. However, on carboxylated surfaces of the PLLA-b-PEO-COOH copolymer, a lower number of initially adhering cells (by 37% than on Falcon dishes, pδ0.05), smaller cell spreading area (by 45% and 37% than on glass and Falcon dishes, respectively, pδ0.01) and longer doubling time (by 49% and 31% than on glass and Falcon dishes, pδ0.001). Thus, surfaces coated by a PLA/PEO-COOH copolymer can be used as minimum background surface to reveal the effect of other more specific adhesion structures.

1. INTRODUCTION

There is a significant effort in development of artificial vascular substitutes to treat various cardiovascular diseases. The use of biodegradable polymers in this field has gained increased attention. Three-dimensional fully or partially resorbable polymeric scaffolds can be colonized by autologous endothelial cells (EC) and vascular smooth muscle cells (VSMC) *in vitro* prior to implantation into the patient's organism, and evolve in fully functioning blood vessels.[1] This strategy is based mainly on designing surfaces promoting fast development of a continuous, mature endothelial layer, which would be naturally thromboresistant, non-immunogenic and semipermeable.[2,3] The role of VSMC in vascular prostheses is more controversial. These cells are prone to excessive migratory and growth response leading to stenosis and even occlusion of the vascular lumen, so they are often considered as an undesirable component of vascular prostheses that should be excluded. One of the most advanced methods for a selective endothelization of prostheses is based on designing its surfaces to bear extracellular matrix-derived amino acid sequences, such as peptides specific for integrin receptors on cells, which would bind selectively the endothelial cells.[4] However, in a more physiologically relevant approach, the VSMC could be considered as a normal, functionally important component of an artificial vascular wall, if we could control their migration and proliferation. Under these conditions, the VSMC cells could become equally beneficial for the function of blood vessel prostheses as they support the endothelization of the prosthesis - better attachment and growth of endothelial cells was observed in regions with underlying VSMC.[1,5] In three-dimensionally-constructed degradable implants, VSMC migrate inside the scaffold, remove it gradually (as cells of mesenchymal origin, they retain a certain degree of phagocytosis ability) and replace it with newly synthesized vascular extracellular matrix (see Bačáková et al.[6] for review).

Therefore, this study concentrates on adhesion and growth behavior of rat aortic smooth muscle cells in cultures on biodegradable polymers with potential use for construction of (1) functional surfaces permissive for cell adhesion but releasing antiproliferative agents, and/or (2) carrying amino acid sequences, known as ligands for integrin cell-membrane receptors, in defined concentration, distribution and cell specificity. The former group of materials is represented poly(L-lactic acid) (PLLA) and poly(DL-lactic acid) (PDLLA), the latter by a block copolymer of lactide with a carboxylated poly(ethylene oxide) segment, PLLA-b-PEO-COOH.

Polylactides are known as good substrates for adhesion and growth of several cell types, including fibroblasts,[7] primary osteoblasts or chondrocytes,[8] and they have been widely studied as materials for drug delivery systems. On the other hand, poly(ethylene oxide) (PEO) based polymers have been used to create inert, non-thrombogenic, non-immunogenic and calcification-resistant surfaces of blood-contacting devices[9] or non-adhesive domains on micropatterned surfaces in order to control protein adsorption and tissue organization on biomaterials.[10] The PEO-containing copolymers may represent a non-adhesive "background" for attachment of defined integrin ligands providing for selective adhesion of a certain cell types or for control of cell proliferation through controlling cell shape, degree of spreading as well as the size, concentration and distribution of focal adhesion plaques on cells.[11]

2. MATERIALS AND METHODS

2.1 Polymeric Substrates

Synhesis of Polymers. The homopolymers poly(L-lactic acid), PLLA, and poly(DL-lactic acid), PDLLA, were synthesized by polymerisation of L and D,L-lactide, respectively, in melt, using Tin(II)-2-ethylhexanoate as a catalyst.[12] The raw polymers were dissolved in chloroform and purified by precipitation into methanol.

A block copolymer composed of poly(L-lactide) and Z-carboxymethyl-poly(ethylene oxide) blocks, PLLA-b-PEO-COOH, was prepared by solution polymerisation of L-lactide in dioxane at 80 °C, using Δ-hydroxy-Z-carboxymethyl-PEO as a macroinitiator and Tin(II)-2-ethylhexanoate as a catalyst.[13] Δ-Hydroxy-Z-carboxymethyl-PEO (PEO-COOH) as macro-initiator for the synthesis of PLLA-b-PEO-COOH copolymer was prepared by anionic polymerisation of ethylene oxide in THF. The polymerisation was initiated by kalium triphenylmethoxide and terminated by addition of 2-brom-terc-butylacetate. The trityl and t-butyl protecting groups were removed in one step by treatment with trifluoroacetic acid and the resulting polymer product was precipitated to diethyl ether. Mono-carboxy-PEO derivative, i.e. A-hydroxy-Z-carboxymethyl-PEO (PEO-COOH), was purified by ion exchange chromatography on DEAE Sephadex (Pharmacia, Uppsala, Sweden) column, dialyzed and lyophilised.

Molecular parameters. Molecular weight of polymers was determined by viscometry in chloroform for PLLA, and by gel-permeation chromatography (GPC) for PDLLA and PLLA-*b*-PEO-COOH. The GPC was in THF carried out using Waters modular HPLC/GPC system using combined PL-Gel SEC columns (Pl-Gel10^3 Å plus Mixed C, Polymer Laboratories, Ltd., England) with WAT410 refraction index detector. The chromatographic data were collected and processed by Data Apex CSW data station (Watrex, Prague). The columns were calibrated by polystyrene and PEO standards (Polymer Laboratories, England) and the calibration was recalculated for polylactide according to universal calibration concept using Mark-Houwink coefficients for polystyrene and polylactide.[14]

Polymer films: Films of polymers were prepared by spin casting of a solution of selected polymer in chloroform on silanized glass coverslips (size 2 x 2 cm, Marienfeld, Germany) The glass coverslips used for film casting were first silanized by treatment with trichlormethyl silane in hexane (0.1 % v/v) to improve the adhesion and long-term stability of the cast polymer films to the glass surface. The film of PLLA-*b*-PEO-COOH copolymer was cast on the top of the PLLA film cast previously. The coverslips with polymer films were placed into polystyrene dishes (diameter 3.5 cm, Falcon, U.S.A.) and sterilized with ultraviolet light irradiation for 2 hours. Uncoated native glass coverslips or Falcon dishes were used as control substrates. The substrates were incubated in phosphate-buffered saline (PBS) for 2 hours, before the cells were seeded.

Contact angle measurements. Dynamic contact angle measurements of the polymer surfaces were carried out by the Wilhelmy-plate method using a KRÜS tensiometer (model K12, Germany). The advancing contact angle (θ_A) and the receding contact angle (θ_R) were measured after incubation of the samples in water for 2 hours.

2.2 Cells

Cells and culture conditions. VSMC were derived by an explantation method from the intima-media complex of the thoracic aorta of young adult male Wistar rats.[15, 16] In passage 5, the cells were seeded onto the polymer samples at the density of 3000 cells/cm^2, i.e. about 30 000 cells/dish, and in 3 ml of Dulbecco-Modified Eagle Minimum Essential Medium (DMEM; Cat. No. 11995-065, Gibco BRL, Life Technologies, U.S.A.), supplemented with 10 % foetal bovine serum (FBS; Cat. No.26140-079, Gibco BRL, Life Technologies, U.S.A.). One day after seeding, the medium was changed to remove non-adhered cells. The cells were cultured for 1, 3 or 7 days at 37°C in humidified air atmosphere containing 5% of CO_2. For each experimental group and time interval, 2 samples were used. At the first two time points, the cells were rinsed in phosphate-buffered saline (PBS, fixed for 5 min in 10% formol (i.e. 3.7 % formaldehyde; Sigma, St. Louis, MO, U.S.A.) in PBS and stained with Gill's haematoxylin and water-soluble eosin Y (both from Fisher Scientific, Fair Lawn, NJ, U.S.A.) using standard protocol provided by the manufacturer, and mounted in Gel/Mount media (Cat. No. M01, Biomeda Corp., Foster City, CA, U.S.A.).

Parameters of cell adhesion and growth. The number of adhering VSMC was counted in 9 randomly selected microscopic fields of 2.7 mm^2 (x10 objective; day 1 after seeding) or 0.17 mm^2 (x40 objective; day 3), homogeneously distributed on each sample. For evaluation of cell shape and size of cell spreading area, images from 5 to 6 regions on samples 1 day after seeding (obj. x10, 2.7 mm^2, 4-26 cells in each region) were captured. A Nikon Eclipse TE 300 microscope (Japan), equipped with cooled CCD camera (CH 360, Photometrics Ltd., U.S.A.), and Image Pro Plus 3.0 software (Media Cybernetics, Silver Spring, MS, U.S.A.), was used for the analysis. Cells forming cell-cell contact were excluded from the evaluation. On day 7 after seeding, when the cell counting in microscopic fields was disabled by a high cell population density and formation of multi-layered areas, the cells were detached by trypsin-EGTA (Sigma, St. Louis, MO, U.S.A.) and counted in Levy's chamber (8 measurements for each sample). The cell population doubling time (DT) was calculated as DT = $(t-t_o)$log 2/log Nt-log Nt_o , where Nt_o and Nt were the numbers of cells per cm^2 at the beginning and the end of the studied culture interval (i.e., between days 1 and 3 or 3 and 7). Four measurements of doubling time for each group of samples and time interval were performed.

Statistics. Data were presented as averages ± SD (Standard Deviation) from 4 to 18 measurements. Statistical significance was evaluated by Student's t-test for unpaired data using a 5% error probability criterion.

3. RESULTS AND DISCUSSION

3.1 Physicochemical Properties of Polymers and Polymer Films

High-molecular-weight homopolymers of semicrystalline PLLA and amorphous PDLLA were prepared with weight average molecular weight of

550,000 and 360,000, respectively. The high molecular weight secures good film-forming properties of polymers. The two-block amphiphilic copolymer PLLA-b-PEO-COOH was composed of hydrophobic PLLA and hydrophilic PEO blocks, both having approximately the same length with M_w of 6300 and 6100, respectively. The film of copolymer was cast on top of the PLLA film, thus allowing for a good adhesion and partial blending of PLLA blocks of the copolymer with chains of the PLLA sublayer, while the hydrophilic PEO segments can form a hydrophilic brush of flexible chains at the surface.[17] Carboxyl groups were introduced to the ends of hydrophilic PEO segments to increase their water propensity and, eventually, to provide for a functional group suitable for further modification.

The contact angle measurements reveal the effect of composition of polymer films on the surface wettability.

Table 1. Advancing (Θ_A) and Receding (Θ_R) Contact Angles (degrees) of the Water-Air Interface on the Polymer Films and Glass Substrates After 2 and 24 Hours of Incubation in Water (n – not determined)

Sample	2 h		24 h	
	Θ_A	Θ_R	Θ_A	Θ_R
PDLLA [1]	80.5	52.5	79	52.7
PLLA [1]	81.5	60.3	80.4	59.5
COOH-PEO-PLLA [2]	41.8	32.0	40.8	29.3
Unmodified glass	54	41	n	n
Silanized glass	89.1	67.9	n	n

[1] The film prepared by spin casting of the homopolymer solution on the silanized glass slide.
[2] The film prepared by spin casting of the copolymer solution on the previously cast PLLA thin film on the silanized glass slide.

3.2 Cell Adhesion and Growth

Initial number of adhering cells. On day 1 after seeding, the cells adhered at population densities ranging from 1549 ± 2532 to 2652 ± 1745 cells/cm^2. On PLLA and PDLLA samples, the densities tended to be lower compared to those on glass coverslips or Falcon dishes (by 10% to 42%). These differences, however, were not statistically significant, which could be due to a relatively high inhomogeneity in cell population density, as indicated by high standard deviations, especially on PLLA surfaces (Fig. 1A). However, on carboxylated surfaces of the PLLA-b-PEO-COOH copolymer, the cell density was significantly lower than that on Falcon dishes (by 37%, p≤ 0.05, Fig. 1A).

Statistically significant differences between the samples of the same experimental group were not found.

Cell Shape and Spreading Area. The VSMC on glass, Falcon dishes and PDLLA were well flattened and mainly polygonal. Their spreading area ranged from 1964 ± 313 to 2235 ± 289 µm^2. In comparison with these cells, VSMC on PLLA films were less spread, and of polygonal or spindle shape. Their spreading was of 1579 ± 179 µm^2, which was by 29% and 20% less than on glass coverslips and Falcon dishes ($p \leq 0.01$ and $p \leq 0.05$), respectively. The lowest degree of cell spreading was found on PLLA-*b*-PEO-COOH copolymer. These cells were often round or spindle-shaped, and the size of their spreading area was only 1236 ± 351µm^2, i.e. by 45% and 37% less than on glass and Falcon dishes, respectively ($p \leq 0.01$; Fig. 1B, 2).

Similarly to cell number, there were no statistically significant differences between samples within the same experimental group.

Cell Population Doubling Time and Density. In the early exponential phase of growth (from day 1 to 3), the doubling times of cells on Falcon dishes, PLLA and PDLLA were similar and ranged from 13.5 ± 4.1 to 14.6 ± 1.0 hours. On glass, the doubling time reached only 12.7 ± 0.6 hours and became significantly shorter than that on Falcon dishes ($p \leq 0.05$). The slowest cell proliferation was found on PLLA-*b*-PEO-COOH samples. The doubling time on this polymer was 19.0 ± 0.4 hours, which was by 49% and 31% longer in comparison to the values obtained on glass and Falcon dishes ($p \leq 0.001$; Tab. 2). As a result, the cell population density on PLLA-*b*-PEO-COOH samples on day 3 after seeding was significantly lower than the values obtained on glass and Falcon dishes, while the densities on PLLA and PDLLA were similar than those found on control substrates (Fig. 3A).

In the late exponential growth phase (from day 3 to 7), the doubling times on both control substrates, i.e. glass and Falcon dishes, were prolonged to 21.9 ± 0.7 and 22.4 ± 0.8 h, respectively. At the same time, the doubling time on PLLA-*b*-PEO-COOH was shortened to 17.7 ± 0.7 h (Tab. 2). Despite of this, the cells on PLLA-*b*-PEO-COOH reached a lower final population density on day 7 (418 000 ± 76 000 cells/ cm^2 vs. 576 000 ± 77 000 cells/cm^2 on glass, $p \leq 0.001$, and 511 000 ± 71 000 cells/cm^2 on Falcon dishes, $p \leq 0.01$). In addition, cells on PLLA-*b*-PEO-COOH were more prone to spontaneous detachment from the growth substrate to the culture media. In contrast, the cells on PLLA and PDLLA reached slightly but significantly higher final population densities than those on Falcon dishes (by 14 and 15%, respectively, $p \leq 0.01$, Fig. 3B).

No significant differences were noted within samples of the same experimental group.

Table 2. Population Doubling Time of Vascular Smooth Muscle Cells on Glass Lactide-Based Polymers in Early (Day 1 to 3) and Late (Day 3 to 7) Exponential Phase of Growth

Sample	Doubling time (h)	
	Day 1 to 3	Day 3 to 7
Glass coverslips	12.7 ± 0.6	21.9 ± 0.7
Falcon dishes	14.6 ± 1.0 *	22.4 ± 0.8
PLLA	13.5 ± 4.1	19.5 ± 2.1
PDLLA	13.6 ± 1.2	20.0 ± 0.9 * ♥♥
COOH-PEO-PLLA	19.0 ± 0.9 *** ♥♥♥	17.7 ± 0.7*** ♥♥♥

Averages ± SD from 4 measurements.
Statistical significance: ***p≤ 0.001 and *p≤ 0.05 compared to glass coverslips;
♥♥♥ p≤ 0.001, ♥♥ p≤ 0.02 and ♥ p≤ 0.05 compared to Falcon dishes.

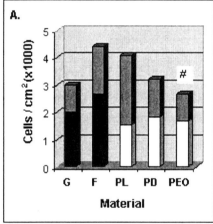 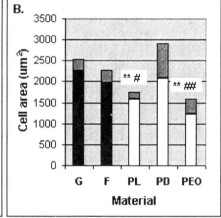

Figure 1. Number (A) and size (B) of the spreading area of VSMC initially adhering to glass coverslips (G), polystyrene Falcon dishes (F), poly(L-lactic acid) (PL) poly(DL-lactic acid) (PD), and a block copolymer PLLA-b-PEO-COOH (PEO) on day 1 after seeding. Averages ± SD from 18 measurements on two independent samples (i.e., 9 on each).
Statistical significance: **p≤ 0.01 compared to glass coverslips; ## p≤ 0.01 and # p≤ 0.05 compared to Falcon dishes.

Smooth Muscle Cells on Lactide-Based Bioactive Polymers 187

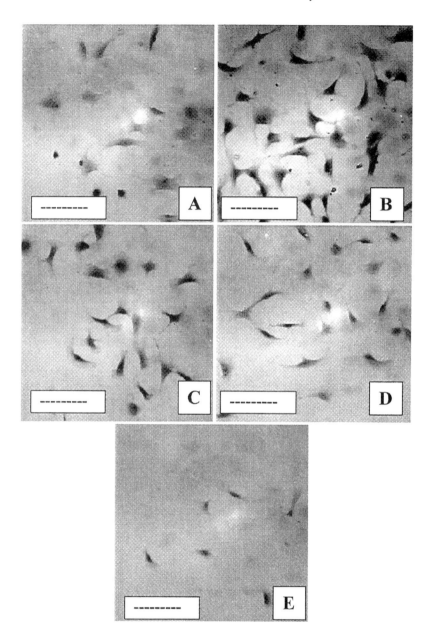

Figure 2. Morphology of VSMC adhering to glass coverslips **(A)**, polystyrene Falcon dishes **(B)**, poly(L-lactic acid), PLLA **(C)**, poly(DL-lactic acid), PDLLA **(D)**, and a block copolymer PLLA-*b*-PEO-COOH **(E)** on day 1 after seeding. Nikon Eclipse TE 300 microscope with Image Pro Plus 3.0 software, obj.10. Bar=100µm.

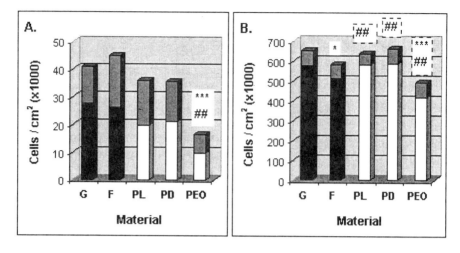

Figure 3. Population density (cells/cm^2) of VSMC on glass coverslips (G), polystyrene Falcon dishes (F), poly(L-lactic acid) (PL) poly(DL-lactic acid) (PD), and a block copolymer PLLA-*b*-PEO-COOH (PEO) on day 3 (**A**) and 7 (**B**) after seeding. Averages ± SD from 18 measurements on two independent samples (i.e., 9 on each).
Statistical significance: ***$p \leq 0.001$ and *$p \leq 0.05$ compared to glass coverslips; ## $p \leq 0.01$ compared to Falcon dishes.

4. CONCLUSION

Both PLLA and PDLLA polymers supported well adhesion and growth of VSMC, while the PLLA-*b*-PEO-COOH copolymer showed significant inhibitory effects on the initial cell adhesion as well as growth. Thus, the PLLA and PDLLA could be used as component of vascular prostheses carrying and releasing humoral factors controlling the VSMC proliferation. The surfaces coated by PLLA-*b*-PEO-COOH copolymer, can serve as background on which the effect of specific ligands controlling the phenotype, migration, growth and differentiation of adhering cells such as oligopeptides specific for integrin receptors (e.g. GREDVY, REDVDY, RGDS) can be evaluated.

ACKNOWLEDGEMENTS

The work was supported by Grant Agency of the Academy of Sciences of the Czech Republic (Grant No. A40500202) and by the program of research centers of the Ministry of Education CR (Grant No. LN00A065).

REFERENCES

1. Greisler, H.P., Tattersall, C.W., Klosak, J.J., Cabusao, E.A., Garfield, J.D., and Kim, D.U., 1991, Partially bioresorbable vascular grafts in dogs, *Surgery* **110**, 645-654,
2. Greisler, H.P., Gosselin, C., Ren, D.W., Kang, S.S., and Kim, D.U., 1996, Biointeractive polymers and tissue engineered blood vessels. *Biomaterials* **17**, 329.
3. Bordenave, L., Remy-Zolghadri, M., Fernandez, P., Bareille, R., and Midy, D., 1999, Clinical performance of vascular grafts lined with endothelial cells. *Endothelium* **6**, 267-275.
4. Holt, D.B., Eberhart, R.C., and Prager M.D., 1994, Endothelial cell binding to Dacron modified with polyethylene oxide and peptide. *ASAIO* **40**, M858-63.
5. Kim, W.G., Park, J.K., Park, Y.N., Hwang, C.M., Jo, Y.H., Min, B.G., Yoon, C.J., Lee, T.Y., 2000, Tissue-engineered heart valve leaflets: an effective method for seeding autologous cells on scaffolds. *Int. J. Artif. Organs* **23**, 624-628.
6. Bačáková, L., Švorčík, V., Rybka, V., Micek, I., Hnatowicz, V., Lisa, V., and Kocourek, F., 1996, Adhesion and proliferation of cultured human aortic smooth muscle cells on polystyrene implanted with N+, F+ and Ar+ ions: correlation with polymer surface polarity and carbonization. *Biomaterials* **17**, 1121-1126.
7. Hsu, S.H., Tseng, H.J., and Fang, Z.K., 1999, Polyurethane blended with polylactides for improved cell adhesion and reduced platelet activation. *Artif. Organs* **23**, 958-961.
8. Noth, U., Tuli, R., Osyczka, A.M., Danielson, K.G., and Tuan, R.S., 2002, *In vitro* engineered cartilage constructs produced by press-coating biodegradable polymer with human mesenchymal stem cells. *Tissue Eng.* **8**, 131-144.
9. Han, D.K., Lee, K.B., Park, K.D., Kim, C.S., Jeong, S.Y., Kim, Y.H., Kim, H.M., and Min B.G., 1993, *In vivo* canine studies of a Sinkhole valve and vascular graft coated with biocompatible PU-PEO-SO3. *ASAIO J.* **39**, M537-M541.
10. Liu, V.A., Jastromb, W.E., and Bhatia, S.N., 2002, Engineering protein and cell adhesivity using PEO-terminated triblock polymers. *J. Biomed. Mater. Res.* **60**, 126-134.
11. Mann, B.K., and West, J.L. (2002). Cell adhesion peptides alter smooth muscle cell adhesion, proliferation, migration, and matrix protein synthesis on modified surfaces and in polymer scaffolds. *J. Biomed. Mater. Res.* **60**, 86-93.
12. Kubies, D., Rypáček, F., Kovářová, J., and Lednický, F., 2000, Microdomain structure in polylactide-*block*-poly(ethylene oxide) copolymer films. *Biomaterials* **21**, 529-536.
13. Rypáček, F., Machová, L., Kotva, R., and Škarda, V., 2001, Polyesters with functional-peptide blocks: synthesis and application to biomaterials. *Polym. Mater. Sci. Eng.* **84**, 817-818.
14. Van Dijk, J.A.P.P., and Smit J.A.M., 1983, Characterization of Poly(D,L-Lactic Acid) by Gel Permeation Chromatography. *J.Polym.Sci.,Part A: Polym.Chem.* **21**, 197-208.
15. Bačáková, L., Mareš, V., and Lisá, V., 1999, Gender-related differences in adhesion, growth and differentiation of vascular smooth muscle cells are enhanced in serum-deprived cultures. *Cell. Biol. Int.* **23**, 643-648.
16. Bačáková, L., and Kuneš, J., 2000, Gender differences in growth of vascular smooth muscle cells isolated from hypertensive and normotensive rats. *Clin. Exp. Hypertens.* **22**, 33-44.
17. Kubies, D., Machová, L., Brynda, E., and Rypáček, F., 2002, Functionalised surfaces of polylactide modified by Langmuir-Blodgett films of amphiphilic block copolymers. *J. Mater. Sci., Mater. Med.* (in press).

BIODEGRADABLE COPOLYMERS CARRYING CELL-ADHESION PEPTIDE SEQUENCES

Vladimír Proks[1,2], Luďka Machová[1], Štěpán Popelka[1,2], and František Rypáček[1]
[1]*Institute of Macromolecular Chemistry, Academy of Sciences of the Czech Republic, Heyrovsky Sq. 2, 162 06 Prague 6, Czech Republic;* [2]*Centre for Cell Therapy and Tissue Repair, 2nd Faculty of Medicine, Charles University, V Úvalu 84, 150 06 Prague 5, Czech Republic*

ABSTRACT

Amphiphilic block copolymers are used to create bioactive surfaces on biodegradable polymer scaffolds for tissue engineering. Cell-selective biomaterials can be prepared using copolymers containing peptide sequences derived from extracellular-matrix proteins (ECM). Here we discuss alternative ways for preparation of amphiphilic block copolymers composed of hydrophobic polylactide (PLA) and hydrophilic poly(ethylene oxide) (PEO) blocks with cell-adhesion peptide sequences. Copolymers PLA-*b*-PEO were prepared by a living polymerisation of lactide in dioxane with tin(II)2-ethylhexanoate as a catalyst. The following approaches for incorporation of peptides into copolymers were elaborated. (a) First, a side-chain protected Gly-Arg-Gly-Asp-Ser-Gly (GRGDSG) peptide was prepared by solid-phase peptide synthesis (SPPS) and then coupled with Δ-hydroxy-Z-amino-PEO in solution. In the second step, the PLA block was grafted to it via a controlled polymerisation of lactide initiated by the hydroxy end-groups of PEO in the side-chain-protected GRGDSG-PEO. Deprotection of the peptide yielded a GRGDSG-*b*-PEO-*b*-PLA copolymer, with the peptide attached through its C-end. (b) A protected GRGDSG peptide was built up on a polymer resin and coupled with Z-carboxy-PEO using a solid-phase approach. After cleavage of the Δ-hydroxy-PEO-GRGDSG copolymer from the resin, polymerisation of lactide followed by deprotection of the peptide yielded a PLA-*b*-PEO-*b*-GRGDSG block copolymer, in which the peptide is linked through its N-terminus.

1. INTRODUCTION

Polymer biomaterials used as templates for implanted cells, or as supports for tissue regeneration must fulfil rather strict requirements, of which two issues become increasingly important: (a) a controlled biodegradability of the polymer matrix, and (b) polymer-cell and/or polymer -tissue interactions.[1,2] In the past decade, significant progress has been made in understanding the ways in which cells interact with their natural environment of extracellular-matrix proteins.[3] This knowledge has laid foundations for the rational design of polymers that could play an active role in tissue regeneration and repair. New polymers and their supramolecular constructs, tailored to provoke a physiological response such as growth and differentiation of cells in a controlled way, are being sought.[4,5]

Aliphatic polyesters obtained by polymerisation of lactones, such as polylactide (PLA), polyglycolide (PGA), Ƭpolycaprolactone (PCL) are often chosen as three-dimensional porous scaffolds in tissue engineering. Through copolymerisation of lactones themselves, polymers with a wide range of structural variations and mechanical properties can be prepared, from loosely associated hydrophilic gels to semicrystalline high-strength materials. On the other hand, the polyesters offer only limited possibilities of chemical modification and formation of functional groups that could be used for binding of bioactive ligands and/or molecular recognition moieties.

Our approach to the design of bioactive surfaces on biodegradable polyester scaffolds is based on the use of block copolymers that could be applied to the polyester surface. Therefore, such block copolymers should contain polyester blocks, which provide for good anchoring copolymer molecules at the surface to the polyester bulk, and one or more hydrophilic blocks, containing functional groups. Through the microphase separation of blocks of copolymers at the polymer/air or the polymer/water interface, the material interface becomes enriched in the functional groups. Polymers with hydrophobic/hydrophilic surface domains[6] or polymer brushes with specific patterns of biospecific groups can be prepared [7].

Suitable amphiphilic block copolymers can be obtained from polylactone and poly(Δ-amino acid)s[8] and/or functionalised (PEO) blocks. In the present work we focus on PLA/PEO block copolymers with functional peptide sequences, derived from the structure of ECM proteins attached to the end of PEO block.

There are two strategies for preparation of PEO-conjugated peptides and further block copolymers of functional PEO-peptide derivatives with polylactide. One is based on the reaction of activated Z-carboxy group of modified PEO using the solid phase peptide synthesis strategy[9]. The advantages of this strategy are high purity of the product, and easy separation of low-molecular-weight compounds On the contrary, disadvantages of this method are a molecular-weight limit for the PEO block that can be efficiently coupled to the resin and the necessity of having a sterically unhindered the N-terminal amino acid of the peptide.[10] This strategy is schematically shown in Figure 1.

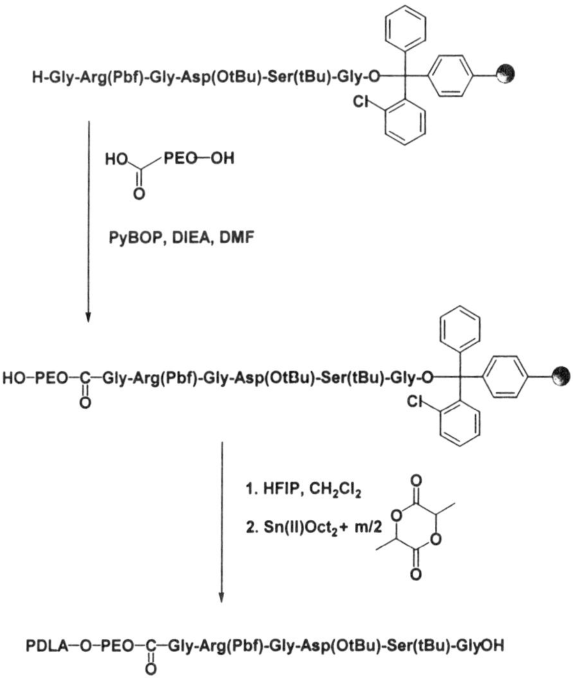

Figure 1. Solid-phase "PEGylation" of GRGDSG peptide and subsequent copolymerisation with lactide in solution.

The second strategy comprises the use of Z-amino substituted PEO to which an activated protected peptide is coupled in solution. The advantage of this strategy is the solution reaction, a short reaction time, and the fact that there's no limitation for the PEO block molecular weight. With excess of the activated peptide we can obtain PEGylated peptide in a good yield. (Fig.2)

Both types of PEO-peptide derivatives can be used as macroinitiators for controlled copolymerisation with lactide, starting on the hydroxy-terminal end of polyethylene oxide.

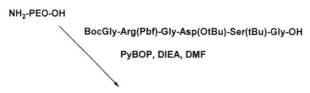

Figure 2. Binding of a peptide to NH$_2$-terminated PEO in solution followed by grafting polymerisation of the PLA block.

2. EXPERIMENTAL SECTION

2.1 Materials

Barlos resin, Fmoc-L-amino acids, Boc- glycine, BOP, PyBOP, 1,1,1,3,3,3-hexafluoropropan-2-ol (HFIP), trifluoroacetic acid and ethyldiisopropylamine (DIEA) were purchased from Aldrich or Fluka, Czech Republic and were used without further purification. DMF, CH$_2$Cl$_2$ and MeOH were obtained from Lachema, Neratovice, Czech Republic. Z-amino poly(ethylene oxide) (Z-NH$_2$-PEO) was obtained from Shearwater Corp., Huntsville, USA. DL-Lactide was synthesized in our laboratory and purified by crystallization from dry toluene prior to polymerization. Sn(II) 2-ethylhexanoate was purchased from Aldrich and purified by vacuum distillation.

The amino acid contents in peptides and copolymer samples were determined by amino acids analysis using the OPA (phthalaldehyde) method. OPA derivatives were separated on a reverse-phase C-18 column in a buffered methanol-gradient HPLC system and determined by UV absorption at 340 nm.

Size-exclusion chromatography (SEC) was carried out on a Waters HPLC-SEC modular system using Plgel 5m Mixed-D column in 0.1 M LiCl solution in DMF.

^{1}H NMR spectra were recorded on a Bruker ACF-300 in CDCl$_3$, DMSO-d_6 or perdeuterated 1,1,1,3,3,3-hexafluoropropan-2-ol with HMDS as internal standard.

2.2 Methods

GRGDSG protected peptides were prepared manually in a stepwise solid-phase peptide synthesis on chlorotrityl (Barlos) resin. One cycle of the synthesis consisted of following operations (10 ml of solvent per gram of the resin). (1) dimethylformamide (DMF) 3 x 2 min, (2) 25% piperidine in DMF 1 x 5 min, (3) DMF 1 x 2 min, (4) 25% piperidine in DMF 1 x 15 min, (5) DMF 4 x 2 min, (6) 1.5 equiv. of Fmoc-AA in DMF, (7) 1.5 equiv. of [(benzotriazol-1-yl)oxy]tripyrrolidinophosponiumhexafluorophospate (PyBOP) with 4 equiv. diisopropylethylamine (DIEA) (45 min).

The coupling efficiency was monitored by visual test with Bromophenol Blue.[11] Incomplete coupling reaction was repeated from steps 5 to 7.

Finally, before cleavage, the resin was washed with 3 x DMF (1 min), 3 x DCM (1 min) and 3 x MeOH (1 min). The cleavage of the protected peptide and the protected peptide-PEO conjugate was performed with 25% hexafluoropropan-2-ol in DCM for 15 min. Deprotection of the peptide was carried out in the 95% TFA.

Δ-(2-Carboxyethyl)-Z-hydroxy-poly(ethylene oxide), (PEO-COOH). In the first step, Δ-(3-oxopropyl)-Z-hydroxy-poly(ethylene oxide) was prepared according to a procedure[12] with a modification as follows: A solution of 3,3-diethoxypropan-1-ol (2 mmole) dissolved in THF was added into polymerisation ampoule under inert conditions together with an equimolar amount of (diphenylmethyl)potassium solution in THF to form potassium 3,3-diethoxypropan-1-olate. After stirring for 10 min and cooling (-78 (C) liquid ethylene oxide (9.6 g) was added from a pressure bottle. The ampoule was cooled in liquid nitrogen and sealed under vacuum. The mixture was allowed to react for 2 days at room temperature. The obtained polymer was precipitated into diethyl ether and collected by filtration. To deprotect the acetal end groups, the polymer was dissolved in water, the solution was acidified to pH 2 with hydrochloric acid and stirred at room temperature for 5 h. The solution of Δ-(3-oxopropyl)-Z-hydroxypoly(ethylene oxide) was finally dialyzed against water. In the second step the aldehyde end groups of the polymer were selectively oxidized. 1.0 g (4.3 mmol) of freshly prepared Ag$_2$O was dispersed in the dialyzed polymer solution and stirred vigorously at 40 (C for 3 h. Silver oxide was separated by filtration through an 0.2) m nylon membrane filter. The dissolved silver was precipitated with 3 ml of saturated sodium chloride. The precipitate was filtered off, the filtrate was slightly acidified and dialyzed. The product was obtained as a white solid after freeze-drying.

Synthesis of the peptide-containing polymers:

Boc-Gly-Arg(Pbf)-Gly-Asp(OtBu)-Ser(tBu)-Gly-NH-PEO

To a solution of Z-NH_2-PEO_{3400} (0.5 g, 0.147 mmol NH_2, 1 equiv.) in 5 ml of DMF, Boc-Gly-Arg(Pbf)-Gly-Asp(OtBu)-Ser(tBu)-Gly-OH (0.1528 g, 0.1625mmol, 1.5 equiv.),BOP (0.0718 g, 0.1625mmol, 1.5 equiv.) and 5 ml DMF were added. The reaction mixture was stirred overnight, then precipitated in to 800 ml of diethyl ether, filtered and the polymer was washed twice with 20 ml of cold ether. Yield: 560 mg (92.5 %)

Boc-Gly-Arg(Pbf)-Gly-Asp(OtBu)-Ser(tBu)-Gly-CONH-PEO-PDLLA

The block copolymer was synthesized by ring-opening polymerization of DL-lactide in toluene in the presence of Boc- Gly-Arg(Pbf)-Gly-Asp(OtBu)-Ser(tBu)-Gly-NH-PEO (dried in vacuum, 2h, 40 °C) as a macroinitiator using tin(II) 2-ethylhexanoate as a catalyst. The polymerization was carried out at 80 θC (18 h) and the reaction components and solvent were dosed in the polymerization reactor under high vacuum/inert gas conditions.

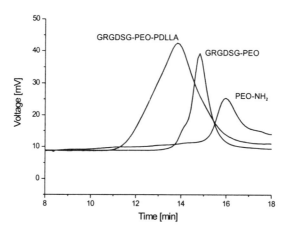

Figure 3. Size-exclusion chromatography of the intermediates and product of the stepwise synthesis of GRGDSG-PEO-PDLLA.

H-Gly-Arg-Gly-Asp-Ser-Gly-NH-PEO-PDLLA

Boc-Gly-Arg(Pbf)-Gly-Asp(OtBu)-Ser(tBu)-Gly-NH-PEO-PDLLA (400 mg) was dissolved in 5 ml of CH_2Cl_2 and added to 20 ml of 95% TFA in CH_2Cl_2. The solution was kept for 3 h at 0 °C. Subsequently, TFA was neutralized with triethylamine and a sample was dialyzed against water to wash out triethylamine trifluoroacetate. The product was concentrated and lyophilised.

Successful deprotection of the peptide part was confirmed by ^{1}H-NMR spectroscopy, based on vanishing of signals of methyl groups at 1.44 ppm (2,2-methyl groups in the *N*-(2,2,4,6,7-pentamethyl-2,3-dihydro-1-benzofuran-5-sulfonyl) protecting group of arginine) and *tert*-butyl protecting group of aspartic acid at 1.42 ppm (see Fig. 4).

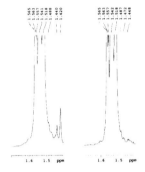

Figure 4. Fragments of the NMR spectra of the peptide containing copolymer: a) protected b) after deprotection.

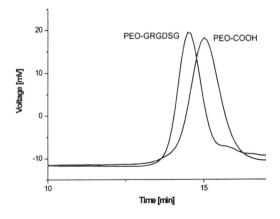

Figure 5. Synthesis of PEO-GRGDSG: size-exclusion chromatograms of starting PEO-COOH and the resulting PEO-peptide conjugate.

HO-PEO-CO-Gly-Arg(Pbf)-Gly-Asp(OtBu)-Ser(tBu)-Gly-OH

H-Gly-Arg(Pbf)-Gly-Asp(OtBu)-Ser(tBu)-Gly-Cl-trityl-resin
(1 g, substitution 0.097 m mol/g) was washed with DMF and coupled with PyBOP-activated (1/3 eq. 0.0209 g) PEO$_{3600}$-COOH (1/3 equiv. 0.1452 g) with 0.027 ml DIEA (4 equiv.) for 5 h, then washed with 3 x DMF, 10 x DCM and 5 x MeOH. The degree of substitution was determined by an increase in resin weight and the coupling step was repeated until a weight increase was observed. Before cleavage with 25% HFIP in DCM, the resin was washed 3 x DMF, 10 x CH$_2$Cl$_2$ and 3 x MeOH. The conjugate was subsequently used for copolymerisation with lactide.

3. RESULTS AND DISCUSSION

Originally, our strategy for the preparation of the PEO-PDLLA copolymers containing a peptide sequence at the end of the PEO block was to synthesize PDLLA-PEO-COOH copolymer with a peptide bound to a Wang resin. In the cleavage step it would be possible to cleave the aduct from the resin and the deprotect its side-chains in the peptide at once. After a simple separation of the unreacted peptide from the copolymer, we could isolate a pure peptide-containing copolymer. This strategy was abandoned due to high steric requirement of the reaction on the solid phase with a PLA/PEO block copolymer used as a reactant.

On the other hand, if we made only the " the peptide PEGylation" step on the solid phase, we were able to obtain the side-chain-protected PEO–peptide intermediate in a good yield, using PEO with a high relatively molecular weight. By subsequent polymerisation of lactide on the terminal hydroxy groups of PEO-peptide, copolymers with the same PLA/PEO ratio but with three-times higher total molecular weight were obtained, in contrast to the original strategy. For surface modification purposes the molecular weight of the polylactide block should be higher compared with the PEO block.

The other strategy prefers the use of Z-amino-substituted PEO and the peptide activated at C-end to ensure effective coupling of the chain-a protected activated peptide in solution and subsequent good purification of polymer-peptide intermediate, which is necessary for obtaining a well-defined block copolymer in final copolymerisation with lactide. The advantage of the reaction in solution is low steric hindrance, which affords shorter reaction times, and, importantly, no molecular weight limitations for the PEO block, at least within a molecular-weight range of up to 20 000. Moreover, using these two strategies, we can obtain two different types of the otherwise identical copolymers. First, in which the peptide is bound through its N-end, and the other, with the peptide bound through the C-end. Using the strategies, which provide copolymers with peptide ligands bonded in a well-defined way, we can evaluate not only the effect on polymer-cell interactions of peptides with different composition (derived from different ECM proteins), but we also can study the role of particular folding and conformation of the surface-exposed peptide sequence. Comprehensive studies of the cell adhesion efficiency and its specificity to different cell types using polymer surfaces modified by patterned brushes of functional block copolymers are under way.

ACKNOWLEDGEMENTS

Support of the Grant Agency of the Academy of the Science of the Czech republic (grant No. A4050202) and Ministry of Education of CR (grant No. LN00A065) is acknowledged.

REFERENCES

1. Ratner, B.D., 1993, New ideas in biomaterials science - a path to engineered biomaterials, *J. Biomed. Mater. Res.* **27**, 837-850
2. Vacanti, J.P., and Langer, R., 1999, Tissue engineering: The design and fabrication of living replacement devices for surgical reconstruction and transplantation, *Lancet* **354**, SI32-SI34.
3. Adams, J.C., 2001, Cell-matrix contact structures, *Cell. Mol. Life Sci.* **58**, 371-392.
4. Langer, R., Cima, L.G., Tamada, J.A., and Wintermantel, E., 1990, Future directions in biomaterials, *Biomaterials* **11**, 738-745.
5. Hubbell, J.A., 1999, Bioactive biomaterials, *Curr. Opin. Biotechnol.* **10**, 123-129.
6. Kubies, D., Rypacek, F., Kovářová, J., and Lednický, F., 2000, *Biomaterials* **21**, 529.
7. Kubies, D., Machová, L., Brynda, E., and Rypacek, F., Functionalised surfaces of polylactide modified by Langmuir-Blodgett films of amphiphilic block copolymers, *J. Mater. Sci., Mater. Med.* (in press).
8. Rypacek, F., Machová, L., Kotva, R., and Škarda, V., 2001, *Polym. Mater. Sci. Eng.* **84**, 817.
9. Houseman, B.T., and Mrksich, M., 1998, *J. Org. Chem.* **64**, 7552.
10. Lu, Y.A., and Felix, A.M., 1994, *React. Polym.* **22**, 221.
11. Krchnak V. *et al.*, 1988, *Int. J. Pept. Prot. Res.* **32**, 415.
12. Nagasaki, Y., Kutsuna, T., Iijima, M., Kato, M., Kataoka, K., Kitano, S., and Kadoma, Y., 1995, *Bioconjugate Chem.* **6**, 231-33.

POLYMER BASED SCAFFOLDS AND CARRIERS FOR BIOACTIVE AGENTS FROM DIFFERENT NATURAL ORIGIN MATERIALS

Patrícia B. Malafaya[1,2], Manuela E. Gomes[1,2], António J. Salgado[1,2], and Rui L. Reis[1,2]
[1]*Department of Polymer Engineering, University of Minho, Campus de Azurém, 4800-058 Guimarães – Portugal;* [2]*3B's Research Group – Biomaterials, Biodegradables and Biomimetics, University of Minho, Campus de Gualtar, 4710-057 Braga, Portugal*

1. INTRODUCTION

The aim of the present chapter is to describe the work developed and ongoing in the 3B's Research Group of the University of Minho regarding tissue engineering applications and our approaches to reach this aim.

It is important to start this chapter by stating that there are multiple clinical reasons to develop bone tissue-engineering alternatives in order to improve quality of life, including the need of better filler materials that can be used in the reconstruction of large orthopaedic defects and the need for orthopaedic implants that are more suitable to their biological environment[1]. As it is now well accepted, a tissue engineered implant is a biological/biomaterials combination in which some component of tissue has been combined with biomaterials to create a device for the restoration or modification of tissue or organ function[2].

In fact, one ideal strategy to help combat serious problems (like transplantation due to the short number of donors tissues and organs) is to enable the self-healing potential of the patient to regenerate body tissue and organs (for instances, bone remodelling). Indeed, tissue engineering can be considered as a new therapeutic trial designed to implement this strategy. The development of this specific approach of tissue engineering is based on several observations: (i) as it was stated before, most of the tissues undergo constant remodelling due to apoptosis and renewal of constituent cells; (ii) isolated cells tend towards forming tissue structures *in vitro* if the conditions are favourable; and (iii) although isolated cells have the capacity to remodel and form the proper tissue structures, they require a template to guide their organization into the proper architecture.[3] At this point, we have defined the main factors necessary to achieve this tissue engineering approach: (i) cells, (ii) growth factors and (iii) their scaffolds. The controlled release concepts can be inherent and be a potential assistant in the three main factors. The 'traditional' drug delivery approach can be applied to encapsulate living cells for incorporation within the scaffolds. In turn, scaffolds can be designed as 'traditional' drug delivery carriers to control a site-and time-specific release profile and also to protect the growth factor.

So, the main factors to achieve this strategy are clear and will be discussed in the further sections in more detail focusing mainly our research work with natural origin materials beginning with scaffolding as the starting point of this approach.

2. SCAFFOLD DESIGN AND FABRICATION

As stated before, the ultimate goal of tissue engineering is to replace, repair or enhance the biological function of damaged, absent or dysfunctional elements of a tissue or an organ. This goal is accomplished using cells that are manipulated through their extracellular environment to develop engineered tissues that can function as living biological substitutes for tissues that are lacking[4]. Many different strategies may be used to develop these engineered tissues. The selection of the best strategy for developing engineered tissues and apply them to the regeneration of a specific tissue defect is determined by several factors, such as the technical feasibility, required properties of the implant, and the interaction of the host with the graft[4].

The selection of the appropriate approach implies the simultaneous selection of an adequate biomaterial design format, which must be able to induce the desired tissue response[4,5]. For example, design formats requiring cell activity on one surface of a device while precluding transverse movement of surrounding cells onto that surface, call for a barrier material, i.e., a membrane[5]. Gels are used to encapsulate and to a more limited extent isolate, cells from surrounding tissues, especially to preclude antibody response to homograft and xenograft cells. Microspheres might also be used to encapsulate cells, growth factors or drugs and deliver them to a specific desired location.

Three-dimensional structures have been recognized since the mid-1970s as important components for the development of engineered tissues[5]. The development of matrices to serve as templates for cell attachment/suspension and delivery has progressed at a tremendous rate in the past years[6].

The materials to be used as scaffolds in tissue engineering must fulfill a number of complex requirements, such as, biocompatibility, appropriate porous structure, mechanical properties and suitable surface chemistry, for example. The selection of the most appropriate polymer to produce the scaffold is a very important step towards the construction of the tissue engineered product since its intrinsic properties will determine in a great extent the properties of the scaffold. However, the selected design and method of producing these scaffolds will deeply influence its final characteristics, as it can dramatically change the type and amount of porosity, the mechanical properties and degradation behaviour, the surface properties (critical for cell adhesion and proliferation) and even the biocompatibility of the scaffold material.

Therefore various processing techniques have and are being developed to fabricate these scaffolds, such as solvent casting[7-10], particulate leaching[7-11], membrane lamination[9,12], fiber bonding[8,9,13], phase separation/inversion[9,14], high pressure based methods[9,15], melt based technologies[8,16,17], and microwave baking and expansion[18].

More recently highly porous 3-D scaffolds have been obtained using advanced textile technologies and rapid prototyping technologies such as fused deposition modelling (FDM) and 3-D printing[19]. These engineering technologies are highly controllable and reproducible and facilitate the manufacture of well-defined 3-D structures[20].

As the demand for new and more sophisticated scaffolds develops, materials are being designed that have a more active role in guiding tissue development. Instead of merely holding cells in place, these matrices are designed to accomplish other functions through the combination of different format features and materials[6].

In this section, it will be described the ongoing work at the 3B's Research Group of the University of Minho concerning the development of templates of different design formats using starch and other natural based polymers to be used in the construction of scaffolds for tissue engineering. This research has been focused in the production of systems based on biocompatible natural origin polymers, which may combine the release of bioactive agents (as discussed in section 3) with appropriate features to allow cell adhesion, proliferation and differentiation as well as tissue matching mechanical properties, aiming at providing a more complete solution towards tissue regeneration. Several materials have been used, namely blends of starch with: ethylene vinyl alcohol (SEVA-C), cellulose acetate (SCA), polycaprolactone (SPCL), polylactic acid (SPLA) as well as protein based materials, chitin and chitosan.

2.1 Fiber Bonding

Fiber meshes consist of individual fiber either woven or knitted into three-dimensional patterns of variable pore size. Fiber meshes can be prepared by several different fiber bonding methods including the use of textile processing techniques[19,21,22]. The advantageous characteristic features of fiber meshes are a large surface area for cell attachment and a rapid diffusion of nutrients in favour of cell survival and growth[8,9,11,23,24]. Obviously, this technique is not the most appropriate for to the fine control of porosity[8,9,23,24]. In addition, this method does not address the problem of creating scaffolds with complex three-dimensional shapes, but it has proven successful for producing hollow tubes that have been proposed for use in intestine regeneration[8,9,23]. Several scaffolds obtained by these methods and from several polymers, have been widely used in tissue engineering research[21,25-31].

For example, a scaffold based on SPCL (a blend of starch with polycaprolactone, 30/70% wt) was obtained by a fiber bonding process[32], in this case consisting in the spinning, cutting and sintering of the fibers. The SPCL scaffolds obtained by this method have a typical fiber-mesh structure, with a fiber diameter around 181μm, with highly interconnected pores and a porosity of about 75% (Figure 1).

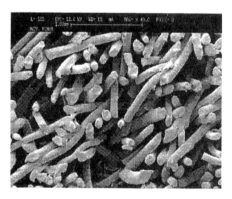

Figure 1. SPCL based scaffold obtained by a fiber bonding process.

Another example is a chitosan-based fiber mesh structure obtained by a wet spinning technique. It was found that interconnected and porous structures of fibrous matrix could allow cell attachment and ingrowth[28]. The typical morphology obtained in these scaffolds is shown in Figure 2. The pore size is in the 100-500 μm range with a fiber mean diameter of 110 μm.

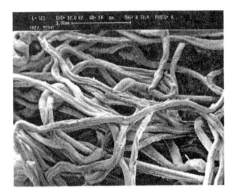

Figure 2. Chitosan based scaffold obtained by a wet spinning technique.

2.2 Solvent-Casting and Particle Leaching

The solvent casting and particle leaching method consists in dispersing sieved mineral (e.g. NaCl) or organic (e.g. saccharose) particles in a polymer solution. This dispersion is then processed either by casting or by freeze-drying in order to produce porous bi- and three-dimensional supports, respectively. The porosity results basically from the selective dissolution of the particles from the polymer/salt (or other porogen agent) mixture, although phase separation of the polymer solution can also contribute to form the porous structure[24]. Therefore the porosity and pore size can be controlled independently by varying the amount and size of the salt particles, respectively. The surface area depends on both initial salt weight fraction and particle size[8,9,23,24]. The disadvantages of this method, as it has been applied so far, include the extensive use of highly toxic solvents and the limitation to produce thin wafers or membranes up to 3mm thick[7-9,19,23,24], as well as the typically rather low mechanical properties of the scaffolds[33].

In our group, we have obtained scaffolds from starch based polymers using the solvent casting and particle leaching methods[34,35], which allowed for the production of an open-porous structure with a good interconnectivity between the pores throughout the entire structure, as shown in Figure 3. It was possible to obtain samples in the shape of discs with up to 1 cm of thickness.

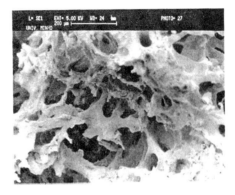

Figure 3. SCA based scaffold obtained by solvent casting-particle leaching method using 65% of salt.

As it should be expected, and was stated before, the mechanical properties of the scaffolds obtained by the solvent casting and particle leaching method are lower when compared to the properties of the samples obtained by melt-based technologies. However, the properties achieved for starch-based polymers using this method may be considered very good when compared to scaffolds obtained from other materials by identical processing methods (proposed for the same type of applications). For example, a PLGA scaffold obtained by the solvent casting and particle leaching method, exhibits a modulus of 1.09 MPa [33].

2.3 Membrane Lamination

The membrane lamination method uses membranes previously prepared by solvent casting and particle leaching. The membranes, with an appropriate shape, are solvent impregnated, then stacked up in a three-dimensional assembly with continuous pore structure and morphology[5]. The bulk properties of the final 3D scaffolds are identical to those of the individual membranes[7,8,23,24].

This method may allow for the construction of 3-D polymer foams with precise anatomical shapes, since it is possible to use computer-assisted modelling to design templates with the desired implant shape[24]. However this fabrication technique is time consuming, because only thin membranes can be used. Another disadvantage is that the layering of porous sheets allows only for a limited number of interconnected pores[19].

There are several ongoing works in our group targeting membrane lamination with chitosan based membranes, chitosan-soybean and chitosan-starch based membranes. For example, TCP/HA particulate composite material was produced using chitosan membranes and fibres as a reinforcing organic material. A compact structure of ceramic material was constructed on a chitosan membrane produced by a solvent casting. This membrane was placed in a specially developed mould, and further supported with chitosan fibres (placed over ceramic-membrane complex). These compact ceramic structures can be fused together to produce a 3-D architecture that might be very useful for guided tissue regeneration/engineering applications.

2.4 Melt Moulding

To our knowledge, melt moulding has not been used by other groups as a single technique to produce scaffolds for tissue engineering. It is normally used in combination with porogen techniques or to produce a pre-shape of the final material, for example in high-pressure based methods.

In the U. Minho group, we have developed a method based on compression moulding combined with salt leaching[34,35]. In this method, a starch based polymer is blended with leachable particles of different sizes, in sufficient amounts to provide a continuous phase of a polymer and a dispersed phase of leachable particles in the blend. The mixture is then compression moulded into discs of 6 cm of diameter and approximately 1cm of height, using a mould specially designed for this purpose. This method allowed to obtain scaffolds with controlled porosity and pore sizes and with good interconnectivity (Figure 4).

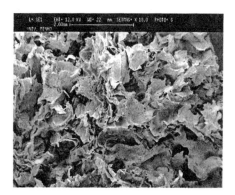

Figure 4. SCA based scaffold obtained by compression moulding-particle leaching method using 65% of salt.

We have also developed melt based technologies to produce scaffolds by means of a single one-step method[16,34,35], such as injection moulding and extrusion with blowing agents (BA). In this process, the polymers are previously mixed with blowing agents, which are previously selected according to their decomposition temperatures, toxicity, etc, prior to processing in an extruder or in an injection moulding machine. For the injection moulding of the scaffolds, a special mould was designed and manufactured, which allows for the injection moulding of the polymeric melt at a much lower pressure. It also allows for an excellent venting of the mould cavity and therefore enables to enhance significantly the expansion inside the mould when compared to a normal mould.

The porous structure of the samples obtained by extrusion or injection moulding of the polymers combined with blowing agents results from the gases released by decomposition of the BA during processing. Therefore, with these melt based methods it is difficult to have full control over the pore size and the interconnectivity between the pores of the materials obtained by these methods. Nevertheless, the subsequent optimisation of processing parameters and of the type and amount of blowing agent, allowed to obtain scaffolds with subsequent higher porosity, interconnectivity between pores and pore sizes that can vary from roughly between 50 up to 1000 µm.

The scaffolds obtained by these melt based methods present a microporosity throughout the whole structure which can play an important role in nutrients flow during the cell culturing and/or the implantation of the scaffolds. A thin layer of solid material surrounds the porous structure of the material obtained with both processes, but this can be removed easily as a final step in the processing of the scaffolds. The structures that are typically obtained are show in Figure 5.

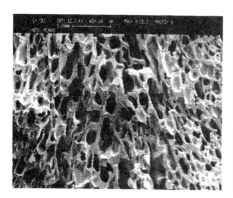 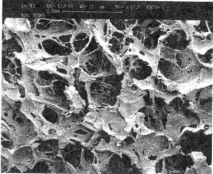

Figure 5. SCA based scaffold obtained by melt based technologies: a) injection moulding with 1% of blowing agent b) extrusion with 2% of blowing agent.

The mechanical properties of the scaffolds obtained by extrusion with blowing agents are very dependent on the type and amount of blowing agent used, exhibiting a compressive modulus that can vary from about 124 up to 230 MPa. Nevertheless, these scaffolds present very promising mechanical properties when compared to other scaffolds, obtained from other biodegradable polymers, and proposed for use in tissue engineering of bone. For example, PLLA/hydroxylapatite composite foams, prepared by a process based on phase separation, presented a compression modulus below 12 MPa [36].

2.5 Freeze-Drying

Phase separation of a polymeric solution may be induced by several ways[14,24]. The basic principle of a freeze-drying process relies on a thermally induced phase separation, which occurs when the temperature of a homogenous polymer solution, previously poured into a mould, is decreased. Once the phase-separated system is stabilized, the solvent-rich phase is removed by vacuum sublimation leaving behind the polymeric foam. The foam morphology is of course controlled by any phase transition that occurs during the cooling step, i.e., liquid-liquid or solid-liquid demixing[14,24]. Current research shows that this method is very sensitive, i.e., the parameters have to be very well controlled[19].

In our group, work has been done on the development of chitosan based porous structures produced by freeze-drying. The properties, such as porosity, of the obtained scaffolds are controlled by the treatments submitted to the scaffolds. These include crosslinking, neutralization with alkali solutions and control of the pH of the initial polymeric solution. It is possible to control the porosity in the 20-1000 µm range and a typical morphology shown in Figure 6. Freeze-drying was also successful on the production of scaffolds from soybean and sodium caseinate protein based matrices.

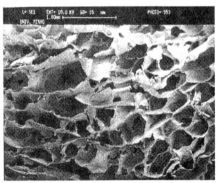

Figure 6. Chitosan based scaffold obtained by freeze-drying methodologies.

2.6 Aggregation of Polymeric Microparticles

Another alternative to produce scaffolds is to use methods based on aggregation of micro/nano particles. The so-called aggregation of polymer microparticles method consists in the aggregation, by physical or chemical means, of microparticles[24]. The porosity is nothing but the interstices between the aggregated microparticles and it is directly related to the microparticles diameter. The possible release of previous encapsulated growth factors from the microparticles is an additional advantage of this technique and for these reason it will be discussed afterwards in this chapter.

2.7 In-Situ Polymerization

All the polymer processing techniques discussed so far are methods that can only be used to manufacture pre-fabricated scaffolds, which may then be used to regenerate the appropriate tissue. However, it is also possible to use polymeric hydrogels that could ideally have the advantage of being injectable. This will allow for the delivery of the construct to be less invasive, thereby reducing surgical risks, reducing pain, and increasing patient comfort. Employment of these types of polymers also ensures delivery of an even distribution of a precise number of cells, as it will be further discussed. They can be configured to provide mechanical support to the cells to maintain their specific phenotype, without inhibiting migration[6].

These materials can be crosslinked at the time of surgery to form solid degradable scaffolds and at the time of the crosslinking reaction it is also possible to incorporate NaCl that provides pores into which new tissue can grow. In this manner, a temporary scaffold may be formed in-situ to replace the mechanical function of the mal-functioning tissue until new tissue, stimulated to form in the scaffold pores, can assume its structural role. During its liquid phase, the hydrogel can be injected or moulded into the defect. It is therefore well suited for this application, since many injuries result in defects, which are relatively inaccessible[8,37]. In addition, the use of this type of materials may represent an important step on the way to eliminate the need for the defect or injured tissue to be exposed to a conventional surgical operation, and instead may lead to a minimally invasive surgery[37]. However, most addition polymerization reactions are exothermic and generate large quantities of heat, which is sufficient to cause some local tissue necrosis.

Starch based (and partially degradable) injectable scaffolds were produced by an in-situ polymerization method that was based on a polymerization process developed in our group in order to obtain materials to be used as bone cements or hydrogels[38,39]. These materials were prepared by adding the liquid phase, constituted by the acrylic monomers (AA, from Merck), and 1% (w/w) of N-dimethylaminobenzyl alcohol (DMOH), which was used as the activator of the initiation process, to the solid phase, which consisted of SEVA-C powder and 2% (wt/wt) of benzoic peroxide (BPO, from Merck), which was used as the radical initiator, after purification by fractional recrystallization from ethanol, mp 104°C BPO. The leachable NaCl particles were added to the liquid or to the solid phase in order o provide the porosity of the structure.

SEM analysis of this scaffolds showed pores ranging in size roughly from 10 to 100 µm in diameter (Figure 7), but once again, the pore size depends on the salt particles used.

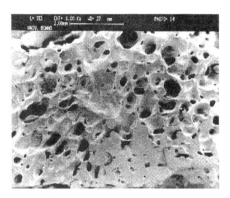

Figure 7. SCA based scaffold obtained by a method based on in-situ polymerization.

The scaffolds obtained by the in-situ polymerization method present the highest water uptake ability, since they have water uptake properties that are typical of hydrogels. Their degradation rates are obviously lower than those presented for the above referred to scaffolds, since this type of scaffolds are composed of a blend of the starch based polymer with acrylic acid. The materials produced by this method are, in fact, not totally degradable, but they might be very useful in situations where it is necessary to ensure a high mechanical strength and/or in situations where the defect or trauma that is necessary to treat is of difficult access, as the use of such type of scaffolds will avoid highly invasive surgery techniques.

2.8 Microwave Based Technique

Another innovative methodology for producing porous biodegradable starch based 3D architectures based on microwave processing was developed in our group[18]. The porous structures produced by microwave technique present an interesting combination of morphological and mechanical properties (matching the compressive behaviour of human cancellous bone), that may find uses in cancellous bone replacement (filling of bone defects) and drug delivery applications, as well as in tissue engineering scaffolds.

Figure 8 shows the typical microstructure of the starch based degradable 3D-architectures produced. Again, it was possible to produce materials with interconnecting pores, and an interesting combination of macroporosity (between 200-900 μm) and microporosity (20-100 μm). The typical density of the biodegradable porous structures was, in this case, in the 0.40-0.50 g/cm^3 range. The measured mechanical properties are in some way remarkable. The best results were a compression modulus of 530 MPa and a maximum compressive strength of 60 MPa. These values, obtained for blowing agent (containing corn starch, sodium pyrophosphate and sodium bicarbonate) amounts of 10%, in the presence of hydrogen peroxide, are very similar to those of the cancellous bone. The better results are obtained in the presence of H_2O_2, due to a partial oxidation of starch molecule. Finally it is very important to stress out that the materials are degradable, and their loss of weight is about 40%, after 30 days of immersion on an isotonic saline solution. The developed morphologies seem to be adequate to be used as tissue engineering scaffolds, or as drug delivery carriers. In this later case the materials water-uptake capability is a very important issue since it is controllable by the porosity as it is discussed further later on this chapter. Work is also ongoing in our group for the development of composites porous structures, using hydroxylapatite as filler, by means of using a similar microwave technique. It is expected that one can improve the mechanical properties and *in-vitro* bioactive behaviour of these porous structures.

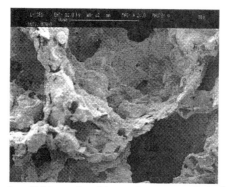

Figure 8. Starch based scaffolds produced by a microwave technique.

3. DELIVERY STRATEGIES FOR TISSUE ENGINEERING

Even if a scaffold possesses optimized characteristics as mentioned in the previous section, it may be not capable of regenerating large critical sized defects in the host tissue. Thus, the ability of a biodegradable scaffold to incorporate and release growth factors in a controlled manner has become a mostly desirable goal together with the capability of encapsulation of living cells, in order to protect and deliver them to a specific desired location.

Probably the simplest method is to supply growth factors directly to the site of regeneration for cell differentiation and proliferation. However, in general, direct injection of growth factors in solution into the regeneration site is rather ineffective, as the injected growth factor is rapidly diffused out from the site, and exerts no effect on bone induction or even in wound healing[40-44]. Therefore, it demands for either extremely higher doses and/or frequent injections. For being clinically used in an efficient manner, these growth factors require a delivery system to guide tissue regeneration and prevent the rapid dispersal of the factors from the site[44,45].

Another important issue is the short biological half-life of growth factors, usually in the order of minutes[46]. Growth factors have poor *in vivo* stability and consequently the biological effects are often unpredictable unless they are administrated via a controlled delivery system[40].

In addition, many therapeutic proteins are large, and penetrate into tissue slowly. As a result of their incorporation into polymeric devices, the protein structure and, thus, biological activity can be stabilized, prolonging the length of time over which activity is release at the delivery site[47]. Frequently, proteins are incorporated into polymers together with other molecules, excipients or co-dispersants, which enhance protein stability in the matrix[46,47]. Often, stabilization is the result of complexation of a charge molecule with the growth factors; the protein is protected from degradation while being complexed[46].

In the protein therapy approach, the growth factor is delivered to the site via an implantable or injectable carrier matrix[48]. There are two main approaches that should be discussed. First, the administration of growth factor alone encapsulated or entrapped, for instances, in micro or nanoparticles and then simply injected at site of regeneration. A second, and a more interesting approach, is to try to incorporate the growth factor in the scaffold and this could be achieved by several different means in a number of scaffolds. The protein could by directly loaded or immobilized on the developed scaffold or by means of combining both approaches, an encapsulated growth factor could be then coupled to the scaffold providing extra means to control both delivery and protein stability. These approaches will be addressed, trying to point out our own research work in this area.

3.1 Micro and Nanoparticles Delivery Systems

To convey a sufficient dose of drug to a particular lesion, suitable carriers of drugs are required. Of the different dosage forms reported, nano and microparticles attained much importance, due to a tendency to accumulate in areas of inflammation within the body[48-51]. In fact, nano and microparticles systems occupy unique position in the drug delivery technology due to their attractive properties. The research in this area is being carried out all over the world at a great pace. Research areas cover novel properties that have been developed increased efficiency of drug delivery, improved release profiles and drug targeting. For this reasons, there are a derivation of methods of controlled release and a range of polymers that are been used for this proposed.

In this section some of the techniques and a range of natural polymers will be better described, focusing in the ongoing work at the 3B's research group of the University of Minho on the field of developing particles (nano and micro) to be used as carriers for different bioactive agents. It is important to stress out that the systems described below can be used to construct scaffolds by means of aggregation of the polymeric particles as discussed in the previous section. An alternative strategy already mentioned can be the coupling of the polymeric particles to the scaffold by means of for instances surface activation.

3.1.1 Starch Microparticles Produced by Emulsion Crosslinking Technique

Starch microparticles were prepared using an emulsion crosslinking technique. Paselli (II) that is a modified starch was used in this study. The native starch is partially hydrolyzed being modified into several modified starches, such as Paselli (II), which is a water-soluble starch. A preliminary study was performed to evaluate the incorporation of a model drug (nonsteroidal anti-inflammatory drug - NSAID) and investigate its release profile as a function of changes in the medium parameters. It was found that the developed microparticles and the respective processing route seem to be appropriate for further studies. In fact, there is some potential for the loading of different growth factors for improving bone regeneration in tissue engineering, especially because the crosslinking reaction of the microparticles takes place at room temperature. The basic idea is to accomplish the delivery in bone tissue engineering applications, as the starch microparticles can be simply injected at site of regeneration or coupled into a porous scaffold.

Using this technique, it was possible to obtain round shape starch microparticles ranging from 3 to 540 μm (of diameter) with a homogeneous particles size distribution. The particles size depends on the conditions of the crosslinking reaction, mainly controlled by the use of surfactant and the stirring rate. Concerning the release of drug from the starch microparticles it was possible to observe that the delivery is very fast in the first 2 hours and independent of medium conditions. However, this behaviour is expected to be slow down in an *in vivo* application due to lower physiological pH. Another interesting fact is that for higher release periods, the increase in the pH increases in some measure the drug release, independently of salt concentration. Concerning the influence of medium ionic strength, it was shown that the drug release was also strongly dependent on salt concentration.

3.1.2 Starch/poly (lactic acid) Microparticles Produced by a Suspension Polymerization Method

Starch-based porous microparticles, based in a polymeric blend of starch with poly(lactic acid) (SPLA), were produced using a suspension polymerization method incorporating acrylic monomers. The obtained microparticles are aimed to be applied as drug delivery carriers. To accomplish this aim, a preliminary study was performed to evaluate the incorporation of a model drug (nonsteroidal anti-inflammatory drug - NSAID) and investigate its release profile as function of changes in the formulations parameters.

Preliminary studies were carried out in the preparation of SPLA-based microparticles by suspension polymerization of acrylic monomers, hydrophobic MMA and hydrophilic DMA and HEMA in the presence of the starch blend. SEM and light scattering analysis show formation of microparticles within the range of 500 to 20 μm, depending on formulation conditions and incorporation of the bioactive agent. It was possible to show the effect of the percentage of surfactant, reactive phase composition and the presence of drug in particles size and respective size distribution. The typical morphology obtained with this methodology is shown in Figure 9. The *in vitro* release profile was found to have a pattern very similar for SPLA-based microparticles independently of particle size and the used monomer.

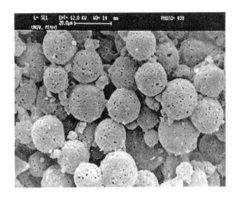

Figure 9. SPLA-based microparticles obtained by a suspension polimerization technique.

3.1.3 Soybean Microparticles Produced by Spray-Drying Technique

A great effort has been devoted to the development of alternative biodegradable polymeric systems for biomedical applications. Among the different types of biodegradable polymers, natural proteins are recognized by their high chemical versatility[52], due to the respective amino acid type structure. Their similarity to human tissue constituents suggests them as ideal templates to be used as biomaterials. Casein and soybean thermoplastics proteins were proposed by our research group for biomedical use, based on the claim that they present an adequate range of mechanical properties and bioactive character (specially when reinforced with bone-like fillers)[53]. Also the good processability, both in the melt and in aqueous media (including the good film forming properties) and the good hydrolytic stability give the soybean proteins a high potential to be used as microparticles

Soybean microparticles were produced using a spray drying technique. The delivery profile showed an initial burst release in the first 12 hours controlled by a diffusion mechanism. For higher immersion periods, it was possible to observe a slower release achieving 90% release after 100 hours in an isotonic saline solution. The versatility of these systems allows for different release profiles depending on the pH of the release environment as well as the crosslinking degree where the 100% release can take several weeks to be achieved.

3.1.4 Chitosan Nanoparticles Produced by Emulsion Crosslinking Technique

Because of biocompatibility, biodegradability, low cost and high loading capability for proteins, chitosan has become a valuable polymer for drug delivery systems. Chitosan nanoparticles are accepted as a suitable biocompatible drug carrier, especially for delivering protein drugs. By means of taking advantage of the polymers cationic properties, proteins can be adsorbed and loaded within the nanoparticles without destroying protein's bioactivity.

Chitosan nanoparticles were produced by a water-in-oil method using cyclohexane as organic medium and Tween 80 as emulsifying agent. With the use of cyclohexane, a smaller size, uniform size distribution, and a smooth surface were obtained. Nanoparticles showed a smooth surface morphology and a size distribution between 500-1000 nm.

Chitosan nanoparticles can be loaded with protein drugs by a passive loading procedure. Chitosan nanoparticles carrying positive charge at neutral pH values can adsorb proteins in high loading values. This mild loading procedure presents an advantage in terms of preserving protein's globular structure, which is essential for their bioactivity. Bovine Serum Albumin (BSA) is an ideal model protein to be used in this type of studies.

Chitosan nanoparticles loaded with BSA showed a burst release at first hours and a slow release of BSA was observed for about two weeks. In order to see prolonged activity of proteins, the release of proteins can be retarded by enclosing microparticles between closed membrane structures. In addition, the release of gentamicin and retinoic acid was also studied, giving raise to similar results.

3.2 Direct Loading or Immobilization in the Porous Scaffolds

3.2.1 Starch Based Porous Scaffolds Loaded with a Model Drug and Produced by a Microwave based Route

A new simple processing route to produce starch based porous materials was developed in the 3B's Research Group, based on a microwave baking methodology, as described in section 2. This innovative processing route was also used to obtain non-loaded controls and loaded drug delivery porous carriers, incorporating a non-steroid anti-inflammatory agent. This bioactive agent was selected as model drug being expected that the developed methodology might be used for other drugs and growth factors. More information can be found in reference[18].

The prepared systems were characterized by ^{1}H and ^{13}C NMR spectroscopy, which permit to study the interactions between the starch based materials and the processing components, namely the blowing agents. The porosity of the prepared materials was estimated by measuring their apparent density and studied by comparing drug loaded and non-loaded porous carriers. The behaviour of the porous structures, while immersed in aqueous media, was studied in terms of swelling and degradation, being intimately related to their porosity. Finally, *in vitro* drug release studies were performed showing a clear burst effect controlled by the porosity, followed by a slow controlled release of the drug during several days depending mainly on the degradation mechanism of the matrix.

3.2.2 Chitosan Based Porous Scaffolds as Potential Drug Delivery Systems

In our point of view, an optimal carrier for bone tissue engineering should be both a controlled release system and a scaffold. As a drug delivery system, the material must prevent rapid factor release and ideally target the growth factor in a predictable manner, allowing therapeutic doses to stimulate desired cells. As a scaffold, the material should act as a favourable site into which bone cells would be attracted to migrate and begin the process of depositing bone matrix. Therefore, the direct incorporation of growth factor in porous scaffolds should be a desirable goal. The inclusion of a bioactive ceramics on the scaffolds design can also confer to the systems a bone bonding behaviour that will guide bone formation. Polymer chitosan and chitosan/hydroxylapatite (HA) bioactive scaffolds have been produced by means of freeze-drying techniques. These structures can be further loaded with several bioactive agents.

These materials were developed by means of using different treatment, such as neutralization in alkali solutions and crosslinking, in order to control the materials performance. The results have shown that the materials' properties can be controlled either by using a crosslinking reaction or by precipitation with NaOH. For instances, the equilibrium hydration degree can be varied from 800% up to 1500%. One interesting fact is that the treatment with alkali solution seems to be more effective in controlling the hydration degree when compared to crosslinking. The result could be related with protonated amine groups of chitosan, which readily dissolve in aqueous medium. It is also important to stress out that the precipitation with NaOH led to a decrease in both macro and microporosity. The developed materials, including those containing HA particles, present a range of properties that might allow for their use on bone engineering applications and as materials for filling bone and dentistry defects. Furthermore, and due to the processing methodology, the developed polymeric and composite chitosan porous structures can be used as porous carriers for drug delivery.

3.3 Starch Based Hydrogels

Hydrogels are of special interested in controlled release applications because of their tissue biocompatibility, the ease with which the drug is dispersed in the matrix and the high control achieved by selecting the physical and chemical properties of the polymeric network. Due to their high versatility in terms chemical and physical properties, hydrogels can be produced to be stimuli-responsive. Smart polymers and hydrogels undergo fast, reversible changes in microstructure from hydrophilic to a hydrophobic state. The driving force behind these transition varies, with common stimuli including the neutralization of charged groups by either a pH shift[54], or the addition of an oppositely charged polymer[55], changes in the efficiency of hydrogen bonding with an increase of temperature or ionic strength[56], and collapse of hydrogels and interpenetrating polymer networks[57,58]. In the particular case of pH-responsiveness, hydrogels have been widely applied[54,59,60]. In networks containing weakly acidic or basic pendent groups, water sorption can result in ionization of these pendent groups depending on the solution pH and ionic composition. For ionic gels containing weakly acidic pendent groups, the equilibrium degree of swelling increases as the pH of external solution increases. Inversely, for gels containing weakly basic pendent groups, the equilibrium swelling degree increases as the pH decreases, being possible in this way to control the release profile of the carrier.

Our group have also been focused on the development of starch-based hydrogels for use as bone cements or drug delivery systems that can be loaded with a biologically active substance[38,39,61]. The design and preparation of novel biodegradable hydrogels developed by the free radical polymerization of acrylamide and acrylic acid, and some formulations with bis-acrylamide, in the presence of a corn starch/ethylene-co-vinyl alcohol copolymer blend (SEVA-C), was studied[39]. The redox system benzoyl peroxide (BPO) and 4-dimethylaminobenzyl alcohol (DMOH) initiated the polymerization at room temperature. Xerogels were characterized by ^{1}H NMR and FTIR spectroscopies. Swelling studies were performed as a function of pH in different buffer solutions determining the water-transport mechanism that governs the swelling behaviour. Degradation studies of the hydrogels were performed in simulated physiological solutions for time up to 90 days, determining the respective weight loss, and analyzing the solution residue by ^{1}H NMR. The mechanical properties of the xerogels were characterized by tensile and compressive tests, as well as by dynamo-mechanical analysis (DMA). Dynamo-mechanical parameters were also studied for hydrated samples. It was possible to produce both thermoplastic and crosslinked hydrogels that can be used on a range of biomedical applications. Some systems exhibit the most desirable kinetic behaviour to be used as controlled release carriers. The hydrogels are also pH sensitive, degradable and present interesting swelling characteristics. The combination of the properties of the developed hydrogels might allow for their application on a range of biomedical applications.

Another work includes the development of new partially biodegradable composite acrylic bone cements based on corn starch/cellulose acetate blends (SCA), prepared by the free radical polymerization of methyl methacrylate and acrylic acid at low temperature[38]. Amounts of biocompatible, osteoconductive and osteophilic mineral component such as hydroxylapatite (sintered and non-sintered), were incorporated in different percentages to confer a bone-bonding character to the bone cements in this type of applications. All cement formulations were characterized by ^{1}H NMR spectroscopy. Curing parameters and mechanical properties were determined finding formulations, which complete the ASTM legislation. Hydration degree, degradation studies, as well as bioactivity tests were performed in all prepared formulations. The developed systems show a range of properties that might allow for their application as self-curing bone cements, exhibiting several advantages with respect to other commercially available bone cements. Composite and partially degradable SCA/HA, acrylic bone cements with controlled balance of hydrophobicity can be formulated from a processed blend of starch and cellulose acetate SCA, and different mixtures of the acrylic monomers AA and MMA, in the presence of hydroxylapatite[38]. Kinetic parameters of the curing formulations activated at low temperature by the system BPO/DMOH, allow the selection of the optimum solid/liquid ratio and the composition of the hydrophilic/hydrophobic AA/MMA components for the design of the most appropriate formulations. The best results are obtained with a solid/liquid ratio of 55/45 and a content in HA of about 20wt%[38]. The optimum balance of hydrophobicity, is attained with a specific composition of MMA and AA. The heterogeneous morphology of the cured cements can be positively applied for the formation of a relatively porous material with a compensation of the contraction of volume after the polymerization and in addition the induction of bioactivity in the presence of the HA component.

3.4 Natural Based Membranes

Another work carried out in the 3B's Research Group involves the development of membranes using several natural origin polymers, such as soybean, casein and chitosan. In fact, membranes have been widely used for biomedical purposes, namely as wound dressings, transdermal drug delivery and as scaffolds for skin tissue engineering[62-67]. In fact, skin acts as a very complex membrane, providing a multifunctional interface between the body and its surrounding. One interesting approach to develop suitable wound dressings and scaffolds for tissue engineering has been focused in proteins present in the extracellular matrix like collagen, elastin and keratin. Several films and membranes with complex 3D porous architecture of these polymers and its composites have been successfully developed[63,66] However, a lot of work has to be done to develop an ideal skin substitute and the recent BSE (Bovine Spongiform Encephalopathy) crises lead to an increasing concern about the use of animal origin proteins in biomedical applications.

Other important application of membranes is the so-called guided bone regeneration (GBR) membrane. In general, bone healing and the formation of new bone are inhibited by the rapid appearance of connective tissue. The concept of GBR primarily consists in barrier membranes that prevent the ingrowth of connective tissue. Furthermore, growth factors can accumulate under the membrane[68]. In addition, a desirable feature is the sustained delivery of bone growth factors incorporated in the polymeric matrix of the membrane.

Our group has been recently working in the development of membranes based on soybean protein isolate (SI) as an alternative protein based polymeric systems for biomedical applications. These systems have demonstrated a pH dependent behaviour when loaded with bioactive agents[69]. The principal advantages of soybean proteins, among other biodegradable polymers and natural proteins, are its non-animal origin, good water resistance and storage stability, being a highly economically competitive material. In this way, SI can be a good candidate to substitute the other protein-based systems described above.

Another non-animal origin polymer that has been widely studied for biomedical applications is chitosan, as it was already mentioned. It is a biocompatible and biodegradable polymer, which can be hydrolyzed by lysozyme (present in human body fluids)[70]. Chitosan is a co-polymer of glucosamine and N-acetylglucosamine obtained by N-deacetylation of chitin. Its healing properties have been reported by several authors[66,67]. On the other hand, it has been observed that glucosamine, a degradation product of chitosan, has a beneficial effect on treatment and symptoms of osteoarthritis as it helps to regenerate joint cartilage[71].

Chitosan membranes have been prepared in our group by solvent casting. Some formulations were crosslinked with glutaraldehyde at various degrees of crosslinking. The aqueous behaviour of such formulations was studied. Properties as the hydration equilibrium degree, the degradation behaviour and mechanical properties were determined with samples immersed in an isotonic saline solution (NaCl 0.154M, pH=7.4) at 37°C. All formulations revealed to be very stable in the simulated aqueous body environment. Secant modulus at 2% of strain ($E_{2\%}$) increased with the degree of crosslinking between 1.5 and 2 GPa for samples in the dry state. $E_{2\%}$ decreased 100 orders of magnitude for chitosan membranes when immersed in the isotonic saline solution. Major differences on the samples mechanical performance (in wet state) could be introduced as function of the degree of crosslinking. Membranes surface was found to be quite smooth and homogeneous. They also exhibit good handling properties.

Blending different biomaterials is an ordinary procedure in the biomedical field. Thus, chitosan and SI membranes were developed by blending these polymers in different ratios of both components, combining chitosan unique properties with those of a protein material. These formulations were found to be stable under an isotonic aqueous environment even without any precipitation/coagulation procedure. These membranes presented an equilibrium hydration degree of about twice of the above described chitosan membranes. Both chitosan and SI possess a pH dependent drug sustained release pattern. However, the different behaviour of these materials can create a narrow pH range in which a bioactive agent can be released. Thus, it is expected that the drug release profile can be tailored, targeting more specified applications. In order to further control membranes properties several methodologies are currently being undertaken, like precipitation of chitosan phase in NaOH solution, crosslinking SI by a heat treatment or crosslinking both phases by E-radiation.

4. CELLS FOR TISSUE ENGINEERING AND THEIR BEHAVIOUR WHEN SEEDED ON NATURAL ORIGIN SCAFFOLDS

When considering tissue engineering applications, the choice of a reliable source of cells is as important as the development of the scaffold itself. These cells should be easily expandable and possess high proliferation rates being non-immunogeneic and have a protein expression rate similar to the tissue to be regenerated[72]. Up to now several sources, from mature bone to bone marrow, of cells were used for bone tissue engineering purposes. From this various sources, the cells obtained from the bone marrow seem to be the most promising. These results come from the fact that within the bone marrow we can find stem cells, which are undifferentiated cells with a high proliferation capability, being able of self-renewal, production of large number of differentiated progeny and regeneration of tissues[73].

Stem cells obtained from bone marrow are known as mesenchymal stems cells (MSC's), and although they posses certain degree of commitment/differentiation, they are still multipotent which means that they can differentiate into cells of mesenchymal origin. These cells were first described by Fridestein *et al.*[74], and are located in the bone marrow around blood vessels (as pericytes), in fat, skin, muscle and other locations[75]. They are isolated through gradient centrifugation[76] and once in culture they grow in colonies having fibroblast like appearance[77]. Although they are present in very small amount in the bone marrow (from 0.001% to 0.01%)[78] they have high proliferation rates, can be expanded over one billion fold in culture making them ideal for the use in tissue engineering[78-80]. Moreover with the use of differentiation factors it is possible to differentiate these cells into osteoblasts[78,79]. The factors commonly used to differentiate MSC's to the osteogenic lineage are dexamethasone and ascorbic acid using E-glycerophosphate as an exogenous source of inorganic phosphate[78,79]. Frequently these factors have influence on the behaviour of cells while being *in vitro* cultured. For instances, it is known that dexamethasone increases the bone forming capability of the cells and ascorbic acid is involved in the activation of the MAPK pathway which will also lead to the expression of the osteogenic phenotype[78-80]. However, the knowledge of how these and other differentiation factors affect mesenchymal stem cells growth and differentiation is still scarce and further basic research is needed to fully understand all the mechanisms involved in the referred phenomena.

4.1 Tissue Engineering Experiments Using Starch Based Scaffolds

In our group, we have been using an osteosarcoma cell line, as model source of cells, to carry out tests with some of the previously described starch based scaffolds. In other work[81], primary cells from human calvarian origin have been used. Some experiments where also performed with rat bone marrow cells[82]. In most of these studies, starch based scaffolds have been studied. For instances, due to the non-toxic properties as well as due to its excellent mechanical properties, SEVA-C scaffolds processed by using a technique based on extrusion with blowing agents have been used with the osteosarcoma cell line. In order that the reader can understand the experiments, the experimental methods will be described in detail below.

4.1.1 Experimental Methods

Human osteosarcoma cells, SaOS-2 cell line obtained from ECACC, were grown as monolayer cultures, in DMEM supplemented with 10%FBS (Biochrome, Germany), 1% antibiotics/antimicotics solution (Sigma, USA), 5 mM β-Glycerphosphate (Sigma, USA) and 50 μM of ascorbic acid (Sigma,USA), until they reach P10 stage. At that time cells were trypsinized, centrifuged and ressupended in culture medium. Aliquots of 20 μl containing 3×10^5 cells were then seeded on top of the porous structures, as described previously[81]. Two hours after cell seeding, 1 ml of culture medium was added to each well and cells/scaffolds constructs were incubated for 2 weeks in a humidified atmosphere at 37°C containing 5% CO_2, with medium changes every 3 to 4 days.

The adhesion of human osteoblast like cells to SEVA-C scaffolds was weekly assessed by SEM. To assess if cells were growing in a 3D manner into the inner regions of the scaffolds, these were cut into equal parts and then observed under the SEM. For that effect cells/scaffolds constructs were washed in 0.15M PBS and fixed in a solution of 2.5% of glutaraldehyde in PBS. After this, the constructs were again washed in PBS, submitted to ethanol series of 50%, 70%, 90%, 100% for 2x15 minutes and finally air dried. Samples were the gold coated in a Sputter Jeol JFC 1100 equipment and viewed in a Leica Cambridge S360 scanning electron microscope.

Cell viability was assessed after 12 hours, 7 and 14 days by using the MTS test as described previously[81]. Cell proliferation of human osteoblast like cells on starch based scaffolds was assessed by means of a total protein assay, the Sedmak method. After the same time periods as for the cell viability assay cells/scaffolds constructs (n=6) were washed in PBS, placed in 750 μl of lysis buffer (20mM Tris, 1mM EDTA, 150mM NaCl and 1% Triton X-100) supplemented with 100 μM phenylmethylsulfonyl fluoride (PMSF, Sigma, USA) and a cocktail of proteinase inhibitors (Chymostatin, Leupeptin, Antpain, Pepstatin) in a final concentration of 1 mg/ml, and finally sonicated at 40 Kv for 3x15 seconds.

After sonication scaffolds were removed and the resulting suspension centrifuged for 10 minutes at 14000 rpm and 4°C, in the end of which the pellet was rejected. Scaffolds without cells but in the same culture conditions were used as blanks. For protein quantification 20 μl of the protein extract were removed, placed in 2ml of Sedmak Reagent (0.06% of Coomassie Blue in 0.3M $HClO_4$) previously diluted in 0.1 N $HClO_4$ in a 1,5:3.5 ratio. The reaction was allowed to occur for 10 minutes, in the end of which absorbance was measured at 620 nm. The results were then plotted against a standard curve made with bovine serum albumin (BSA) ranging from 0 to 25 µg. Total protein was then calculated by extrapolation for the 750 µl of protein extract solution.

Osteopontin expression was weekly screened by western blot. For this purpose, protein was weekly extracted and quantified as described previously. Aliquots containing equal amounts of protein (20 µg) were then loaded into a 4% stacking polyacrilamide gel and a 10% running gel, subjected to electrophoresis and electrotransferred to a Hybond P membrane (Amersham, USA). Blots were then further incubated for 1 hour, at room temperature, with primary antibody against osteopontin (University of Iowa, USA) in a 1:200 dilution. After washing with 1% milk TBS-T solution, blots were further incubated for 1 hour with anti-mouse IgG antibody coupled to horse radish peroxidase. The immune complex was detected by incubation with ECL system (Amersham) and visualized by chemiluminescence.

4.2   Results

The mechanism that dominates initial cell attachment to biomaterials surface *in vitro* is the adsorption of proteins from cell culture medium serum on its surface[83,84]. This film of protein acts *in vitro*, as the matrix synthesized *in vivo* by bone forming cells and, its nature, extent and stability is to a large extent determined by the surface properties of the material and is thus a reflection of the substrate characteristics[83,84]. When cells are seeded on porous biomaterials for tissue engineering, they will first interact with this film protein through specific receptors present on the plasma membrane, being the interaction of these receptors with the protein film the responsible, in a first stage, for cell attachment, and, latter on, for cell migration within the scaffolds.

Regarding the present experiment, SEM observation allowed to see that osteoblast like cells were well adhered to the SEVA-C based scaffolds after 1 week in culture (Figure 10a). Cells were mainly adhered to the bars of the scaffolds, showing at the same time that they were able to span across pores, being demonstrated in this way the adequacy of the pore size developed (Figure 10a). Furthermore, an observation made into the inner regions of the scaffolds (Figure 10b), as referred in the methods section, showed that cells were also capable of colonizing the referred areas, being this colonization smaller when compared to the one on the scaffolds' surface. By week 2 it was possible to observe a high degree of colonization both on the surface of the material (Figure 10c) and inner regions of the scaffolds (Figure 10d), accompanied by collagen production by the cells (Figure 10d).

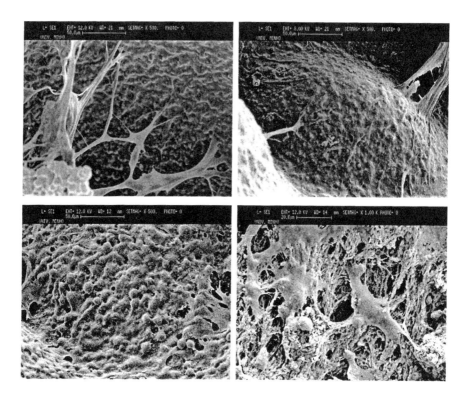

Figure 10. Human osteoblast like cells seeded after 1 (a,b) and 2 (c,d) weeks on porous SEVA-C scaffolds.

Regarding cell viability tests, a constant increase of the optical density (OD) was registered during the two weeks of the experiment, this meaning that human osteoblast like cells were producing large amounts of a brown formazan which is an indicator of normal metabolism (Figure 11). This fact shows that cells were able to incorporate and metabolize MTS and hence indicates their perfect viability. Cell proliferation assays (Figure 12) corroborate the results from SEM observation and demonstrate that cells were able to grow within the 3D structure during the two weeks of growth. Furthermore, the fact that cells were still growing clearly shows that they were not confluent and still had places where to grow. Together with the data obtained from SEM analysis we can clearly state that the developed porous structure was adequate for sustaining cell growth.

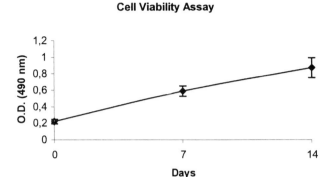

Figure 11. Cell viability was weekly assessed by means of a total protein assay. Cell density used was 3x10⁵cells/scaffold. Cells were kept in culture for 2 weeks in complete culture medium supplemented with 5 mM β-glycerophosphate, 50 µM ascorbic acid.

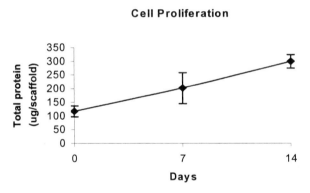

Figure 12. Cell proliferation was weekly assessed by means of a total protein assay. Cell density used was 3x10⁵cells/scaffold. Cells were kept in culture for 2 weeks in complete culture medium supplemented with 5 mM β-glycerophosphate, 50 µM ascorbic acid.

During the course of bone formation, osteoblasts produce a series of proteins, which will make part of the bone ECM, being osteopontin one of them[85]. Regarding the present experiment, western blot analysis clearly shows that osteopontin was being expressed by the cells previously seeded on the scaffolds, during the four weeks of the experiment as shown in Figure 13. This fact, associated with the collagen deposition observed by SEM (Figure 10d), clearly shows that active deposition of bone extracellular matrix was happening as well as its probable mineralization.

W1　　　　W2　　■■ 75 KD

Figure 13. Western blot analysis of osteopontin expression of SaOS-2 cells seeded on starch based scaffolds. Expression of the referred protein was detected for the four weeks (w1, w2), indicating the deposition of bone extracelullar matrix (ECM).

5. CONCLUSIONS

The research carried out by the 3B's Group has led to the development of scaffolds systems that can accomplish different functions in the regeneration of tissue by means of tissue engineering strategies. This was achieved by the development of several processing techniques, which enable to obtain a range of scaffolds design, with tailorable properties. All this research has been based on taking advantage of the versatility of natural origin polymers such as starch based matrices, chitin and chitosan, and proteins such as soybean and casein.

The present chapter clearly shows the different possibilities for producing scaffolds and carriers by an all range of processing methods. It is possible to design scaffolds and carriers, or both in one single system, with a range of properties that are specifically targeting a particular biomedical application.

Finally, it could be shown, by means of some examples, the adequability of some of the developed systems not only to sustain cell adhesion and proliferation but more important to promote the formation of some extracellular matrix.

REFERENCES

1. Burg, K.J.L., Porter, S., and Kellam, J.F., 2000, Biomaterial developments for bone tissue engineering. *Biomaterials* **221**, 2347-2359.
2. Langer, R., and Vacanti, J.P., 1993, Tissue engineering. *Science* **260**, 920-926.
3. Langer, R., 1999, Selected advances in drug delivery and tissue engineering. *J. Control. Rel.* **62**, 7-11.
4. Hardin-Young, J., Teumer, J., Ross, R.N., and Parenteau, N.L., 2000, Approaches to transplanting engineered cells and tissues. In: Lanza R, Langer R, Vacanti J, editors, Principles of Tissue Engineering (2nd Ed), Academic Press, New York, pp. 281-291.
5. Pachence, J.M., and Kohn, J., 1997, Biodegradable polymers for tissue engineering. In: Lanza R, Langer R, Chick W, editors, Principles of Tissue Engineering: Academic Press, New York, pp. 273-293.
6. Vacanti, C.A., Bonassar, L.J., and Vacanti, J.P., 2000, Structural Tissue Engineering. In: Lanza R, Langer R, Vacanti J, editors, Principles of Tissue Engineering (2nd Ed): Academic Press, New York, pp. 671-68.

7. Agrawal, C.M., Athanasiou, K.A., and Heckman, J.D., 1997, Biodegradable PLA-PGA polymers for tissue engineering in orthopaedics. *Mater. Sci. Forum* **250**, 115-228.
8. Thomson, R., Yaszemski, M., and Mikos, A., 1997, Polymer scaffold processing. In: Lanza R, Langer R, Chick W, editors, Principles of Tissue Engineering: Academic Press, New York, pp. 263-272.
9. Lu, L., and Mikos, A., 1996, The importance of new processing techniques in tissue engineering. *MRS Bulletin* **21**, 28-32.
10. Mikos, A.G., Thorsen, A.J., Czerwonka, L.A., Bao, Y., Langer, R.B., 1994, Preparation and characterization of poly(l-lactid acid) foams. *Polymer*,1068 –1077.
11. Langer, R.,1999, Selected advances in drug delivery and tissue engineering. *J. Contr. Rel.* **62**, 7-11.
12. Mikos, A.G., Sarakinos, G., Leite, S.M., Vacanti, J.P., and Langer, R., 1993, Laminated three-dimensional biodegradable foams for use in tissue engineering. *Biomaterials* **14**, 323-330.
13. Mikos, A.G., Bao, Y., Cima, L.G., Ingber, D.E., Vacanti, J.P., and Langer, R.B., 1993, Preparation of poly(glycolic acid) bonded fiber structures for cell attachment and transplantation. *J. Biomed. Mater. Res.* **27**, 183-189.
14. Hinrichs, W., 1992, Porous polymer structures for tissue regeneration. PhD Thesis. Univ. Twente, The Netherlands.
15. Mooney, D.J., Baldwin, D.F., Suh, N.P., and Vacanti, J.P., 1996, Novel approach to fabricate porous sponges of poly(d,l-lactido-co-glycolic acid) without the use of organic solvents. *Biomaterials* **17**, 1417-1422.
16. Gomes, M.E., Ribeiro, A.S., Malafaya, P.B., Reis, R.L., and Cunha, A.M., 2001, A new approach based on injection moulding to produce biodegradable starch-based polymeric scaffolds: morphology, mechanical and degradation behaviour. *Biomaterials* **22**, 883-889.
17. Thompson, R.C., Yaszemski, M.J., Powders, J.M., 1995, Fabrication of biodegradable polymer scaffolds to engineer trabecular bone. *J. Biomat. Sci.-Polym. Edn.* **7**, 23-28.
18. Malafaya, P.B., Elvira, C., Gallardo, A., San Roman, J., and Reis, R.L., 2001, Porous starch-based drug delivery systems processed by a microwave route. *J. Biomat. Sci: Polym. Edn.* **12**, 1227-1241.
19. Hutmacher, D.W., 2000, Scaffolds in tissue engineering bone and cartilage. *Biomaterials* **21**, 2529-2543.
20. Hutmacher, D.W., Teoh, S.H., Zein, I., Renawake, M., and Lau, S., 2000, Tissue engineering Research: the engineer's role. *Med. Dev. Tech.* **1**, 33-39.
21. Langer, R., and Vacanti, J., 1999, Tissue engineering: the challenges ahead. *Sci. Amer.* **280**, 62-65.
22. Guidoin, M., Marois, Y., Bejui, J., Poddevin, N., King, M., and Guidoin, R., 2000, Analysis of retrived polymer fiber based replacements for the ACL. *Biomaterials*, 2461-2474.
23. Thomson, R.C., Wake, M.C., Yaszemski, M., and Mikos, A.G., 1995, Biodegradable polymer scaffolds to regenerate organs. *Adv. Polym. Sci.* **122**, 247-274.
24. Maquet, V., and Jerome, R., 1997, Design of macroporous biodegradable polymer scaffolds for cell transplantation. *Mater. Sci. Forum* **250**, 15-42.
25. Vunjak-Novakovic, G., Obradovic, B., Martin, I., Bursac, P., Langer, R., and Freed, L.E. Dynamic cell seeding of polymer scaffolds for cartilage tissue engineering. *Biotech. Progr.* **14**, 193-202.
26. Freed, L.E., Hollander, A., Martin, I., Barry, J., Langer, R., and Vunjak-Novakovic, G.,1998, Chondrogenesis in a cell-polymer-bioreactor system. *Exp. Cel. Res.* **240**, 58-65

27. Holder, W., Gruber, H., Moore, A., Culberson, C., Anderson, W., Burg, K., and Mooney, D., 1998, Cellular ingrowth and thickness changes in poly-L-lactide and polyglycolide matrices implanted subcutaneously in the rat. *J. Biomed. Mater. Res.* **41**, 412-421
28. Gao, J., Niklason L., and Langer, R., 1998, Surface hydrolysis of poly(glycolic acid) meshes increases the seeding density of vascular smooth muscle cells. *J. Biomed. Mater. Res.* **42**, 417-424
29. Aigner, J., Tegeler, J., Hutzler, P., Campoccia, D., Pavesio, A., Hammer, C., Kastenbauer, E., and Naumann, A., 1998, Cartilage tissue engineering with novel nonwoven structured biomaterial based on hyaluronic acid benzyl ester. *J. Biomed. Mater. Res.* **42**, 172-181.
30. Rotter, N., Aigner, J., Naumann, A., Planck, H., Hammer, C., Burmester, G., and Sittinger, M., 1998, Cartilage reconstruction of resorbable polymer scaffolds for tissue engineering of human septal cartilage. *J. Biomed. Mater. Res.* **42**, 347-356.
31. Sittinger, M., Reitzel, D., Dauner, M., Hierlemann, H., Hammer, C., Kastenbauer, E., Plank, H., Burmester, G., Bujia, J., 1996, Resorbable polyesters in cartilage engineering: affinity and biocompatibility of polymer fiber structures to chondrocytes. *J. Biomed. Mater. Res.* **33**, 57-63.
32. Mendes, S.C., Bezemer, J., Classe, M.B., Grypma, D.W., Bellia, G., Innocenti, F.D., Reis, R.L., van Blitterswijk, C,A, and de Bruijn, J.D., 2002, Evaluation of two biodegradable polymeric systems as substrates for bone tissue engineering. *Tissue Eng.* (in press).
33. Nam, Y.S., Yoon, J.J., and Park, T.G., 2000, A novel fabrication method of macroporous biodegradable polymer scaffolds using gas foaming salt as a porogen additive. *J. Biomed. Mater. Res.: Appl. Biomater.* **53**, 1-7
34. Gomes, M.E., Godinho, J.S., Tchalamov, D., Cunha, A.M., and Reis, R.L., 2002, Design and processing of starch based scaffolds for hard tissue engineering. *J. Appl. Med. Polym.* (in press).
35. Gomes, M.E., Godinho, J.S., Tchalamov, D., Cunha, A.M., and Reis, R.L., 2002, Alternative tissue engineering scaffolds based on starch: processing methodologies, morphology, degradation and mechanical properties. *Mat. Sci. Eng. C* **20**, 19-26.
36. Zhang, R., and Ma, P.X., 1999, Poly(Δ-hydroxyl acids)/hydroxyapatite porous composites for bone-tissue engineering.i.preparation and morphology. *J. Biomed. Mater. Res.* **44**, 446-455.
37. Temenhoff, J.S., and Mikos, A.G., 2000, Injectable materials for orthopaedic tissue engineering. *Biomaterials* **21**, 2405-2412.
38. Espigare,S.I., Elvira, C., Mano, J.F., San Román, J., and Reis, R.L., 2002, New biodegradable and bioactive acrylic bone cements based on starch blends and ceramic fillers. *Biomaterials* **23**, 1883-1895.
39. Elvira, C., Mano, J.F., San Román, J., and Reis, R.L., 2002, Starch based biodegradable hydrogels with potential biomedical applications as drug delivery systems, *Biomaterials* **23**, 1955-1966.
40. Tabata,Y., 2000, The importance of drug delivery systems in tissue engineering. *PSTT* **3**, 80-89.
41. Bessho, K., 1996, Ectopic osteoinductive difference between purified bovine and recombinant human bone morphogenetic protein. In: Lindholm TS, editor, Bone morphogenetic proteins: biology, biochemistry and reconstructive surgery, RG Landes Co, Georgetown, pp.105-111.

42. Hotz, G., 1998, Delivery systems for osteoinductive proteins. In: Stark GB, Horch R, Tanczos E, editors, Biological matrices and tissue reconstruction, Springer, Berlin, pp.207-213.
43. Goodman, G.R., Dissanayake, I.R., Bowman, A.R., Pun, S., Ma, Y., Jee, W.S.S., Bryer, H.P., and Epstein, S., 2001, Transforming growth factor-E administration modifies cyclosporine A-induced bone loss. *Bone* **28**, 583-588.
44. Maeda, M., Kadota, K., Kajihara, M., Sano, A., and Fujioka, K., 2001, Sustained release of human growth hormone (hGH) from collagen film and evaluation on wound healing in db/db mice. *J. Control. Rel.* **77**, 261-272.
45. Li, R.H., and Wozney, J.M., 2001, Delivering on the promise of bone morphogenetic proteins. *Trends Biotech.* **19**, 255-265.
46. Baldwin, S.P., and Saltzman, W.M., 1998, Materials for protein delivery in tissue engineering. *Adv. Drug Deliv. Rev.* **33**, 71-86.
47. Anseth, K.S., Metters, A.T., Bryant, S.J., Martens, P.J., Elisseeff, J.H., and Bowman, C.N., 2002, In situ forming degradable networks and their application in tissue engineering and drug delivery. *J. Control. Rel.* **78**, 199-209.
48. Li, R.H., and Wozney, J.M., 2001, Delivering on the promise of bone morphogenetic proteins. *Trends Biotech.* **19**, 255-265.
49. Dieplod, R., Kreuter, J., Guggenbuhl, P., and Robinson, P., 1989, Distribution of poly-hexyl-2-cyano-[3-^{14}C] acrylate nanoparticles in healthy and chronically inflamed rabbit eyes. *Int. J. Pharm.* **54**, 149-153.
50. Illum, L., Wright, J., and Davis, S.S., 1989, Targeting of microspheres to sites of inflammation. *Int. J. Pharm.* **52**, 221-224.
51. Alpar, H.O., Field, W.N., Hyde, R., and Lewis, D.A., 1989, The transport of microspheres to from the gastro-intestinal tract to inflammatory air pouches in the rat. *J. Pharm. Pharmacol.* **41**, 194-196.
52. Paetau, I., Chen, C.Z., and Jane, J.L., 1994, Biodegradable plastic made from soybean products. 1. Effect of preparation and processing on mechanical properties and water absorption. *Ind. Eng. Chem. Res.* **33**, 1821-1827.
53. Vaz, C.M., Mano, J.F., Fossen, M., Van Tuil, R.F., de Graaf, L.A., Reis, R.L., and Cunha, A.M., 2000, Mechanical, dynamic-mechanical and thermal properties of soy-protein thermoplastics with potential biomedical applications. *J. Macromol. Sci. B* **41**, 33-46.
54. Risbud, M.V., Hardikar, A.A., Bhat, S.V., and Bhonde, R.R., 2000, pH-sensitive freeze-dried chitosan-polyvinyl pirrolidone hydrogels as controlled release systems for antibiotic delivery. *J. Control. Rel.* **68**, 23-30.
55. Chenite, A., Chaput, C., Wang, D., Combes, C., Buschmann, M.D., Hoemann, C.D., Leroux, J.C., Atkinson, B.L., Binette, F., and Selmani, A., 2000, Novel injectable neutral solutions of chitosan form biodegradable gels *in situ*. *Biomaterials* **21**, 2155-2161.
56. Kim, M.R., and Park, T.G., 2002, Temperature-responsive and degradable Hyaluronic acid/pluronic composite hydrogels for controlled release of human growth hormone. *J. Control. Rel.* **80**, 69-77.
57. Melekaslan, D., and Okay, O., 2000, Swelling of strong polyelectrolyte hydrogels in polymer solutions: effect of ion pair formation on the polymer collapse. *Polymer* **41**, 5737-5747.
58. Ilavsky, M., Mamytbekov, G., Hanykov, L., and Dusek, K., 2002, Phase transition in swollen gels 31. swelling and mechanical behaviour of interpenetrating networks composed of poly(1-vinyl-2-pyrrolidone) and polyacrylamide in water/acetone mixtures. *Eur. Pol. J.* **38**, 875-883.

59. Park, S.B., You, J.O., Park, H.Y., Haam, S.J., and Kim, W.S., 2001, A novel pH-sensitive membrane from chitosan-TEOS IPN; preparation and its drug permeation characteristics. *Biomaterials* **22**, 323-330.
60. Alvarez-Lorenzo, C., and Concheiro, A., 2002, Reversible adsorption by a pH- and temperature-sensitive acrylic hydrogel. *J. Control. Rel.* **80**, 247-257.
61. Pereira, C.S., Cunha, A.M., Reis, R.L., Vazquez, B., and San Roman, J., 1998, New starch-based thermoplastic hydrogels for use as bone cements or drug-delivery carriers. *J. Mater. Sci.: Mater. Med.* **9**, 825-833.
62. Naik, A., Kalia, Y.N., and Guy, R.H., 2000, Transdermal drug delivery: overcoming the skin's barrier function. *Pharm. Sci. Tech. Today* **3**, 318-326.
63. Hafemann, B., Ensslen, S., Erdmann, C., Niedballa, R., Zuhlke, A., Ghofrani, K., and Kirkpatrick, C.J., 1999, Use of a collagen/elastin-membrane for the tissue engineering of dermis. *Burns* **25**, 373-384.
64. Balasubramani, M., Kumar, T.R., and Babu, M., 2001, Skin substitutes: a review. *Burns* **27**, 534-544.
65. Sai, K., and Babu, M., 2000, Collagen based dressings - a review. *Burns* **26**, 54-62.
66. Ishihara, M., Nakanishi, K., Ono, K., Sato, M., Kikuchi, M., Saito, Y., Yura, H., Matsui, T., Hattori, H., Uenoyama, M., and Kurita, A., 2002, Photocrosslinkable chitosan as a dressing for wound occlusion and accelerator in healing process. *Biomaterials* **23**, 833-840.
67. Howling, G.I., Dettmar, P.W., Goddard, P.A., Hampson, F.C., Dornish, M., and Wood, E.J., 2001, The effect of chitin and chitosan on the proliferation of human skin fibroblasts and keratinocytes in vitro. *Biomaterials* **22**, 2959-2966.
68. Ueyama, Y., Ishikawa, K., Mano, T., Koyama, T., Nagatsuka, H., Suzuki, K., and Ryoke, K., 2002, Usefulness as guided bone regeneration membrane of the alginate membrane. *Biomaterials* **23**, 2027-2033.
69. Vaz, C.M., deGraft, L.A., Reis, R.L., and Cunha, A.M., 2002, pH-sensitive soy protein hydrogels for the controlled release of an anti-inflammatory drug. *J. Mater. Sci.: Mater. Med.* (in press).
70. Nordtveit, R.J., Varum, K.M., and Smidsrod, O., 1996, Degradation of partially N-acetylated chitosans with hen egg white and human lysozyme. *Carbohydrate Polym.* **29**, 163-167.
71. Fenton, J.I., Chlebek-Brown, K.A., Peters, T.L., Caron, J.P., and Orth, M.W., 2000, The effects of glucosamine derivatives on equine articular cartilage degradation in explant culture. *Osteoarthritis Cartilage* **8**, 444-451.
72. Heath, C.A., 2000, Cells for tissue engineering. *TIBTECH* **18**, 17-19.
73. Blau, H.M., Brazelton, T.R., and Weimann, J.M., 2001, The evolving concept of a stem cell: entity or function. *Cell* **105**, 829-841.
74. Friedenstain, A.J., 1973, Determined and inducible osteogenic precursor cells. In: Hard Tissue Growth, Repair and Remineralization, Elsevier, Amsterdam, pp.169-185.
75. Caplan, A.I., and Bruder, S.P., 2001, Mesenchymal stem cells: Building blocks for molecular medicine in the 21st century. *Trends in Mol. Med.* **7**, 259-264.
76. Haynesworth, S.E., Goshima, J., Goldberg, V.M., and Caplan, A.I., 1992, Characterization of cells with osteogenic potential from human marrow. *Bone* **13**, 81-88.
77. Jaiswall, N., Haynesworth, S.E., Caplan, A.I., and Bruder, S.P., 1997, Osteogenic differentiation of purified, culture-expanded human mesenchymal stem cell *in vitro*. *J. Cell Biochem.* **64**, 295-312.

78. Pittinger, M.F., Mackay, A.M., Beck, S.C., Jaiswal, R.K., Douglas, R., Mosxca, J.D., Moorman, M.A., Simonetti, D.W., Craig, S., and Marshak, D.R., 1999, Multilineage potential of adult mesenchymal stem cells. *Science* **284**, 143-147.
79. Bruder, S.P., Jaiwal, N., and Haynesworth, S.E., 1997, Growth kinetics, self renewal, and the osteogenic potential of purified human mesenchymal stem cells during extensive subcultivation and following cryopreservation. *J. Cell Biochem.* **64**, 278-294.
80. Jaiswal, R.K., Jaiswal, N., Bruder, S.P., Mbalaviele, G., Marshak, D.R., and Pittenger, M.F., 2000, Adult human mesenchymal stem cell differentiation to the osteogenic or adipogenic lineage is regulated by mitogen-activated protein kinase. *J. Biol. Chem.* **275**, 9645-9652.
81. Salgado, A.J., Gomes, M.E., Chou, A., Coutinho, O.P., Reis, R.L., and Hutmacher, D.W., 2002, Preliminary study on the adhesion and proliferation of human osteoblasts on starch based scaffolds. *Mater. Sci. Eng. C: Biomimetic and Supramolecular Systems* **20**, 27-33.
82. Gomes, M.E., Sikavitsas, V.I., Behravesh, E. , Reis, R.L., and Mikos, A.G., 2002, Effect of flow perfusion on the osteogenic differentiation of bone marrow stromal cells cultured on starch based three-dimensional scaffolds. *J. Biomed. Mater. Res.* (submitted).
83. Steele, J.G., Dalton, B.A., Thomas, C.H., Healy, K.E., Gengenbach, T.R., and McFarland, C.D., 1999, Underpaying mechanisms of cellular adhesion in vitro during colonization of synthetic surfaces by bone-derived cells. In: Davies JE, editor, Bone engineering, em square, Toronto, pp.225-231.
84. Horbett, T.A., Cooper, K.W., Lew, K.R., and Ratner, B.D., 1998, Rapid postadsorptive changes in fibrinogen adsorbed from plasma to segmented polyurethanes. *J. Biomater. Sci.: Polym. Ed.* **9**, 1071-1087.
85. Sodek, J., Ganss, B., McKee, M.D., 2000, Osteopontin. *Crit. Rev. Oral Biol. Med.* **11**, 279-303.

PREPARATION AND CHARACTERIZATION OF NATURAL/SYNTHETIC HYBRID SCAFFOLDS

Gilson Khang[1], Sang Jin Lee[2], Chang Whan Han[3], John M. Rhee[1], and Hai Bang Lee[2]
[1]*Department of Polymer Science and Technology, Chonbuk National University, 664-14, Dukjin, Chonju 561-756, Korea;* [2]*Biomaterials Laboratory, P. O. Box 107, Korea Research Institute of Chemical Technology, Yuseong, Deaejon 305-600, Korea;* [3]*Department of Orthopedics, Catholic University, Medical College, 520-2 Deaheungdong, Jungku, Daejeon 301-723, Korea*

1. INTRODUCTION

It has been recognized that tissue engineering offers an alternative technique to whole organ and tissue transplantation for diseased, failed or malfunctioned organs. To reconstruct new tissues, cells which are harvested and dissociated from the donor tissue including nerve, liver, pancreas, cartilage, and bone, and scaffold substrates which cells are attached and cultured resulting in the implantation at the desired site of the functioning tissue is needed. Recently, the family of poly(Δ-hydroxy acid)s such as polyglycolide (PGA), polylactide (PLA) and its copolymer like poly(lactide-*co*-glycolide) (PLGA) which are among the few synthetic polymers approved for human clinical use by FDA are extensively used or tested for the scaffold materials as a bioerodible material due to good biocompatibility, controllable biodegradability, and relatively good processability.[1] These polymers degrade by nonspecific hydrolytic scission of their ester bonds. The hydrolysis of PLA yields lactic acid which is a normal byproduct of anaerobic metabolism in human body and is corporated in the tricarboxylic acid (TCA) cycle to be finally excreted by the body as carbon dioxide and water. PGA biodegrades by a combination of hydrolytic scission and enzymatic (esterase) action producing glycolic acid which can either enter the TCA cycle or be excreted in urine and be eliminated as carbon dioxide and water. The degradation time of PLGA can be controlled from weeks to over a year by varying the ratio of monomers and the processing conditions.[2] It might be a suitable biomaterial for use in tissue engineered repair systems[3-6] in which cells are implanted within PLGA films or scaffolds and in drug delivery systems[7-8] in which drugs are loaded within PLGA microspheres.

However, it is more desirable to endow with new functionality for the PLA, PGA and PLGA scaffold for the applications of cell and tissue engineering.[3-6] For example, hydrophobic surfaces of PLA, PGA, and PLGA possess high interfacial free energy in aqueous solutions, which tend to unfavorably influence their cell-, tissue- and blood-compatibility in initial stage of contact, so, it might be more favorable to hydrophilic surface resulting in more uniform cell seeding and distribution. Another example, the bioactive materials impregnated scaffolds might be better for the cell proliferation, differentiation, and migration due to the stimulation of cell growing from the sustained release of cytokine molecules such as nerve growth factor and vascular endothelial cell growth factor (VEGF).

One of the significant natural bioactive materials is demineralized bone particle (DBP) which is a powerful inducer of new bone growth. Urist[9] described firstly the sequence of bone induction using demineralized cortical bone matrix and reported that bone morphogenetic protein acts as local mitogen to stimulate proliferation of mesenchymal stem cells.[10] Another natural material is the small intestine submucosa (SIS) powder.[11] Badylak *et al.* described systematically that an acellular resorbable scaffold material derived from the SIS has been shown to be rapidly resorbed, support early and abundant new blood vessel growth, and serve as a template for the constructive remodeling of several body tissue including musculoskeletal structures, skin, body wall, dura mater, urinary bladder and blood vessels. The SIS material consists of naturally occurring extracellular matrix (ECM) that has been shown to be rich in components which support angiogenesis such as fibronectin, glycosaminoglycans including heparin, several collagens including Types I, III, IV, V and VI, and angiogenic growth factors such as basic fibroblast growth factor and VEGF.

Microporous biodegradable polymeric scaffolds impregnated with bioactive materials have been prepared by several techniques including solvent casting/salt leaching, phase separation, solvent evaporation, and emulsion freeze drying method in order to maximize cell seeding, attachment, growth, extracellular matrix production, vascularization and tissue ingrowth.[1,12]

In this study, we developed the novel natural/synthetic composite scaffold like DBP impregnated PLA (DBP/PLA), and SIS impregnated PLA and PLGA (SIS/PLA and SIS/PLGA, respectively) scaffolds for the possibility of the application for tissue engineered bone and cartilage. DBP/PLA and SIS/PLA scaffolds were prepared by solvent casting/salt leaching method, respectively. Scaffolds were characterized by scanning electron microscopy (SEM) and mercury intrusion porosimeter. Also the effect of DBP and SIS on bone formation from the DBP/PLA and SIS/PLA scaffolds was observed by the implantation onto the athymic nude mouse.

2. DBP/PLA SCAFFOLDS FOR THE TISSUE ENGINEERED BONE

In order to endow with new bioactive functionality from DBP as natural source to PLA synthetic biodegradable polymer (molecular weight: 110,000 g/mole, Resomer® L206, Boehringer-Ingelheim, Ingelheim, Germany), porous DBP/PLA as natural/synthetic composite scaffolds were prepared for the possibility of the application of tissue engineered bone and cartilage. It has been recognized that DBP contains many kinds of osteogenic and chondrogenic cytokines as bone morphogenetic protein and widely used as a filling agent for bone defects in clinic due to improved availability through the growing tissue bank industry. Fig. 1 shows the pulverized DBP using freezer mill that the size decreased from 100 ~ 300 µm to 10 ~ 20 µm for the improvement of dispersivity into PLA matrix.

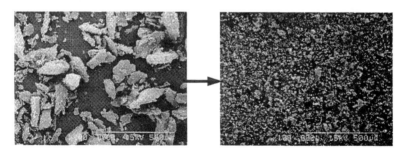

Figure 1. SEM microphotographs before and after pulverized DBP (original magnification; × 100).

SEM microphotographs of DBP/PLA scaffolds with control, 20, 40 and 80% DBP by means of solvent casting/salt leaching method are shown in Fig. 2. 20 w/v% of PLA concentration and 90 w/w% of PLA to ammonium bicarbonate were fixed and then DBP content were varied 20, 40 and 80 w/w% to PLA. All of the surface, cross sections, and sides of DBP/PLA scaffolds were highly porous with good interconnections between pores in which can support the surface of cell growth, proliferation and differentiation. Particularly, a uniform distribution of well interconnected pores from the surface to core region. It can be observed that the pore size was almost same, however, in the order of 81 µm (PLA control) > 76 µm (20% of DBP) > 74 µm (40% of DBP) > 69 µm (80% of DBP). Porosities as well as specific pore areas also were almost same from 97.8 % of PLA control to 94.4 % of 80% DBP and 68.3 m^2/g of PLA control to 62.75 m^2/g of 80% DBP, respectively, even though the amount of DBP increased.

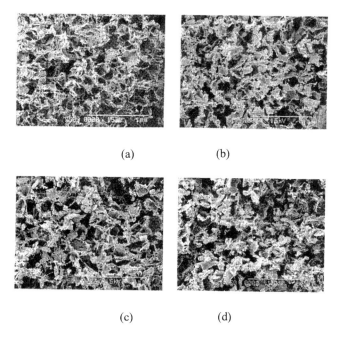

(a)   (b)

(c)   (d)

Figure 2. SEM microphotographs of DBP/PLA scaffolds by means of the solvent casting/salt leaching method (original magnification, × 50); (a) PLA, (b) 20 % DBP, (c) 40 % DBP, and (d) 80 % DBP.

The DBP/PLA scaffolds were utilized to transplant and applied as a template guiding the formation of a bone and cartilage structures from the induction of osteogenesis and chondrogenesis. Scaffolds of PLA alone, DBP/PLA of 40 and 80%, and DBP powder were implanted on the back of athymic nude mouse to observe the effect of DBP on the induction of cell proliferation for 8 weeks. In PLA scaffold (Fig. 3(a)), fibroblast-like cells (f) and vascular capillary (v) were observed between pore interconnection of the undegradaded PLA (l), however, there was no evidence of new bone formation. In DBP powder implants (Fig. 3(b)), we can observe the evidence of calcification (c) around DBP (bp) from the undifferentiated stem cells in the subcutaneous sites and other soft connective tissue sites having a preponderance of stem cells. It might be suggested that bone morphogenetic protein in the DBP stimulates osteogenesis. Urist[9,10] explained by the experiment of subcutaneous implant in allogenic recipients that by day 5, mesenchymal stem cells differentiate, and by day 7 chondroblast developed with osteoblasts appearing at day 9. Angiogenesis ensues around day 11, and this correlates with chondrolysis. New bone formation occurs between 12 and 18 days postimplantation. Finally, ossicle development replete with hematopoietic marrow lineage occurs by day 21.

In DBP/PLA scaffolds of 40 and 80 % DBP (Figs. 3(c) and 3(d), respectively), the evidence of calcified region (c) around DBP (bp) as well as fibroblast-like cells (f) and vascular capillary (v) between pore interconnection of the undegradaded PLA (l) were observed. We conclude that the effect of DBP/PLA scaffolds on bone induction are stronger than PLA scaffolds, even though the bone induction effect of DBP/PLA scaffold might be lowered than only DBP powder, that is to say, in the order of DBP only > DBP/PLA scaffolds of 40 and 80% DBP > PLA scaffolds only for osteoinduction activity. In summary, it seems that DBP plays an important role for bone induction in DBP/PLA scaffolds.

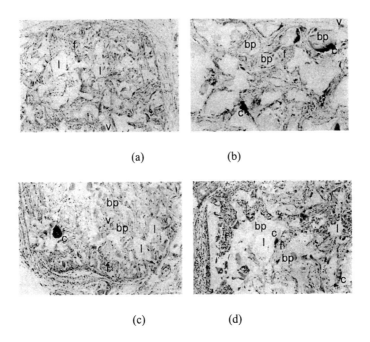

Figure 3. Photomicrographs from H & E histological sections of implanted (a) PLA scaffold, (b) DBP powder, (c) DBP/PLA scaffolds with 40% of DBP, and (d) DBP/PLA scaffolds with 80% of DBP.

3. SIS/PLA SCAFFOLDS FOR THE TISSUE ENGINEERED BONE

In order to endow with new bioactive functionality from SIS as natural source to PLA and PLGA synthetic biodegradable polymer, porous SIS/PLA and SIS/PLGA as natural/synthetic composite scaffolds were prepared for the possibility of the application of tissue engineered bone and cartilage. It has been recognized that SIS contains naturally occurring many kinds of secreted, circulating, and extracellular matrix-bound growth factors as platelet derived growth factor, epidermal growth factor, transforming growth factor, basic fibroblast growth factor and VEGF, and extracellular matrix as fibronectin, glycosaminoglycans including heparin, as well as several collagens including Types I, III, IV, V and VI.[11] Also, SIS was widely used and tested for skin substitutes, a filling matrix for cartilage defects in clinic due to the improvement availability through the commercialization by DePuy and Cook. Fig. 4 shows the pulverized SIS using freezer mill that the size of 10 ~ 20 μm for the enhancement of dispersivity into PLA matrix.

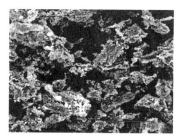

Figure 4. SEM microphotographs after freezer-milled SIS (original magnification; × 100).

SEM microphotographs of SIS/PLA scaffolds with 1:10, 1:12 and 1:14 of the ratio of polymer to SIS by means of solvent casting/salt leaching method are shown in Fig. 5. SIS (0.4 g) and PLA or PLGA (1 g) to ammonium bicarbonate were fixed and then ammonium bicarbonate contents were varied with 10 g (L1), 12 g (L3) and 14 g (L4). All of surface, cross section, and side of SIS/PLA scaffolds were highly porous with good interconnections between pores in which can support the surface of cell growth, proliferation and differentiation. Particularly, it was observed a uniform distribution of well interconnected pores from the surface to core region due to the characteristics of salt leaching method. It can be observed that the pore size was almost same like 175.8 μm for L1, 144.4 μm for L3, and 156.1 μm for L4.

Fig. 6 shows the effect of different salt content on pore size distribution of PLA/SIS scaffolds analysed by mercury porosity meter. It was observed almost same pore size distribution and in the range of 10 μm as the smallest to 450 μm as the largest pore size. Porosities also were almost same around 88 ~ 92%, that is to say, the variation of the salt amount from 10 g to 14 g on the basis of 1 g of PLA did not affect the pore size and pore size distribution.

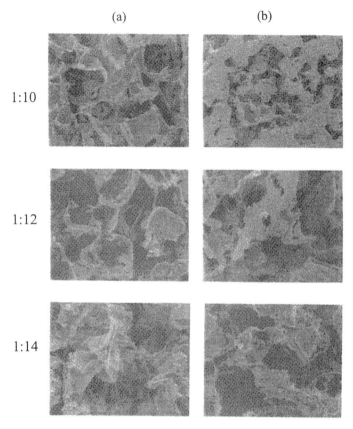

Figure 5. SEM microphotographs of (a) cross section and (b) surface for SIS/PLA scaffolds with different salt contents. (1:10, 1:12 and 1:14 by weight ratio of polymer to salt, respectively) (original magnifications × 100).

Also, we observed that the size distribution of SIS/PLA and SIS/PLGA scaffolds was constantly uniform since the size distribution of a porogen as ammonium bicarbonate was also same resulting in relatively large surface area per volume, higher porosity, almost same interconnective structure between pore, more uniform the pore size and pore size distribution, no change pore size and distribution varied with SIS contents, and less processing variables compared with other preparing methods. The scaffolds fabricated by the solvent casting/salt leaching methods were utilized to transplant and applied as a template guiding the formation of a bone and cartilage structures from the induction of osteogenesis and chondrogenesis by SIS.

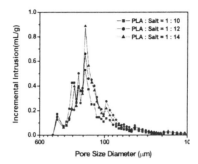

Figure 6. Effect of different salt content on pore size distribution of SIS/PLA scaffolds by means of the solvent casting/salt leaching method.

Fig. 7 shows the wetting property of SIS impregnated PLGA and PLA scaffolds. As shown in figure, the drop of blue dye solution was easily wetted in SIS/PLGA and PLA scaffolds within second due to more hydrophillized surface by collagen SIS powder. From these results, it might be expected more fast penetration of cell culture medium, better uniform cell seeding and distribution, and better cell migration and growth.

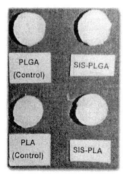 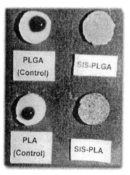

Figure 7. The wetting experiment by the drop of blue dye solution.

Five groups as PGA nonwoven mesh without GA treatment (Fig. 8(a)), PLA scaffold without (Fig. 8(b)) or with GA treatment (Fig. 8(c)), and 0.5:1 SIS/PLA without (Fig. 8(d)) or with GA treatment (Figs. 8(e) and (f)), were implanted on the back of athymic nude mouse to investigate the effect of SIS on the induction of cells proliferation for 8 weeks as shown in Fig. 8 for the each microphotograph of von Kossa staining sections. In PGA scaffold (Fig. 8(a)), the calcified bone stained by von Kossa was observed around PGA scaffolds, however, there was no evidence of new bone formation at the inner part of PGA scaffolds. It might be suggested that the hydrophobicity of PGA nonwoven could not permit to migrate the undifferentiated stem cells at the subcutaneous sites into PGA scaffold resulting in the bone formation of the vicinity of scaffolds. In addition, it was observed that there was no evidence of new bone formation at PLA scaffold without or with GA treatment as shown in Figs. 8(b) and (c) due to no biological activity and functionality of PLA. However, we can observe the evidence of calcification by the bioactivity of SIS/PLA and SIS/PLGA scaffolds from the undifferentiated stem cells in the subcutaneous sites and other soft connective tissue sites[4] having a preponderance of stem cells compared with PLA only and PGA only as shown in Figs. 8(d) and (e) for von Kossa staining and Fig. 8(f) for H and E staining. (Data of SIS/PLGA were not shown.) We can observe the more complete bone formation with GA treated SIS/PLA hybrid scaffold compared with no GA treatment. Possible explanation is the exposure of SIS to GA resulted in significant calcification as well as peri-implant fibrosis due to covalent bonding between collagen molecule by crosslinking reaction. It has been recognized that these peri-implant fibrosis can be altered the healing characteristics of SIS. Advantages of GA treatment for SIS are the reduction of the potential xenogenic and allogenic biomaterials and the improvement of the preserving strength of the devices as well as the controlling resorption time. Badylak et al.[13] have successfully carried out the isolation and the identification of many kinds of secreted, circulating, and extracellular matrix-bound growth factors from SIS. So, it might be explained that these growth factors have significantly affected the critical processes of tissue development and differentiation, that is to say, the osteogenesis and chondrogenesis of the undifferentiated stem cells in the subcutaneous sites and other soft connective tissue sites having a preponderance of stem cells. In summary, it seems that SIS plays an important role for bone and cartilage induction in SIS/PLA scaffolds rather than only synthetic polymer.

4. CONCLUSION

The physical and chemical requirements of ideal scaffolds for cell/tissue ingrowth are[1,12] (i) biocompatibility, (ii) promotion of cell adhesion, (iii) enhancement of cell growth, (iv) retention of differentiated cell function, (v) large surface area per volume, (vi) high porosity to provide adequate space for cell seeding, growth and extracellular matrix production, and (vii) a uniformly distributed and interconnected pore structure. In terms of these requirements of scaffolds, natural/synthetic hybrid scaffolds have positive effects for the differentiation of undifferentiated stem cell for the application of tissue engineering due to the bioactivity of natural biomaterials.

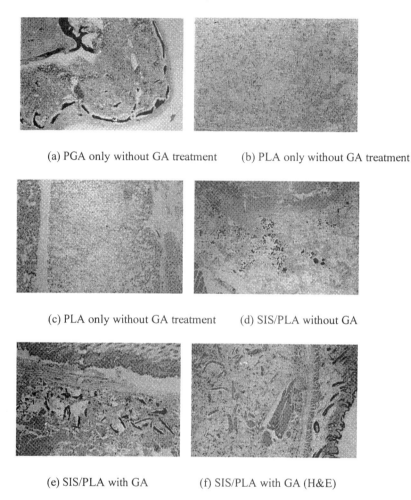

Figure 8. Photomicrographs of von Kossa and H&E histological sections of implanted (a) PGA nonwoven, (b) PLA scaffold only without GA treatment, (c) PLA scaffold only with GA treatment, (d) SIS/PLA scaffold without GA treatment, (e) SIS/PLA scaffold with GA treatment and (f) SIS/PLA scaffold with GA treatment (H&E). (original magnifications × 100).

ACKNOWLEDGEMENTS

This work was supported by a grant from Korea Ministry of Health and Welfare and Ministry of Information and Communication (IMT-2000 Research Program, 01-PJ11-PG9-01NT00-0011).

REFERENCES

1. Khang, G., and Lee, H.B., 2001, Chapter 67, Cell-synthetic surface interaction: Physicochemical surface modification. In *Methods of Tissue Engineering* (A. Atala and R. Lanza, eds.), Academic Press, New York, pp. 771-780.
2. Perrin, D.E., and English, P.E., 1997, Chapter 1, Polyglycolide and polylactide. In *Handbook of Biodegradable Polymers* (A. J. Domb, J. Kost and D. M. Wiseman, eds.), Harwood Academic Publishers, The Netherlands, pp. 3-28.
3. Khang, G., Park, C.S., Rhee, J.M., Lee, S.J., Lee, Y.M., Choi, M.K., and Lee, H.B., 2001, Preparation and characterization of dimineralized bone particle impregnated PLA scaffold. *Macromolecular Research* **9**, 267-276.
4. Khang, G., Shin, P., Kim, I., Lee, B., Lee, S.J., Lee, Y.M., Lee, H.B., and Lee, I., 2002, Preparation and characterization of small intestine submucosa particle impregnated PLA scaffold: The application of tissue engineered bone and cartilage, *Macromolecular Research* **10**, 158-167.
5. Lee S.J., Khang, G., Lee, Y.M., and Lee, H.B., 2002, Interaction of human chondrocyte and fibroblast cell onto chloric acid treated poly(Δ-hydroxy acid) surface, *J. Biomater. Sci., Polym. Ed.*, **13**, 197-212.
6. Khang, G., Choee, C.W., Rhee J.M., and Lee, H.B., 2002, Interaction of different types of cells on physicochemically treated PLGA surface. *J. Appl. Polymer Sci.* **85**, 1253-1262.
7. Choi, H.S., Khang, G., Shin, H.C., Rhee, J.M., and Lee, H.B., 2002, Preparation and characterization of fentanyl-loaded PLGA microspheres; *In vitro* release profiles. *Int. J. Pharm.* **234**, 195-203.
8. Seo, S.A., Choi, H.S., Khang, G., Rhee, J.M., and Lee, H.B., 2002, Characteristics of biodegradable PLGA wafer containing fentanyl. *Int. J. Phar.* **239**, 93-101.
9. Urist, M.R., 1965, Bone: formation by autoinduction, *Science* **150**, 893-899.
10. Mizuno, S., and Glowacki, J., 1996, Three-dimensional composite of demineralised bone powder and collagen for *in vitro* analysis of chondroinduction of human dermal fibroblast, *Biomaterials* **17**, 1819-1825.
11. Badylak, S.F., 1989, Small intestinal submucosa as a large diameter vascular graft in the dog, *J. Surg. Res.* **15**, 678-689.
12. Ishaug S.L., Yasemski, M.J., Bizios, R., and Mikos, A.G., 1994, Osteoblast function on synthetic biodegradable polymers, *J. Biomed. Mater. Res.* **28**, 1445-1453.
13. Voytik-Harvin, S.L., Brightman, A.O., Kraine, M.R., Waisner, B., and Badylak, S.F., 1997, Identification of extractable growth factors from small intestine submucosa. *J. Cell. Biochem.* **67**, 478-491.

POLYHIPE POLYMER: A NOVEL SCAFFOLD FOR *IN VITRO* BONE TISSUE ENGINEERING

Maria Bokhari[1,2], Mark Birch[2], and Galip Akay[1]
[1]*School of Chemical Engineering and Advanced Materials, University of Newcastle, Newcastle upon Tyne, NE1 7RU, U.K.;* [2]*School of Surgical and Reproductive Sciences (Trauma & Orthopaedics), Medical Faculty, University of Newcastle, Newcastle upon TyneNE2 4HH, U.K.*

1. INTRODUCTION

During the past decade exciting new approaches have emerged that could potentially revolutionise the treatment of patients suffering from failure of vital tissues and organs. Tissue engineering is a multidisciplinary field that applies the knowledge of engineering, life sciences, and the clinical sciences to solve the critical medical problems of tissue loss and organ failure. This rapidly expanding area of research is where new materials and techniques are continually being sought. The aim is to produce a biomaterial scaffold that enables the production of tissue that closely matches healthy cellular structures and has good functionality[1].

In the last few years, the use of 3D polymer scaffolds has shown increasing potential for bone tissue regeneration. In particular, they can be designed and fabricated into structures that present increased area for cell anchorage and growth and provide adequate mechanical stability. Bone metabolism is a complex process that involves the resorption of existing bone by osteoclasts and the subsequent formation of a new bone matrix by osteoblasts. These activities are essential for bone remodelling, regeneration and repair. For tissue engineering applications, 3D bone biomaterials must be capable of supporting the functional properties of osteogenic cells. 3D polymeric scaffolds act as shape guidance templates for *in vitro* and *in vivo* tissue development[2].

The major objective of this study is to evaluate the biocompatibility of a new class of micro-cellular polymers known as PolyHIPE polymer, PHP [3] and its ability to support osteoblast growth and differentiation.

2. RESULTS

2.1 Characterisation of PolyHIPE Polymer

PolyHIPE Polymer is a porous material prepared through a high internal phase emulsion (HIPE) polymerisation route. The pore volume can be as high as 97%. As illustrated in Figure 1 PolyHIPE polymers have a highly porous structure in which the pore size (D) and interconnecting hole size (d) can be controlled to obtain average pore and interconnect sizes in the range of $0.5~\mu m \leq D \leq 1000~\mu m$ and $0 \leq d/D \leq 0.5$. Recently, it has been shown that the cell differentiation is pore size dependent when chondrocytes are cultured *in vitro*[3]. In this study two PolyHIPE polymers with different pore sizes were compared. Both polymers had an average porosity of 95%, whilst Polymer A had a median pore diameter of 40 microns and Polymer B, 100 microns. The manufacturing process allows for the size of the pores and the interconnecting holes to be changed independently within certain geometric constraints. The elasticity and phase volume of the microporous polymer can be tailored, while the surface chemistry and characteristics can be modified either during or after polymerisation. In this study the surface of the pore walls of PolyHIPE polymer were coated with hydroxyapatite (10 % wt) in order to make the scaffold more biocompatible and to encourage new bone formation. Energy dispersive x-ray analysis (EDAX) was used to determine the incorporation of hydroxyapatite within polyHIPE polymer (data not shown).

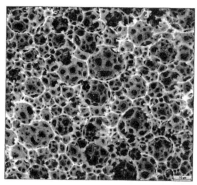

Figure 1. Scanning electron micrograph of PolyHIPE polymer.

2.2 Osteoblast Growth on PolyHIPE

Rat osteoblast cells were cultured on the polymers for 48 hours and then analysed by the spectrophotometric MTT assay using 3-[4,5-dimethylthiazol-2-yl]-2,5-diphenyl tetrazolium bromide (MTT). The dark purple MTT formazan product released by viable cells was measured at a wavelength of 560nm. The differences in the optical densities were used to estimate the number of viable cells. This assay was carried out to ensure that the polymers did not have a toxic effect on the cells. As shown in Figure 2, there was no evidence of cytotoxicity in response to the polymers.

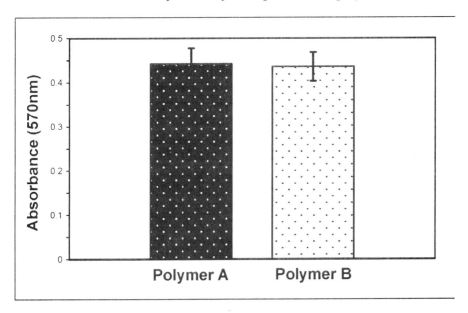

Figure 2. The graph shows the comparison of Rat osteoblast proliferation under the same culture conditions. Error bars= standard deviation of the mean. Students t-test gave p=>0.05.

2.3 *In Vitro* Analysis of the Polymer-Cell Construct

Osteoblasts that were seeded onto Polymers- A and -B attached to the porous surfaces and continued to grow over the 35 day (Figure 3). Osteoblasts grew and penetrated more rapidly in polymer-B (100μm). The osteoblasts were seeded at the same density of 300×10^5 cells/well. Cell penetration within polymer-A (40 μm) was more time dependent. Due to the larger diameter of the pores of polymer-B, cells, when seeded, might have dropped rather than remained on the surface and migrated in a time dependent fashion.

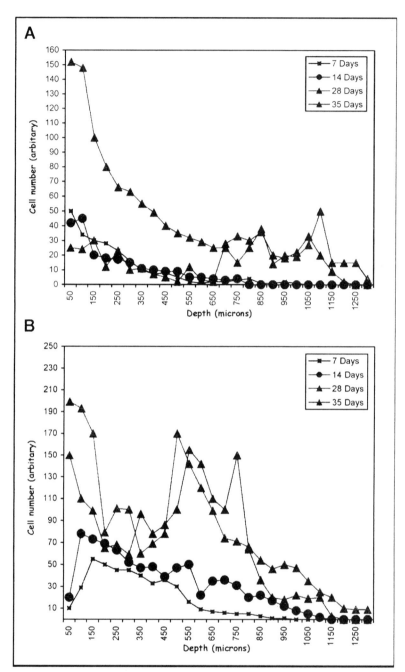

Figure 3. (a) Graph shows cell number in Polymer A against depth during the 35 day time period. (b) Graph shows cell number in Polymer B against depth during the 35 day culture period.

2.4 Investigation of Cell Morphology and Adhesion

Scanning electron microscopy demonstrated the presence of cells on PolyHIPE polymer. Osteoblasts cultured on PolyHIPE showed numerous filopodia which is suggestive that they are specifically interacting with their environment (Figure 4a, below). The osteoblasts demonstrated morphological characteristics associated initially with an anchorage stage, and subsequently with an attachment phase. The osteoblasts contacted the scaffold by means of numerous filopodia and fiber like processes. After 14 days in culture, cells were anchored to the polymer by multiple lamellipodia (Figure 4b). Finally they spread onto the scaffold forming confluent cellular multilayers by day 28 (Figure 4c).

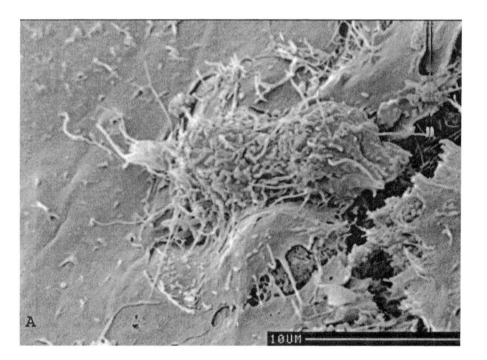

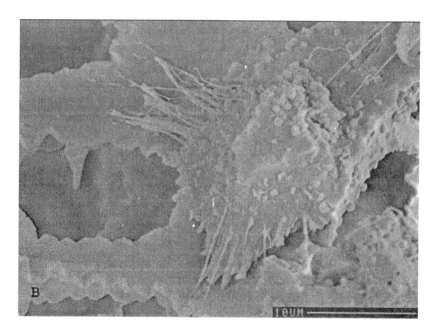

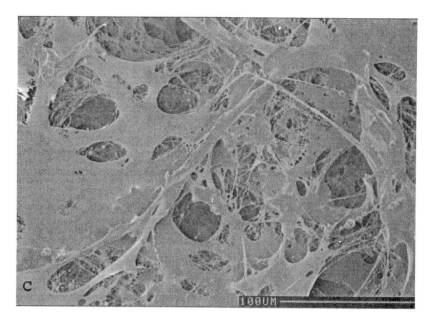

Figure 4. SEM images of osteoblasts cultured on PolyHIPE Polymer. (a) 7 days after seeding, spherical osteoblasts contacting the polymer. (b) after 14 days in culture, cells firmly attached to the polymer by multiple lamellipodia. (c) after 28 days in culture, cells appear to be well spread on the surface of the polymer in a confluent manner.

2.5 Osteoblast Differentiation and Bone Formation *In Vitro*

Bone nodules consist of differentiated osteoblasts, extracellular matrix and related minerals, and their formation characterizes functionally mature osteoblasts[4]. Several lines of evidence suggest that their presence is a good model of osteogenesis[3,4,5]. Figure 5 shows the formation of bone nodules on the scaffold after 35 days in culture.

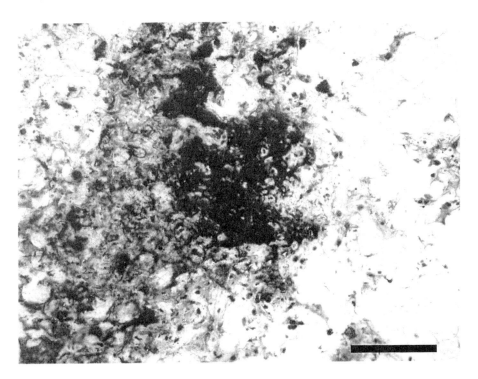

Figure 5. A histological section 7 µm of the surface of PolyHIPE cultured with rat osteoblastic cells for 35 days. Cells were stained with H & E and bone nodules stained with Von Kossa. Long arrow indicates a bone nodule, the short arrow indicates PolyHIPE polymer. The bar represents 0.1mm.

3. CONCLUSION

The ideal biomaterial for bone should be porous to allow cellular ingrowth and new bone formation but for bone also possess mechanical and interlocking properties. We have shown that a microcellular polymer such as PolyHIPE, has the ability to support the growth and mineralization of osteoblast like cells in vitro and previous work has shown this scaffold to have good mechanical properties suited for load bearing tissues[3]. We believe this material is an ideal candidate in the tissue engineering of bone both *in vitro* and *in vivo*.

ACKNOWLEDGEMENTS

This work was funded by Engineering and Physical Sciences Research Council (UK). We would like to thank Brian Mawhinney and Linda Wragg for their technical help.

REFERENCES

1. Risbud, M.V., and Sittinger, M., 2002, Tissue engineering: Advances *in vitro* cartilage generation. *TRENDS in Biotechnology*, **20** (8), 9-14.
2. Honda, M., et al., 2000, Cartilage formation by cultured chondrocytes in a new scaffold made of poly(L-lactide-epsilon-caprolactone) sponge. *J. Oral Maxillofac. Surg.* **58**,767-775.
3. Akay, G., Downes, S., and Price, V.J., 2000, Microcellular polymers as cell growth media and novel polymers. *World Intellectual Property Organization Publication*, WO 00/34454, pp. 53.
4. Beresford, J.N., Graves, S.E., and Smoothy, C.A., 1993, Formation of mineralised nodules by bone derived cells *in vitro*: A model of bone formation. *Am. J. Med.. Genetics,* **45**, 163-178.
5. Malaval, L., Modrowski, D., Gupta, A.K., and Aubin, J.E., 1994, Cellular expression of bone-related proteins during the *in vitro* osteogenesis in rat bone marrow stromal cell cultures. *J. Cell Physiol.* **158**, 555-572.

PANCREATIC ISLET CULTURE AND TRANSPLANTATION USING CHITOSAN AND PLGA SCAFFOLDS

Y. Murat Elçin[1], A. Eser Elçin[1,2], Reinhardt G. Bretzel[3], and Thomas Linn[3]
[1]*Ankara University, Faculty of Science, Tissue Engineering and Biomaterials Laboratory, and Biotechnology Institute, Ankara 06100, Turkey;* [2]*Gazi University, GEF, Biology Division, Ankara 06100, Turkey;* [3]*Medical Clinic and Policlinic III, Justus-Liebig University, Giessen 35392, Germany*

1. INTRODUCTION

Transplantation of pancreatic islets has been a therapeutic approach to cure type I diabetes [1-3]. One of the major obstacles faced during this approach is the rejection of allogeneic islets if they are not immunosuppressed or made tolerant to donor-induced side effects [4,5].

In vitro cultured pancreatic islets can be less immunogenic, probably related to the elimination of passenger leukocytes and other Ia+ (antigen) presenting cells within the isolates [6]. By culturing the islets prior to transplantation, it may be possible to achieve long-term acceptance [7-9]. However, islets cultivated in petri dishes gradually disintegrate in a time-dependent way, presumably related to the free-floating conditions. Under free-floating culture conditions, some islets disperse as single cells, and some others transform into beta cell aggregates, thus adhering to the culture dishes. Due to disintegration and spontaneous dispersion, the retrieval rate of transplanted islets from culture dishes is usually dampened [6,10].

Several studies have shown that immunoisolation of islets using permselective hollow membranes can prevent the rejection following transplantation [11-13], however problems such as, hypoxia (formation of central hypoxemic clusters, necrotic cores) and fibrosis (induced by the release of oxygen radicals and nitric oxide) still exist. Another approach of immunoisolation has been the immobilization of islets within micro- or macrospheres made up of insolubilized viscous hydrogels. By this way, disintegration of islets is usually prevented, but the hypoxia within the devascularized islets, leading to lactacidosis, is still a matter of concern[10].

It seems likely that it is helpful to use some sort of support for islets to be cultured, and further transplanted. Porous and biodegradable polymeric scaffolds represent potential for use in isolated islet studies. The hypothesis is that by using scaffolds, the survival of isolated islets may be achieved if proper cell signalling mechanisms can be triggered. Such open polymeric scaffolds do not immunoisolate the islets, but have a higher potential to guide neovascularization when transplanted. If immunogenic cells are eliminated during *in vitro* culture, there is the possibility that islets can reorganize into neovascularized islet clusters (organoids).

In this study, we have compared the efficiency of two types of polymeric materials to house isolated rat pancreatic islets: (*i*) chitosan ($>$1o 4$\cong$linked 2-amino-2-deoxy-E-D-glucopyranose)-based hydrogel fibers, and (*ii*) macroporous poly (DL-lactide-co-glycolide) (PLGA) scaffolds. The first polymer is a natural polyaminosaccharide having structural similarity to glycosaminoglycans; the second one is a synthetic α-hydroxy acid polymer. Both are known to be relatively biocompatible and are biodegradable, and have been used in many biomedical applications including tissue engineering and drug delivery [14-17]. Our findings demonstrate that isolated rat pancreatic islets on both substrates do survive and respond to glucose stimulation with the return to basal secretion thereafter, for a period of at least three weeks under culture conditions. Islets within the scaffolds maintain some level of insulin activity when transplanted subcutaneously to rats, especially if they are supported by VEGF-induced neovascularization.

2. EXPERIMENTAL PROCEDURES

2.1 Islet Isolation

Islets were isolated from 300-325 g adult male Wistar rats (Charles River Wiga GmbH, Sulzfeld, Germany) by ductal distension and collagenase (1,6-2,0 mg collagenase/ml, activity: 0.9 PZ U/mg; Serva, Heidelberg, Germany) digestion technique, described elsewhere in detail[18]. Islet purification was performed on a discontinuous three-phase density gradient made up of Histopaque (Sigma, St. Louis, USA) and Ficoll (Biocoll™,

Biochrom, Berlin, Germany). The islets were cultured in TCM-199 (with L-glutamine and 5.5 mM glucose; Gibco Europe GmbH, Karlsruhe, Germany) supplemented with heat-inactivated FCS (5%; Biochrom), HEPES (10 mM; Biochrom), penicillin-streptomycin (100 IU/ml and 100 µg/ml, respectively; Biochrom), ciproflaxin (20 µg/ml; Bayer, Leverkusen, Germany) and gentamycin (40 µg/ml; Brahms, Wiesbaden, Germany). Viability of the islets was assessed by MTT (thiazolyl blue, Sigma) and dithizon (Sigma) stainings. The isolation yield routinely averaged 500±120 islets/rat.

2.2 Scaffolds

2.2.1 Chitosan fibers

Preparation of the chitosan fibers are explained elsewhere in detail[15,16]. Briefly, 2% (w/v) chitosan ([1→4] linked 2-amino-2-deoxy-β-D-glucopyranose) chloride (viscosity= 72 mPa, deacetylation= 95%, Protasan CL 214, Pronova, Oslo, Norway) solution was blended with 2% (w/v) albumin (fraction V, bovine origin, Sigma) in 7:3 ratio, to improve porosity and surface roughness of the resulting hydrogel. Then, this mixture was extruded with a high flow rate into an alkaline solution consisting of 0.5 M NaOH and methanol through a 25 G syringe. The formed hydrogel fibers were allowed to stabilize in the solution for 30 minutes, then successively washed with deionized water and ethanol, and molded into plastic rings to form cylinders (height=8 mm, ϕ=5 mm). The molded fibers were exposed overnight to UV for sterilization and kept at 4°C until islet seeding.

2.2.2 PLGA sponges

Macroporous PLGA sponges were fabricated by a solvent casting and particulate leaching technique described elsewhere[19]. Briefly, the raw copolymer with a MW distribution of 90,000-126,000 (85:15, Sigma) in dichloromethane (10%; w:v) was loaded into a mold packed with NaCl particles sieved to a size between 250-400 µm. The solvent was allowed to evaporate; residual solvent was removed by vacuum drying for an additional 24 h. Dry polymer/salt sponges were then placed into distilled deionized water for 48 h to leach out salt particles with water changes at every 6 h. The sponges were then dried in a vacuum oven and cut with a cork borer into cylinders (ϕ=6 mm, height=4 mm). To improve the hydrophilicity, the sponges were coated with 1% (w/v) poly(vinyl alcohol) solution (MW= 10.000, Sigma). Then, they were stored under nitrogen atmosphere over anhydrous $CaSO_4$ at 4°C until use. The sponges were UV-sterilized, prior to islet seeding.

2.3 Islet Seeding and Culture

Sterile polymer scaffolds were prewetted in culture medium containing 5% FCS (37°C) for 30 min prior to cell seeding. Hundred islets of ca. 150 µm-size were hand-picked under a dissecting microscope and transferred into prewetted scaffolds placed in 35 mm-culture dishes using a microsyringe. After 30 min, 2 mL of TCM-199 medium was added carefully into each dish. Islet-polymer costructs were maintained in the medium at 37°C, 90% humidity, 5% CO_2 / 95% air, with daily medium changes for 3 weeks. The medium was routinely checked for detached islets.

2.4 Functional Tests

Static incubation of islets at different glucose concentrations was performed to evaluate islet response to glucose. On Days 7/8/9 and 14/15/16, insulin secretion was assessed. Briefly, the bioartificial constructs containing 100 islets were incubated at 37°C for 24 h in 2 ml complete TCM-199 medium containing 5.5 mM glucose, then 24 h in 2 ml complete medium containing 16.5 mM glucose, and then 24 h in 2 ml medium containing 5.5 mM glucose again. The amount of insulin released into the culture medium was assayed using an ELISA developed for rat insulin (Mercodia, Sweden). Medium was daily checked for any displaced islet and substracted from the initial islet number. Insulin secretion of islets under standard culture conditions was also determined (controls). When the medium was exchanged, waste medium was collected as sample for a period of 3 wk. The insulin secretion data were calculated as µU per 24 h per islet and expressed as means±SD. Data analysis were performed with Microsoft Excel.

2.5 Transplantation

Islet-polymer constructs were subcutaneously transplanted into rat epigastric groin fascia after 24-48 h of culture (n=18). Some of the transplantation sites had previously been neovascularized by VEGF (1 µg)-activated polymers[15]. At set time points, the constructs were removed and evaluated by histology and insulin extraction from the explants.

2.6 Insulin Extraction

The explants were kept frozen at –20°C, until use. For processing, the samples were repeatedly minced and frozen in liquid nitrogen, placed in acid-alcohol/IRI buffer and centrifuged. The supernatant was analysed for insulin using ELISA (Mercodia).

2.7 Histology

For light microscopy, islet-chitosan samples were fixed in Bouin's solution and the paraffin sections were stained with H&E. Islet-PLGA samples were cryo-fixed and sectioned before H&E staining. Viability of the islets was also assessed by staining the islets with MTT (thiazolyl blue, Sigma) and dithizon (Sigma). Islets cultured without using scaffolds served as the controls.

3. RESULTS AND DISCUSSION

The number of detached islets from both of the polymer scaffolds was very low (<5%). Hematoxyline & eosin, MTT- and dithizon-stainings showed that the islets on both substrates survived for the duration of *in vitro* experiments, while chitosan was found to provide a better environment for islets (Figures 1 and 2; *islet-PLGA photos not given*). Chitosan has structural similarity to glycosaminoglycans. Findings indicate that glycosaminoglycans are involved in the modulation of cell attachment, differentiation and morphogenesis[15,17]. Chitosan forms hydrogels with good properties for the controlled release of macromolecules (*e.g.* growth factors)[15,17]. PLGA is a hydrophobic polymer; however, permits the easy construction of macroporous scaffolds with controlled pore size that have better mechanical properties, compared to chitosan hydrogels. On the other hand, the control group (floating islets) showed a faster decrease in viability, compared with the islets on scaffolds, for the duration of experiments.

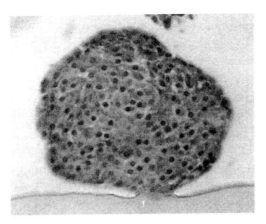

Figure 1. A representative micrograph showing hematoxylin-eosin stained rat pancreatic islet on chitosan scaffold after 24 h in culture. Chitosan scaffold can be seen at the bottom of the image.

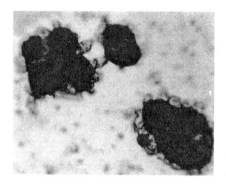 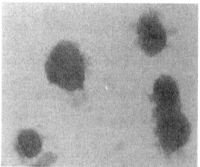

Figure 2. MTT- (left) and dithizone- (right) stained rat pancreatic islets on chitosan scaffold after 2 weeks in culture.

Functional tests showed that the islets on polymer supports responded to glucose stimulation with the return to basal secretion (Figure 3). At low glucose concentration (5.5 mmol/l) insulin release from islet-chitosan (IC) and islet-PLGA (IP) constructs were 3.69 ± 0.47 and 3.02 ± 0.57 µU/ml/h/islet at day 7, and 3.43 ± 1.61 and 2.91 ± 1.30 µU/ml/h/islet at day 14, respectively. At high glucose concentration (16.5 mmol/l) insulin release was 6.14 ± 1.25 and 5.25 ± 0.81 µU/ml/h/islet at day 8, and 6.97 ± 1.29 and 4.37 ± 1.82 µU/ml/h/islet at day 15, from IC and IP, respectively. A prompt decrease in insulin release was observed at days 9 and 16, when the islets were returned back to low glucose concentration (4.42 ± 0.88 and 3.07 ± 0.83 µU/ml/h/islet at day 9, and 3.59 ± 0.47 and 2.18 ± 1.14 µU/ml/h/islet at day 16, respectively for IC and IP) (Figure 3). The control group (floating islets) responded to glucose stimulation performed at Days 7/8/9; however, the response at Days 14/15/16 was very low compared with that of islets on scaffolds (Figure 3; compare A with B and C). It seems likely that by housing the islets on polymer scaffolds, an upregulation of glucose response has been achieved, *in vitro*.

Histological analysis of transplanted islets on scaffolds showed a disintegration into single cells in time (Figure 4). The disintegration of the explants that were neovascularized with VEGF was slower than the explants that did not receive VEGF (Figure 4, left and right images).

Isolation procedure disrupts islets from surrounding tissues. Complete re-vascularization of transplanted islets needs a certain period of time. Until re-vascularization, islets depend on diffusion for oxygen and nutrient supply. However, insulin extraction data exhibited that the grafts still contained some insulin activity after 3 weeks of transplantation, especially in VEGF-treated group (Table 1).

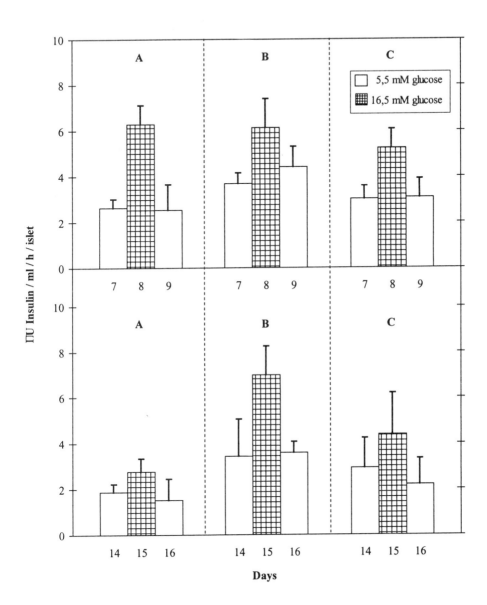

Figure 3. Static glucose challenge of cultured rat pancreatic islets on polymer scaffolds at Days 7/8/9 and 14/15/16. A: Control group (floating islets); B: Islets on chitosan scaffolds; C: Islets on PLGA scaffold.

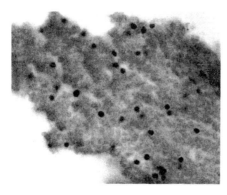 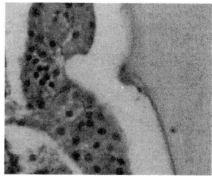

Figure 4. Light micrographs showing islet-chitosan constructs at one week-post transplantation. Left: Explant that did not receive any VEGF-neovascularization support; Right: Explant supported with VEGF-neovascularization. Note the disintegration level of the islet shown at the left panel is higher than that of the islet shown at the right panel.

Table 1. Insulin Extraction Data of Rat Pancreatic Islet-Polymer Constructs Explanted from Rat Subcutaneous Tissue

	VEGF	Day 3	Day 7	Day 14	Day 21
Islets-Chitosan	(-)	NA	9.41	NA	NA
	(+)	NA	19.5	25.9	NA
Islets-PLGA	(-)	0.63	NA	0.97	NA
	(+)	3.18	NA	8.55	7.78

Explants minced and frozen repeatedly in liquid nitrogen, transferred to acid-alcohol/IRI buffer and centrifuged; supernatants analysed using ELISA for rat insulin (pg/ml/islet). VEGF (-): transplantation to subjects without neovascularization; VEGF (+): transplantation to subjects with 1 μg/ml VEGF-induced neovascularization. NA: data not available.

4. CONCLUSION

Biodegradable polymer scaffolds can be used as solid supports to maintain a suitable three-dimensional environment for rat islets *in vitro*. Compared to controls (floating islets in culture), islets on both polymer scaffolds had a longer-term response to *in vitro* glucose stimulation, including a return to basal secretion after the glucose stimulus was discontinued. *In vivo* studies demonstrated that islet-chitosan constructs were able to retain a low, but some level of insulin activity if they were supported by recombinant VEGF-induced neovascularization. Additionally, a short-term immuno-suppression may be useful to increase the graft viability. Finally, further studies including the transplantation of higher number of islets to diabetic animals needs to be tested to show the practical applicability of the given islet-scaffold systems, *in vivo*. Such studies are currently ongoing in our laboratory.

ACKNOWLEDGEMENTS

Y. Murat Elçin, Ph.D., acknowledges the support of Ankara University Biotechnology Institute, and the Turkish Academy of Sciences (EA-TÜBA-GEBİP/2001-1-1), Ankara, Turkey.

REFERENCES

1. Bretzel, R.G., Hering, B.J., Eckhard, M., Ernst, W., Friemann, S., Padberg, W., Weimar, B., Brandhorst, H., Brandhorst, D., Federlin, K., and Brendel, M.D., 1997, Simultaneous and after kidney transplantation of islets of Langerhans at Giessen University in patients with insulin-dependent diabetes mellitus (IDDM): A one-year follow up study. *Acta Diabetol* **34**, 121.
2. Hering, B.J., Schultz, A.O., Geier, C., Bretzel, R.G., and Federlin, K., 1996, Newsletter No.7, International Islet Transplant Registry, Dept. Medicine, JLU, Giessen.
3. Kendall, D.M., and Robertson, R.P., 1996, Pancreas and islet transplantation in humans. *Diabetes Metab* **22**, 157-163.
4. Lanza, R.P., Sullivan, S.J., and Chick, W.L., 1992, Perspectives in diabetes: Islet transplantation with immunoisolation. *Diabetes* **41**, 1503-1510.
5. Barrou, B., Sylla, C., Suberbielle, C., Autran, B., Debre, P., and Bitker, M.O., 1996, Pancreatic islet transplantation: isolation techniques and *in vitro* immunomodulation. *Prog Urol* **6**(6), 871-877.
6. Chao, S.H., Peshwa, M.V., Sutherland, D.E.R., and Hu, W-S., 1992, Entrapment of cultured pancreas islets in three-dimensional collagen matrices. *Cell Transplantation* **1**, 51-60.
7. Bowen, K.M., and Lfferty, K.J., 1980, Reversal of diabetes by allogenic islet transplantation without immunosuppression. *Aust J Exp Biol Med* **58**, 441-449.
8. Keddinger, M.F., Haffen, K., Greiner, S., and Eloy, R., 1977, *In vitro* culture reduces immunogenicity of pancreatic islets. *Nature* **270**, 736-737.
9. Lacy, P.E., Davie, J.M., and Finke, E.H., 1979, Prolongation of islet allograft survival following *in vitro* culture (24°C) and single injection of ALS. *Science* **204**, 312-313.
10. Velten, F., Laue, C., and Schrezenmeir, J., 1999, The effect of alginate and hyaluronate on the viability and function of immunoisolated neonatal rat islets. *Biomaterials* **20**, 2161-2167.

11. Lanza, R.P., Hayes, J.L., and Chick, W.L., 1996, Encapsulated cell technology. *Nat Biotechnol* **14**, 1107-1111.
12. Suzuki, K., Bonner-Weir, S., Trivedi, N., Yoon, K.H., Hollister-Lock, J., Colton, C.K., and Weir, G.C., 1998, Function and survival of macroencapsulated syngeneic islets transplanted into streptozocin-diabetic mice. *Transplantation* **66**, 21-28.
13. Kroencke, K.D., Kolb-Bachofen, V., Berschick, B., Burkart, V., and Kolb, H., 1991, Activated macrophages kill pancreatic syngenic islet cells via arginine-dependent nitric oxide generation. *Biochem Biophys Res Com* **175**, 752-758.
14. Elçin, Y.M., Dixit, V., and Gitnick, G., 1998, Hepatocyte attachment on modified chitosan membranes: In vitro evaluation for the development of liver organoids. *Artif Organs* **22**, 837-846.
15. Elçin, Y.M., Dixit, V., Lewin K., and Gitnick, G., 1999, Xenotransplantation of fetal porcine hepatocytes in rats using a tissue engineering approach. *Artif Organs* **23**(2), 146-152.
16. Elçin, A.E., Elçin, Y.M., and Pappas, G.D., 1998, Neural tissue engineering: adrenal chromaffin cell attachment and viability on chitosan scaffolds. *Neurol Res* **20**, 648-654.
17. Elçin, Y.M., Dixit, V., and Gitnick, G., 1996, Controlled release of endothelial cell growth factor from chitosan-albumin microspheres for localized angiogenesis: *in vitro* and *in vivo* studies, *Art Cells, Blood Subs and Biotechnol* **24**(3), 257-271.
18. Linn, T., Romann, D., Voges, S., and Federlin, K., 1992, Abdominal testis transplantation prevents rejection of islet allografts in low dose streptozotocin induced diabetes. *Transplantion Proceedings* **24**, 998-1003.
19. Mikos, A.G., Thorsen, A.J., Czerwonka, L.A., Bao, Y., and Langer, R., 1994, Preparation and chracterization of poly (L-lactic acid) foams. *Polymer* **35**, 1068-1077.

CHALLENGES AND PROSPECTS FOR TARGETED TRANSGENESIS IN LIVESTOCK
Practical Applications of Gene Targeting

Margarita M. Marques*†, Alison J. Thomson†, and Jim McWhir
Department of Gene Expression and Development, Roslin Institute, Roslin, Midlothian, Scotland EH 25 9PS, U.K.

1. INTRODUCTION

Until recently the only ways of making transgenic livestock were by pronuclear injection or, more controversially, by sperm mediated DNA transfer. Both techniques usually result in multiple copies of the transgene at a random site within the genome. This is associated with unpredictable transgene expression often due to gene silencing. In the mouse, this problem has been addressed by directing single copy transgenes to particular sites in the genome[1,2] (gene targeting). This has been possible because of the availability, in that species, of embryo-derived stem cells (ES cells)[3] which can be modified *in vitro* and then used to create transgenic mice. Despite considerable research effort, however, ES cells are not available for any livestock species. ES-like cells have been derived from sheep, pigs and cattle that can contribute to the formation of chimaeras but they do not contribute to the germline (reviewed by McWhir[4]).

Cloning livestock by nuclear transfer from somatic cells[5] has allowed the development of gene targeting. The key steps in producing a targeted farm animal are depicted in Fig. 1. First, it is necessary to generate a DNA

---

* Current address: Instituto de Desarrollo Ganadero. Universidad de León, León, España.
† These two authors contributed equally to this work.

construct, comprising a selectable marker gene flanked by regions of homology to the target locus. This 'targeting vector' is transfected into the cells, frequently by electroporation. After selecting for cells that have integrated the construct (either by homologous recombination or more frequently by random integration), a screen must be carried out to identify the targeted clones. Finally, cultured somatic cells carrying the desired genetic modifications are used as nuclear donors in cloning experiments.

Initial interest in animal cloning was linked to the production of large numbers of genetically superior livestock. However, gene targeting has also opened up the possibility of introducing targeted genetic changes into livestock to engineer biomedically useful animals. For example, genes involved in immune-rejection have been disrupted by gene targeting to generate livestock whose organs may eventually prove to be protected from hyperacute rejection following transplantation into patients[6,7].

In the longer term, targeted transgenesis may be used to manipulate desirable agricultural traits related to growth rate, meat or wool production, reproduction, etc. However, such applications relate to the production of low value commodities and will depend upon improvement in the efficiency of production of transgenic animals. Biomedical applications are likely to be taken up far more rapidly.

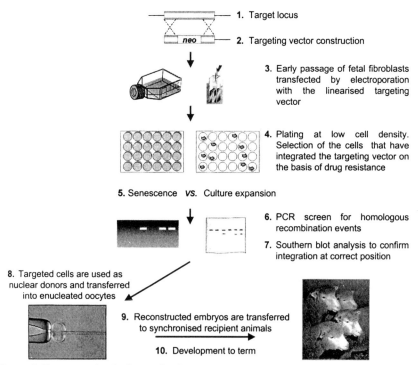

Figure 1. Gene targeting in farm animals.

2. PROSPECTS

2.1 Using Animals as "Bioreactors" to Produce Pharmaceutical Proteins

One of the most promising applications of transgenic animals is large-scale, low cost production of therapeutically relevant proteins and peptides in the body fluids such as milk and blood. The production of transgenic proteins in animals has been successfully achieved for many therapeutic proteins including growth hormone[8], lactoferrin[9], erythropoietin[10] and Insulin-like growth factor 1[11]. PPL Therapeutics have expressed human alpha-1-antitrypsin (hAAT) in the milk of transgenic sheep[12] at levels sufficient for large-scale production. Indeed recombinant hAAT has been purified from these sheep and has been used in Phase II Clinical trials for the treatment of hereditary emphysema (alpha-1-antitrypsin deficiency) and cystic fibrosis. In another example transgenic pigs have been engineered to express human haemoglobin in their blood for use in producing blood substitutes[13]. More recently, Kuroiwa and colleagues reported the generation of cloned calves that produce human immunoglobulins in their blood[14]. Such work leads the way to generating animals with a humanised immune system that, upon immunisation, produce human antibodies to treat diseases or infections. For example, tumour-specific antigens could be used to raise antibodies against cancers.

The transgenic approaches discussed above involved random integration of the transgene at an unknown chromosomal location. As the position of integration of a transgene strongly influences the observed level of expression[15], many of the transgenic lines generated do not produce sufficient amounts of the transgenic protein, making it necessary to screen several lines for appropriate levels of expression. This is a serious consideration when producing transgenic livestock since the relatively long generation length makes the process both expensive and time consuming. Gene targeting allows the precise placement of a transgene at a selected chromosomal location that is predicted to provide reliable high level expression of the transgene – the so called 'knock-in' approach. Encouraging preliminary data for this approach has been obtained from the first lambs generated from targeted cells. In this experiment a transgene, containing the hAAT cDNA inserted into the first exon of the ovine β-lactoglobulin (*BLG*) gene, was targeted to the ovine alpha1(I) procollagen gene (*COL1A1*)[16]. When one of the lambs was induced to lactate, hAAT protein was detected in the milk at higher levels than previously observed with sheep carrying multiple copies of the same transgene randomly integrated[17].

Another advantage of the knock-in approach is that it can be used to place a transgene under the control of an endogenous promoter of a tissue-specific gene. For example, placing transgenes at a milk protein locus, to provide high level, mammary-specific transgene expression. The primary advantage is that all of the controlling elements necessary for appropriate expression need not be characterized, as these are provided by the recombination event. This approach may get round the problem of "leaky" inappropriate expression that has been reported for some transgenic animals containing randomly integrated transgenes[18]. Inappropriate expression of transgenes is undesirable as it may, depending on the protein, lead to adverse health effects on the animals. Targeting the transgene to a mammary-specific gene, such that integration brings it under the control of the endogenous promoter might reasonably be expected to provide tighter tissue-specific regulation. Finally, as there is a limit to the amount of total protein that can be secreted into the milk, knocking out expression of one of the milk protein genes will be advantageous for "making room" for more of the pharmaceutical protein. For example, E-casein deficient mice are perfectly healthy suggesting that the loss of this milk protein is unlikely to debilitate the animal[19]. In addition to the production of pharmaceuticals in milk, targeted transgenesis can also be used to modify the industrial or nutritional properties of milk[20] (see Fig. 2).

2.2 Generation of Disease Resistant Livestock

Disease is a major factor limiting livestock productivity. Improving disease resistance by transgenic means will not only be of benefit in terms of animal welfare, but will also be of great economic importance. In addition, it will contribute to achieving guaranteed quality of disease-free animal products for human use.

As reviewed by Müller and Brem[21], transgenic disease-resistance strategies include the modification of genes known to modulate immune response, the introduction into the genome of specific resistance genes, and the targeted disruption of genes causing disease. One of the best examples of the latter strategy is the inactivation of the prion protein gene PrP, directly linked to spongiform encephalopathies. The experiments performed with knock-out mice[22] showed that animals lacking PrP were resistant to infection, and remained free of the symptoms of disease after inoculation with mouse scrapie prions. Thus, the removal of this gene in sheep may result in animals resistant to scrapie without detrimental side effects. A cautionary warning, however, is provided by data in knock-out mice that suggest an association with changes in sleep and learning behaviour[23,24]. Targeted disruption of the PrP gene in cultured sheep fetal fibroblasts has been reported[25]. However, the majority of targeted clones were either a mixture of targeted and non-targeted cells or senescent. From the four live-born lambs, three died soon after birth and the other survived for only 12 days.

Transgenesis may be useful in enhancing resistance to mastitis, the most prevalent infection of dairy cattle. In this case livestock would be engineered that expressed antibacterial proteins in the mammary gland. Preliminary work carried out with mice demonstrated antibacterial activity in the milk of animals engineered to produce human lysozyme[26]. Kerr and colleagues[27] showed that transgenic production of lysostaphin by the lactating mammary gland confers substantial resistance to experimental challenge with *Staphylococcus aureus*.

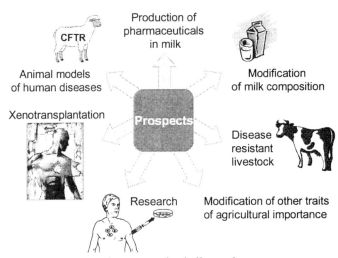

Figure 2. Potential applications of gene targeting in livestock.

2.3 Development of Animal Models for Human Diseases

Many mouse models of human disease have been generated using gene targeting in ES cells and these have been of great scientific value. However, in many cases livestock would make a better model system as they are closer to humans in size and physiology. Mouse models of the disease cystic fibrosis are a case in point. This disease is caused by mutations in the cystic fibrosis transmembrane conductance regulator gene. The most common human mutation is at amino acid position 508. In the mouse, introduction of this mutation by gene targeting does not produce the lung disease exhibited in patients[28] and it has been argued that a sheep model would more closely mimic the human pathology, due to similar lung physiology and longer life span[29].

2.4 Xenotransplantation

The severe shortage of human organs for transplantation has generated great interest in cross-species transplantation (xenotransplantation). The use of animals as organ donors has been the subject of intense debate for both ethical and safety reasons. The ethical debate is centred upon the morality of modifying animals to meet human needs, though arguably this is no different from conventional animal breeding. The safety issues are associated with porcine endogenous retroviruses (PERVs) which have been shown to recombine with human viruses when cocultured with human cells[30].

Pigs have been the focus of research in xenotransplatnation mainly because of their compatible size and physiology. However, the application of xenotransplantation has been blocked by severe immunological barriers[31]. The main barrier occurs at the interface of the pig organ and the human blood supply, triggering hyperacute rejection of the graft. The key xenoantigen is the carbohydrate galactose-Δ-1,3-galactose or Δ-gal epitope[32], expressed on the surface of almost all mammalian cells. Synthesis of Δ-gal is catalysed by the enzyme Δ(1,3)galactosyltransferase (*GGTA1* gene). Old World monkeys, apes and humans lack this enzyme and consequently the Δ-gal epitope. However, they produce large amounts of natural antibody in response to continuous antigenic stimulation by gastrointestinal bacteria.

A first attempt to inactivate the *GGTA1* gene by homologous recombination was carried out successfully in sheep fibroblasts in culture[25]. At the beginning of 2002, three independent groups[6,7,33] published the successful generation of targeted pig cells, with live piglets being born in the first two cases. Recently, PPL Therapeutics have announced the production of the world's first double gene knock-out piglets at the GGTA1 locus, demonstrating an encouraging step towards solving the problem of the waiting lists for transplants. Indeed, the same approach has been tried in knock-out mice[34] and cells from these animals have shown a reduced binding to, and activation of, human serum. However, this is not the complete answer and additional problems of acute rejection remain unsolved. After bypassing hyperacute rejection, there is still the obstacle of acute vascular rejection. In this case, the anti-donor antibodies are not directed exclusively against the Δ-Gal epitope and the involvement of the complement system is far more subtle[35].

3. CHALLENGES

3.1 Overcoming Senescence

Since the work of Hayflick and colleagues in the 1960s[36], it has been known that normal somatic cells propagated in culture withdraw from the cell cycle after a finite number of divisions and enter an irreversible arrest designated replicative senescence. Studies performed with sheep foetal fibroblasts[37] have set this number between 40 and 120 divisions. From the physiological point of view, senescence seems to be correlated with a block in the cell cycle in late G1 phase near the G1/S boundary[38]. Phenotypically, cells become enlarged, acquire a flattened and irregular shape (see Fig. 3) and show an increased cytoplasmic granularity. Changes in ultrastructural characteristics and molecular marker expression[39,40] have also been described.

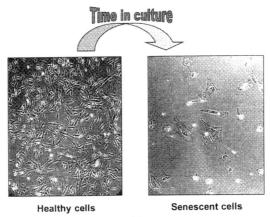

Healthy cells   **Senescent cells**

Figure 3. Cell morphology of ovine fetal fibroblasts.

The triggering of senescence appears to be linked to telomere length. Telomeres are the ends of chromosomes and comprise repeat DNA sequences and associated proteins. The maintenance of telomere length requires expression of the telomerase gene. As most cultured somatic cell types have little to no detectable levels of telomerase activity, telomeres get shortened after each population doubling. Eventually, when the telomeres become critically short, the cells stop dividing. Currently, a question of major interest is the extent to which replicative senescence in culture provides insights about senescence *in vivo*[41,42].

What is the importance of senescence for extending the scope of applications for gene targeting in livestock?. Gene targeting involves a series of *in vitro* manipulations (Fig.1) during the course of which, cells can senesce, possibly compromising their capability as nuclear donors. However, nuclear transfer studies performed with cells subjected to long-term culture[43] (up to 445 population doublings) showed that cells could be competent for nuclear transfer after many passages. However, an associated challenge is to identify clones in which homologous recombination has taken place before the cells stop dividing. This becomes a crucial point when considering that the cells have to grow (for ovine fibroblasts) at least up to a confluent 25cm^2-flask in order to get enough genomic DNA for Southern blot analysis.

Several options have been proposed to avoid or retard the appearance of senescence. As senescence may be associated with a reaction of the cells to a stressful environment in culture, the first obvious way to deal with this problem is to reduce the stress associated with "*in vitro*" manipulations. A dilution plating targeting protocol to get an average of 1-3 clones per well of a series of 24 well plates (see Fig.1) has proved successful in our hands[44]. Unlike ring cloning methods, this procedure has the advantage that clones remain vigorous and can provide sufficient DNA for Southern blot analysis. It has the disadvantage, however, that some of the resulting clones are mixed and candidate targeted clones may also contain non-targeted cells.

Forced expression of the human telomerase catalytic protein subunit (hTERT) may be one solution to this problem[45,46]. Recent studies in sheep fibroblasts[47] have shown that stable transfection with hTERT, reconstituted telomerase activity and extended the proliferative lifespan of these cells. Another possibility is what has been called "rejuvenating" the fibroblasts through nuclear transfer[48]. This involves the use of cells close to senescence as nuclear donors, followed by recovering the resulting foetuses and isolating new fibroblast cell lines. This possibility may enable consecutive rounds of targeting.

Perhaps the ideal solution to the problem of senescence would be the isolation in farm animal species of cells in which the telomerase gene is already active and which do not normally senesce - ES cells. The increase in our knowledge of ES cell isolation, particularly after the characterisation of human ES cells, has produced a renewed interest in isolating ES cells from livestock. The development of nuclear transfer from somatic cells has not entirely eliminated interest in establishing ES cells in farm animals. Irrespective of their potential for generating chimaeras, their greatest value may be for use as nuclear donor cells in nuclear transfer.

3.2 Enrichment for Targeted Events in Somatic Cells

Homologous recombination is a rare phenomenon in mammalian cells. As the frequency of homologous recombination events is far lower than for random integration, methods to enrich for the desired events have been developed. To date, only genes that are transcriptionally active in nuclear donor cells have been successfully modified by gene targeting in farm animals[6,7,16,25,33]. Targeting a transcriptionally active gene offers the advantage of using an enrichment method referred to as the promoter trap (*PT*) strategy. *PT* targeting vectors (represented in Fig. 4A) are designed to use the transcriptional activity of the endogenous target promoter to drive the expression of a positive selectable cassette[49]. Hence, the *PT* vector contains a promoterless selectable cassette, for example a *neo* gene (conferring resistance to the neomycin analogue G-418), which either splices into the 5′untranslated region of the target gene or generates a fusion protein. Following transfection with the targeting vector and selection with G418, cells that survive are those in which the selectable cassette acquires an active promoter by homologous recombination into the target locus. The majority of random integrations will be silent and the resistance gene will not be expressed (unless the vector integrates fortuitously by random insertion close to a promoter that allows sufficient expression to generate drug-resistance). A promoter trap enrichment procedure is not possible with a non-expressed gene and the high background of random integrants complicates significantly the identification of the targeted clones.

To address the question of whether a non-promoter trap vector can be used for successful gene targeting in somatic cells, we compared the efficiency of the promoter trap (*PT*) and non-promoter trap (*NPT*) strategies to target the ovine *COL1A1* gene. For this purpose, the promoterless-*neo* targeting vector[16], as well as the fetal fibroblast line PDFF2 previously used in nuclear transfer, were obtained from PPL Therapeutics. As displayed in Fig. 4B, the targeting vector was modified by introduction of a second selectable cassette (blasticidin resistance gene driven by SV40 viral promoter) and was electroporated into PDFF2 cells. Transfected cells were subjected to dilution plating in 24-well plates (10^3 cells/well; see Fig. 4C), and treated 48 hours after transfection, either with G418 (*PT*) or blasticidin (*NPT*). PCR screen and Southern blot analysis shown in Fig. 4C confirmed the presence of targeted cells with both strategies, indicating that, at least at an expressed locus, gene targeting may be achieved without a promoter trap[50]. Harrison *et al.*[34] have reported successful gene targeting at the porcine *GGTA1* gene using a non-promoter trap strategy, although in this case, enrichment by positive-negative selection was applied.

3.3 Targeting Non-Expressed Genes

Using similar protocols we have also performed experiments to target a transgene to the milk protein gene *β-casein*.

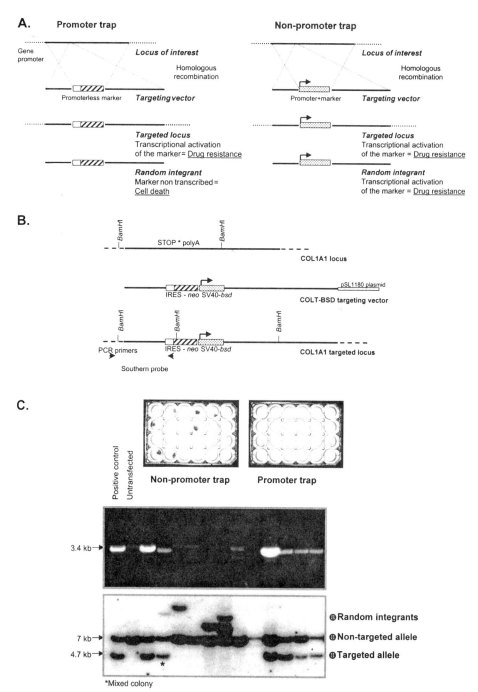

Figure 4. Comparison of promoter trap and non-promoter trap strategies to target the ovine *COL1A1* locus.

As the β-casein gene is inactive in the ovine fetal fibroblasts used, we employed a non-promoter trap strategy and screened over 700 colonies. Although an initial PCR screen identified candidate targeted clones, none of these were confirmed by Southern Blot analysis[51]. It is likely that the original clones were a mixture of targeted and non-targeted cells[25,50] and that the non-targeted cells had a growth advantage. One possible explanation for this growth advantage is that the chromatin structure at the inactive β-casein gene locus may have prevented long-term expression of the drug resistance gene. Hence the targeted cells, lacking drug resistance, either senescenced or died leaving the non-targeted cells to take over the culture. This possibility points to the potential importance of experimental details, such as level of drug selection, in the outcome of a targeting experiment. Similar problems were reported by Smithies et al.[52], in one of the first papers published on gene targeting. They observed that although homologous recombination occurred at the β-globin locus in cells that did not express the gene they could not isolate targeted clones whereas targeted clones could be isolated when cells with an active β-globin gene were used.

In addition to the problem that targeted cells at a non-expressed locus may be lost, non-expressed genes may be less amenable to homologous recombination due to chromatin structure. It is known that the chromatin state is altered at non-expressed versus expressed loci[53,54] and this may effect the frequency of homologous recombination by rendering homologous sequence unavailable for recombination. The study of elements which affect chromatin structure may point to novel ways of attacking this problem.

4. CONCLUSION

Although the potential applications of targeted transgenesis in livestock are numerous, several technical improvements are required to allow its routine use. In the short term this is likely to limit commercial applications to high value products such as pharmaceuticals and animal models of human diseases such as cystic fibrosis. Methods to increase the efficiency of gene targeting and to enrich for targeted cells are urgently required. Protocols to retard the onset of cellular senescence also need to be further developed. If the technical hurdles can be overcome, then targeting non-expressed genes in livestock will increase the applicability of gene targeting both for high level protein production (eg. Knock-in at the β-casein locus) and animal models (eg. Knock out at the CFTR locus). The development of novel methods of gene targeting is likely to have other applications out with the field of farm animal transgenesis, such as gene therapy.

REFERENCES

1. Bronson, S.K., Plaehn, E.G., Kluckman, K.D., Hagamann, J.R., Maeda, N., and Smithies, O., 1996, Single-copy transgenic mice with chosen-site integration. *Proc. Natl. Acad. Sci. USA*, **93**, 9067-9072.
2. Wallace, H., Ansell, R., Clark, J., and McWhir, J., 2000, Pre-selection of integration sites imparts repeatable transgene expression. *Nucleic Acids Res.* **28**, 1455-1464.
3. Evans, M.J., and Kaufman, M.H., 1981, Establishment in culture of pluripotential cells from mouse embryos. *Nature* **292**, 154-156.
4. McWhir, J., 1999, Biomedical and Agricultural Applications of Animal Transgenesis. In Transgenesis Techniques (A. R. Clarke, ed), Humana Press, Totowa, N.J.
5. Campbell, K.H., McWhir, J., Ritchie, W.A., and Wilmut, I., 1996, Sheep cloned by nuclear transfer from a cultured cell line. *Nature* **380**, 64-66.
6. Dai., Y., Vaught, T.D., Boone, J., Chen, S-H., Phelps, C.J., Ball, S., Monahan, J.A., Jobst, P.M., McCreath, K.J., Lamborn, A.E., Cowell-Lucero, J.L., Wells, K.D., Colman, A., Polejaeva, I.A., and Ayares, D.L., 2002, Targeted disruption of the α-1,3-galactosyltransferase gene in cloned pigs. *Nature Biotechnol.* **20**, 251-255.
7. Lai, L., Kolber-Simonds, D., Park, K-W., Cheong, H-T., Greenstein, J.L., Im, G-S., Samuel, M., Bonk, A., Rieke, A., Day, B.N., Murphy, C.N., Carter, D.B., Hawley, R.J., and Prather, R.S., 2002, Production of α-1,3-galactosyltransferase knockout pigs by nuclear transfer cloning. *Science* **295**, 1089-1092.
8. Devinoy, E., Thepot, D., Stinnakre, M. G., Fontaine, M. L., Grabowski, H., Puissant, C., Pavirani, A., and Houdebine, L. M., 1994, High level production of human growth hormone in the milk of transgenic mice: the upstream region of the rabbit whey acidic protein (WAP) gene targets transgene expression to the mammary gland. *Transgenic Res.* **3**, 79-89.
9. Platenburg, G.J., Kootwijk, E.P., Kooiman, P.M., Woloshuk, S.L., Nuijens, J.H., Krimpenfort, P.J., Pieper, F.R., de Boer, H.A., and Strijker, R., 1994, Expression of human lactoferrin in milk of transgenic mice. *Transgenic Res.* **3**, 99-108.
10. Massoud, M., Attal, J., Thepot, D., Pointu, H., Stinnakre, M. G., Theron, M. C., Lopez, C., and Houdebine, L. M., 1996, The deleterious effects of human erythropoietin gene driven by the rabbit whey acidic protein gene promoter in transgenic rabbits. *Reprod. Nutr. Dev.* **36**, 555-563.
11. Zinovieva, N., Lassnig, C., Schams, D., Besenfelder, U., Wolf, E., Muller, S., Frenyo, L., Seregi, J., Muller, M., and Brem, G., 1998, Stable production of human insulin-like growth factor 1 (IGF-1) in the milk of hemi- and homozygous transgenic rabbits over several generations. *Transgenic Res.* **7**, 437-447.
12. Wright, G., Carver, A., Cottom, D., Reeves, D., Scott, A., Simons, P., Wilmut, I., Garner, I., and Colman, A., 1991, High level expression of active human alpha-1-antitrypsin in the milk of transgenic sheep. *Biotechnology (NY)* **9**, 830-834.
13. Swanson, M.E., Martin, M.J, O'Donnell, J.K., Hoover, K., Lago, W., Huntress, V., Parsons, C.T., Pinkert, C.A., Pilder, S., and Logan, J.S., 1992, Production of functional human hemoglobin in transgenic swine. *Biotechnology (NY)* **10**, 557-559.
14. Kuroiwa, Y., Yoshida, H., Ohshima, T., Shinohara, T., Ohguma, A., Kazuki, Y., Oshimura, M., Ishida, I., and Tomizuka, K., 2002, The use of chromosome-based vectors for animal transgenesis. *Gene Ther.* **9**, 708-712.
15. Dobie, K.W., Lee, M., Fantes, J.A., Graham, E., Clark, A.J., Springbett, A., Lathe, R., and McClenaghan, M., 1996, Variegated transgene expression in mouse mammary gland is determined by the transgene integration locus. *Proc. Natl. Acad. Sci. USA* **93**, 6659-6664.

16. McCreath, K.J., Howcroft, J., Campbell, K.H., Colman, A., Schnieke, A.E., and Kind, A. J., 2000, Production of gene-targeted sheep by nuclear transfer from cultured somatic cells. *Nature* **405**, 1066-1069.
17. McClenaghan, M., Archibald, A.L., Harris, S., Simons, J.P., Whitelaw, C.B.A., Wilmut, I., and Clark, A.J., 1991, Production of Human alpha1-antitrypsin in the milk of transgemic sheep and mice: Targeting expression of cDNA sequences to the mammary gland. *Animal Biotechnology* **2**, 161-176.
18. Carver, A., Wright, G., Cottom, D., Cooper, J., Dalrymple, M., Temperley, S., Udell, M., Reeves, D., Percy, J., Scott, A., et al., 1992, Expression of human alpha 1 antitrypsin in transgenic sheep. *Cytotechnology* **9**, 77-84.
19. Kumar, S., Clarke, A.R., Hooper, M.L., Horne, D.S., Law, A.J., Leaver, J., Springbett, A., Stevenson, E., and Simons, J.P., 1994, Milk composition and lactation of beta-casein-deficient mice. *Proc. Natl. Acad. Sci. USA* **91**, 6138-6142.
20. Clark, A.J. 1996, Genetic modification of milk proteins. *Am. J. Clin. Nutr.* **63**, 633S-638S.
21. Müller, M., and Brem, G., 1994, Transgenic strategies to increase disease resistance in livestock. *Reprod. Fertil. Dev.* **6**, 605-613.
22. Büeler, H., Aguzzi, A., Sailer, A., Greiner, R.-A., Autenried, P., Aguet, M., and Weissmann, C., 1993, Mice devoid of PrP are resistant to scrapie. *Cell* **73**, 1339-1347.
23. Tobler, I, Gaus, S. E., Deboer, T., Achermann, P., Fischer, M., Rulicke, T., Moser, M., Oesch, B., McBride, P.A., and Manson, J.C., 1996, Altered circadian activity rhythms and sleep in mice devoid of prion protein. *Nature* **380**, 639-642.
24. Nishida, N., Katamine, S., Shigematsu, K., Nakatani, A., Sakamoto, N., Hasegawa, S., Nakaoke, R., Atarashi, R., Kataoka, Y., and Miyamoto, T., 1997, Prion protein is necessary for latent learning and long-term memory retention. *Cell Mol. Neurobiol.* **17**, 537-545.
25. Denning, C., Burl, S., Ainslie, A., Bracken, J., Dinnyes, A., Fletcher, J., King, T., Ritchie, M., Ritchie, W.A., Rollo, M., de Sousa, P., Travers, A., Wilmut, I., and Clark, A.J., 2001, Deletion of the alpha(1,3)galactosyl transferase (GGTA1) gene and the prion protein (PrP) gene in sheep. *Nat. Biotechnol.* **19**, 559-562.
26. Maga, E.A., Anderson, G.B., and Murray, J.D., 1995, The effect of mammary gland expression of human lysozyme on the properties of milk from transgenic mice. *J. Dairy Sci.* **78**, 2645-2652.
27. Kerr, D.E., Plaut, K., Bramley, A.J., Williamson, C.M., Lax, A.J., Moore, K., Wells, K,D., and Wall, R.J., 2001, Lysostaphin expression in mammary glands confers protection against staphylococcal infection in transgenic mice. *Nature Biotechnol.* **19**, 66-70.
28. Snouwaert, J.N., Brigman, K.K., Latour, A.M., Malouf, N.N., Boucher, R.C., Smithies, O., and Koller, B.H., 1992, An animal model for cystic fibrosis made by gene targeting. *Science* **257**, 1083-1088.
29. Harris, A., 1997, Towards an ovine model of cystic fibrosis. *Hum. Mol. Genet.* **6**, 2191-2194.
30. Patience, C., Takeuchi, Y., and Weiss, R. A., 1997, Infection of human cells by an endogenous retrovirus of pigs. *Nature Med.* **3**, 282-286.
31. Logan, J.S., 2000, Prospects for xenotransplantation. *Curr. Opin. Immunol.* **12**, 563-568.
32. Galili, U., 2001, The α-gal epitope (Galα1-3Galβ1-4GlcNAc-R) in xenotransplantation. *Biochimie* **83**, 557-563.
33. Harrison, S.J., Guidolin, A., Faast, R., Crocker, L.A., Giannakis, C., d'Apice, A.J.F., Nottle, M.B. and Lyons, I., 2002, Efficient generation of α (1,3) galactosyltransferase knockout porcine fetal fibroblasts for nuclear transfer. *Transgenic Res.* **11**, 143-150.
34. Tearle, R.G., 1996, The the α-1,3-galactosyltransferase knockout mouse. Implications for xenotransplantation. *Transplantation* **61**, 13-19.
35. Platt, J.L., 2002, Knocking out xenograft rejection. *Nature Biotechnol.* **20**, 231-232.

36. Hayflick, L., 1965, The limited in vitro lifetime of human diploid cell strains. *Exp. Cell Res.* **37**, 614-636.
37. Denning, C., Dickinson, P., Burl, S., Wylie, D., Fletcher, J., and Clark, A.J., 2001, Gene targeting in primary fetal fibroblasts from sheep and pig. *Cloning and Stem Cells* **3**, 221-231.
38. Lanza, R.P., Cibelli, J.B., Blackwell, C., Cristofalo, V.J., Francis, M.K., Baerlocher, G.M., Mak, J., Schertzer, M., Chavez, E.A., Sawyer, N., Lansdorp, P.M., and West, M.D., 2000, Extension of cell life-span and telomere length in animals cloned from senescent somatic cells. *Science* **288**, 665-669.
39. Cristofalo, V.J., and Pignolo, R.J., 1996, Molecular markers of senescence in fibroblast-like cultures. *Exp. Gerontol.* **31**, 111-123.
40. Frippiat, C., Chen, Q.M., Zdanov, S., Magalhaes, J-P., Remacle, J., and Toussain, O., 2001, Subcytotoxic H_2O_2 stress triggers a release of transforming growth factor-E1, which induces biomarkers of cellular senescence of human diploid fibroblasts. *J. Biol. Chem.* **276**, 2531-2537.
41. Sedivy JM., 1998, Can ends justify the means?: telomeres and the mechanisms of replicative senescence and immortalization in mammalian cells. *Proc. Natl. Acad. Sci. USA* **95**, 9078-9081.
42. Rubin H., 2002, The disparity between human cell senescence in vitro and lifelong replication in vivo. *Nature Biotechnol.* **20**, 675-681.
43. Kubota, C., Yamakuchi, H., Todoroki, J., Mizoshita, K., Tabara, N., Barber, M., and Yang, X., 2000, Six cloned calves produced from adult fibroblast cells after long-term culture. *Proc. Natl. Acad. Sci. USA* **97**, 990-995
44. Thomson, A.J., Marques, M.M., and McWhir, J., 2002, Gene targeting in livestock. *Reproduction*, (in press).
45. Bodnar, A.G., Oullette, M., Frolkis, M., Holt, S.E., Chiu, C.P., Morin, G.B., Harley, C.B., Shay, J.W., ,Lichtsteiner, S., and Wright, W.E., 1998, Extension of life-span by introduction of telomerase into normal human cells. *Science* **279**, 349-352.
46. Rubio, M.A., Kim, S-H., and Campisi, J., 2002, Reversible manipulation of telomerase expression and telomere length. Implications for the ionizing radiation response and replicative senescence of human cells. *J. Biol. Chem.* **277**, 28609-28617.
47. Cui, W., Aslam, S., Fletcher, J., Wylie, D., Clinton, M. and Clark, A.J., 2002, Stabilization of telomere length and karyotypic stability are directly correlated with the level of hTERT gene expression in primary fibroblasts. *J. Biol. Chem.* **277**, 38531-38539.
48. Cibelli, J.B., Stice, S.L., Golueke, P.J., Kane, J.F., Jerry, J., Blackwell, C., Ponce de León, A., and Robl, J.M., 1998, Cloned transgenic calves produced from nonquiescent fetal fibroblasts. *Science* **280**, 1256-1258.
49. Sedivy, J.M., and Dutriaux, A., 1999, Gene targeting and somatic cell genetics: a rebirth or a coming of age?. *TIG* **15**, 88-90.
50. Marques, M.M., Thomson, A.J., McCreath, K.J., and McWhir, J., (manuscript in preparation).
51. Thomson, A.J., Marques, M.M., and McWhir, J., (manuscript in preparation).
52. Smithies, O., Gregg, R.G., Boggs, S.S., Koralewski, M.A., and Kucherlapatti, R.S., 1985, Insertion of DNA sequences into the human chromosomal E-globin locus by homologous recombination. *Nature* **317**, 230-234.
53. Felsenfeld, G., Boyes, J., Chung, J., Clark, D., and Studitsky, V., 1996, Chromatin structure and gene expression. *Proc. Natl. Acad. Sci. USA* **93**, 9384-9388.
54. Gregory, P.D., and Horz, W., 1998, Chromatin and transcription-how transcription factors battle with a repressive chromatin environment. *Eur. J. Biochem.* **251**, 9-18.

CONTROLLED RELEASE OF BIOACTIVE AGENTS IN GENE THERAPY AND TISSUE ENGINEERING

Dilek Şendil Keskin[1] and Vasıf Hasırcı[2]
[1]*Department of Engineering Sciences, and* [2]*Department of Biological Sciences, Biotechnology Research Unit, Middle East Technical University, Ankara, 06531, Turkey*

1. INTRODUCTION

Even though the drugs are effective in the treatment of some diseases, they may be inefficient or incapable of solving the problem in some other diseases. It is known that some diseases have genetic causes and therefore the search for a therapy in these cases is intense. The solutions involving either direct application of a gene or its basic product, proteins, especially the growth factors, are often contemplated. Gene therapy is a novel approach to treating diseases based on modifying the expression of a person's genes toward a therapeutic goal. While genes and proteins offer a great opportunity for the treatment of many diseases their administration require critical consideration of the structure and conditions. When the conventional methods of drug administration is adopted for the administration of genes and proteins the results are not successful. Genetic material and the proteins are too labile or unstable due to their fragile 3-D structures and this makes their administration to a medium for long periods in unprotected form impossible. For gene delivery in vivo, additional problems have to be overcome, including the anatomical size constraints, protection from non-specific interactions with body fluids, extracellular matrix and nontarget cells.

A similar problem is faced with when tissue engineering is considered. Tissue engineering involves seeding of human cells on biodegradable carriers of appropriate chemistry and morphology, allows the cells to proliferate and differentiate before eventually implanting them into the appropriate human target site. In order to achieve proper proliferation, differentiation and development of vasculature continuous availability of hormones and growth factors are required. Thus application of these proteinaceous compounds in tissue engineering emerges as a difficult problem. Both genes and proteins necessitate their administration within a protective carrier structure that will also provide their controlled delivery. Gene therapy and tissue engineering era are becoming more important with the advance in biotechnology achieved through various studies including the results of the Human Genome Project.

2. GENE THERAPY AND CONTROLLED DELIVERY

Although gene therapy is mostly considered in treating lethal or disabling diseases it has a preventative potential, too. There is evidence that gene therapy may be effective in the treatment of certain single gene deficiency diseases[1,2]. The fundamental challenge to gene therapy is to develop approaches for delivering genetic material to the target cells in the patient in a way that is efficient, specific and safe.

2.1 Why Gene Therapy is Needed?

Although some proteins are shown to be effective in the treatment of certain diseases when administered via direct injections or within controlled release systems, some others are known to be ineffective under these administration conditions owing to their limited half life, low stability in vivo, need for continuous and controlled administration, rapid clearance. Besides, their fragile structures can be affected by the temperature, moisture or degradation products of the delivery systems. Gene therapy can offer a solution if the genetic material could be delivered taking these conditions into consideration.

> Uses of gene therapy
> Replace missing or defective genes,
> Provide genes that help destruction of cancer cells,
> Supply genes that revert the cancer cells to normal,
> Deliver genes as a form of vaccination,
> Provide genes that promote or impede the growth of new tissues,
> Provide genes that stimulate the healing of damaged tissues.

Inborn errors of metabolism, cardiovascular diseases, cancer, central nervous system degenerative diseases etc. are among the diseases that constitute the main application of gene therapy[2].

It is known that several methods like surgery, chemotherapy, radiation are the common methods used to treat cancers. The patients who can not be helped by these methods still stand a chance: gene therapy. Specific applications of gene therapy for cancer treatment can be carried out in various ways. Treatment might be possible by correcting an abnormality in a tumor suppressor gene with the inserting a copy of the wild type gene, by enhancing immunogenicity of the tumor via introducing genes that encode foreign antigens, by inserting a sensitive or suicide gene into tumor, by blocking the expression of oncogenes, or by killing tumor cells by inserting toxin genes under tumor specific promoters. The first application in a cancer case was in 1990 and since then application of gene therapy in cancer increased more than any other method of treatment[3].

Another example of gene therapy is the development of nebulized recombinant human deoxyribonuclease for delivery directly to the lungs of patients suffering from cystic fibrosis.

3. TISSUE ENGINEERING AND CONTROLLED DELIVERY

Localized delivery may also be important when considering the use of potent growth factors, such as fibroblast growth factor (FGF), vascular endothelial growth factor (VEGF), and bone morphogenic proteins (BMP)[4]. Growth factors are required to promote tissue regeneration. For example, they might be provided to induce vascularization, for the much needed provision of oxygen and nutrients to the cells. They are also essential for tissue formation and play an important role in tissue engineering[5]. Strategies for the growth factor delivery in tissue engineering[6]:
1. Delivery of the protein directly to target cells
2. Delivery of the DNA encoding the growth factor to cells in the body.
3. Ex vivo gene therapy (achieve the same outside the body)
4. Delivery of the protein itself via some carrier matrix

4. TYPES OF MACROMOLECULE CARRIERS USED IN GENE THERAPY AND TISSUE ENGINEERING

In order for the delivery of genes to the nuclei of the cells a delivery vehicle called a vector is needed. Many vectors in use now are based on either viruses with some modifications or non-viral vectors. Of the several types of viral vectors that are in clinical trials, the major ones are retroviruses, adenoviruses, and herpes viruses[7]. The non-viral vectors could be DNA, protein (has capacity to bind to specific cell receptors), polycation complexes, or lipid complexes (facilitate passage across the cell membrane[8]. Other than these the transfections or transport of macromolecules could be achieved via bombardment, ultrasound transfection, or naked DNA transfection. However, practical applications for such methods are limited especially for *in vivo* gene transfer.

4.1 Viral Vectors

Viral vectors, while providing a natural way for gene therapy, are also the associated with certain problems.

Retroviruses, for example, can exhibit insufficient gene transfer capability because of their low transduction into nondividing cells. They are, however, less immunogenic as they are incapable of inducing host cell expression of viral proteins.

The disadvantage of the adenovirus vectors include the transient gene expression because they do not integrate into the host chromosome, immunological reactions such as neutralizing antibody response, dissemination of the vectors from the site of the local injection. In case of clinical application safety is highly important. The first case of fatality induced by infusion of adenovirus vectors into hepatic artery was recently reported. Thus, development of new generation AV is absolutely necessary for the clinical uses of the vector for gene therapy applications like Rheumatoid arthritis[9].

Adenoviruses were reported to evoke immune response in vivo because they retained some of their own genes[10]. Significant immunogenicity was reported with single direct i.m. application of adenoviral mediated gene therapy formulation for the formation ectopic bone[7]. The rapid immune clearance and the leading issues of pathogenicity and safety should also be considered when the use of viruses in gene delivery is considered.

Baltzer, tried adenovirus (carrying a marker gene for luciferase production) infection at bone defects and harvested tissues from liver, spleen, and lung to determine whether distal sites were transduced[11]. They have found only transient activity in liver.

4.2 Non-Viral Vectors

For the controlled release of BMP or a macromolecule like DNA the carrier must prevent rapid factor clearance and ideally release in a predictable manner allowing therapeutic doses to be available for an appropriate duration. The scaffold material should act as a permissive environment into which cells would be encouraged to migrate and begin the process of depositing tissue in the carrier template. In the case osteoblasts for tissue engineering applications, in addition to osteprogenitor cells the endothelial cells must also be able to migrate into or near the matrix and form vascular beds to nourish the newly formed tissue. Additional requirements for the carrier include the ease of manufacture (physical scale up of batch processes), cost effectiveness, biocompatibility, malleability (to fit into various defect sites). Clinicians would like a material that can be injected percutaneously. However, once in vivo, the carrier must be cohesive and should not flow from the defect site. Moreover, materials with optimal scaffolding properties (such as high porosity and large continuous micropores) are typically unable to hold a large reservoir of protein and are not capable of retaining the protein at the site for a prolonged period of time. Biocompatibility is also essential for the medical implant materials and the most cell friendly materials are found in nature. However, materials that are well characterized, easy to manufacture, cost efficient, predictable and easy to sterilize are synthetic polymers and not those derived from natural sources. Furthermore, cells usually prefer hydrophilic surfaces but it is hydrophobic materials that typically have longer residence times in vivo. In the ideal situation good selection leads to a synergistic effect with the growth factor.

Scaffold properties : the carrier scafollding properties are defined by the specific internal and external microarchitecture of the material. The presence of interconnected pores large enough (>100 microns) for cell infiltration, neovascularizationa and diffusion of nutrients in, and vast products out, is esential.

Degradation rate of the carrier matrix is another major parameter in determining the suitability of the carrier for gene therapy and tissue engineering. It should be in synchrony with the rate of bone regeneration. If the matrix degrades too slowly it will inhibit bone growth and retard the modeling process. Carriers with insufficient interconnecting pores and a slow degradation rate run the risk of encapsulation by a bony shell, and therafter become isolated from the repair process. If the carrier matrix degrades too quickly, the risk is that the defect shape will no longer be dictated by the matrix, which often serves as a template for new tissue and is shaped carefully by the surgeon to a particular geometry. As materials displaced and degraded (i.e. collagen and calcium phosphate) they can potentially serve as building blocks for cells regenerating the new tissue. Others, such as the break down products of PLGA, can potentially be toxic by causing an acidic microenvironment if not removed quickly.

Virtually all carriers can be classified into one of four categories: inorganic materials, synthetic polymers, natural polymers, or composites of these.

Non-viral vectors as proteins are receiving increasing attention because of the several advantages such as the ease of manipulation, biocompatibility, biodegradation, stability, low cost, safety, and high flexibility regarding to the size of transgene delivered.

For the delivery of macromolecules from such systems the selection of the polymer and formulation are very important in order to achieve efficient incorporation and sustained delivery reproducibly. Poly(lactic acid-co-glycolic acid) (PLGA) is a synthetic polyester that can be designed to exhibit varying degradation rates, and can have varying physical forms. In a recent study, DNA was incorporated into a PLGA scaffold that was formed via gas foaming process to avoid the use of organic solvents[12]. In another study DNA was release from these scaffolds could be achieved in a controlled manner[9]. The amount of DNA encapsulated in PLGA microsphere has been controlled by varying the molecular weight of the PLGA[10]. In another study referred to in the same manuscript, sustained delivery of DNA from injectable alginate hydrogels was reported. Collagen, on the other hand, is a suitable natural material but its mechanical and degradation properties are difficult to control.

Due to low transfection efficiency for some cell types like glioma cells during direct gene therapy applications, normally a high concentration of virus is required. At such high doses, viruses usually induce a potent immune response that further reduces the efficiency of gene transfer. Thus, to overcome this problem Beer, have developed a method in which the recombinant adenovirus was encapsulated within a biodegradable polymeric microsphere, made of PLGA[13]. This design enabled a low dose, prolonged release eliminating repeated administration for increasing the tranfection efficiency and also the immunogenicity.

In another approach designed by considering immunogenicity with viral gene therapy, Partridge have transfected the osteoprogenitors ex vivo with the adenovirus carrying Human BMP-2 gene and then seeded them onto a PLGA scaffold designed for bone tissue engineering[14]. The in vivo application of the system showed successful bone tissue formation.

In a study by Laurencin, a biodegradable PLGA-Hydroxyapatite composite was combined with ex vivo retroviral tranfected BMP-2 producing cells and used to demonstrate the bone regeneration efficiency[15]. The transfected cells rapidly attached and adapted to the scaffold in vitro. The primary advantage of this approach when compared to the delivery of BMP alone is that the continuous production of BMP by cells grown and the support that the biodegradable matrix may lead to the much needed long term osteoinductive effect which results in clinically significant bone formation. However, the synthesis of adenoviral gene products stimulated an immune response towards the infected cells and this has been found to result in a loss of therapeutic gene expression 1-2 weeks after injection[15].

The multilamellar structure of cationic lipid-DNA complexes used in clinical nonviral gene delivery consist of DNA monolayers sandwiched between lipid bilayers with cationic and neutral head groups. New factors can be incorporated to facilitate the release of the DNA inside the cells. Ongoing research is focused also on the relationship between the physical and chemical properties of the complex and the transfection efficiency[16].

4.3 The Form of the Carrier

The form of the carrier is as important as the chemistry and the origin of the material. Depot delivery systems that can provide continuous protein delivery after a single administration can be designed in different forms such as microspheres and microcapsules, nanospheres and nanocapsules (Fig. 1), rods (Fig. 2), foams, films, laminar structures, injectable solutions or gels. Among them the most common form for construction of a tissue engineering matrix is the foam (Fig. 3). The main reason for this is that tissue engineering generally involves foams as cell carriers due to the excessively high void volumes and loading of growth factors into the same structures is reasonable. However, this type of carrier is disadvantageous due to easy accessibility of the pores that leads to rapid release from these structures. This is especially valid for the lower molecular weight compounds such as drugs[17]. For the rod type implants, however, it is possible to obtain a slower release and a more controlled release can be obtained by varying certain parameters such as comonomer ratio, hydrophilicity of the polymeric material, etc. (Fig. 4). For the genetic material delivery there is no predetermined structure and, therefore, the form that would provide highest protection and most efficient transfection is chosen. This generally is a micro- or nanocapsule. The major problem associated with these structures is the exposure of the genetic material to the organic solvents needed during formation of the capsules.

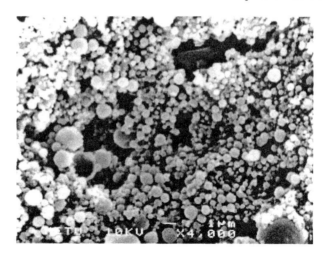

Figure 1. SEM of asparaginase loaded polyhydroxybutyrate-co-hydroxyvalerate (PHBV8) microspheres (x 4000) (from Baran et al[18]).

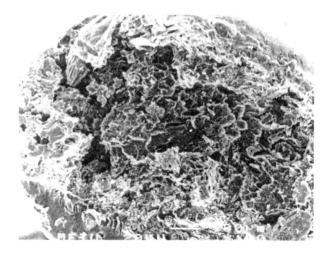

Figure 2. SEM of analgesic loaded polylactide-co-glycolide (PLGA 85:15) rod (cross section) (x 100) (from Sendil et al[19]).

BMPs are a highly potent group of proteins in healing bone, require a specific design for the delivery system that would be applied to the site of repair. Thus for treating large bone defects, a large volume, appropriate size and shape, mechanically competent construct would be needed as both carrier for the controlled release of BMPs and as a scaffold for the new tissue formation[3,5]

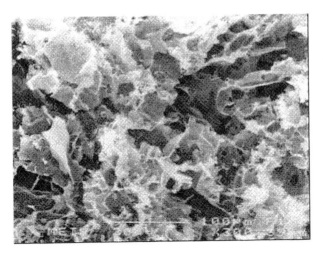

Figure 3. SEM of tetracycline loaded polyhydroxybutyrate-cohydroxyvalerate (PHBV7) foam (x 300) (from Sendil et al[17]).

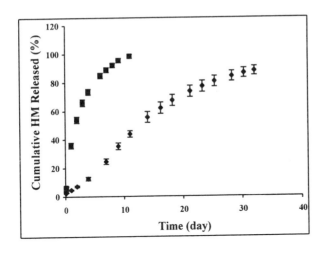

Figure 4. Hydromorphone release from PLGA rods with different comonomer ratios. (♦) PLGA (85:15), (■)PLGA (50:50) (from Sendil et al[19]).

4.4 Smart Polymers

Recent advances in the design of stimuli responsive polymers that show changes in the shape, dimension, surface characteristics, or solubility have created possibilities for tissue engineering and gene therapy applications.

A thermosensitive chitosan-glycerol phosphate system was investigated for the protein delivery, gene delivery, and tissue engineering applications[21]

This system exhibited reverse thermogelling properties: it was a sol at room temperature and gelled at the body temperature.

Similarly pH sensitive polymers have been gaining interest. Poly(propyl acrylic acid) and poly(ethacrylic acid) are also examples of pH sensitive polymers applied in gene delivery[20]. Both undergo a conformational change at ca. pH 5-6.

4.5 Polyplexes

In another major area of nonviral gene delivery, chemicals such as cationic lipids or polymers are used to condense DNA into particles. These major non-viral gene therapy systems are called polyplexes (complexes of DNA with polycations) [21,22]. The size of the particles tend to be in the range 100-300 nm. The transport of these complexes into the cell was through receptor mediated endocytosis. Much of gene therapy is done with complementray DNA (cDNA), which is reverse transcripted from messenger RNA, because the actual genomic sequences are too large. For example, the factor VIII gene has about 185 000 base pairs but the cDNA has only 9000 base pairs simply because all the noncoding regions (introns) have been removed. The problem with using cDNA is that cells have complexes (splicosome) that take RNA, and splice out the introns. Even though the cDNA is a pure coding sequence, the splicosome still looks for recognition sequences on the RNA and splices that.

Poly(L-lysine), poly(ethylene imine) have also been investigated for this purpose. Pluronic block copolymers, are very valuable for gene delivery in skeletal muscle.[23]

Despite their low efficiency in gene transfer, lipid based gene transfer vehicles (lipoplexes-genosomes) are characterized with certain advantages even over viral ones: they are less toxic and immunogenic, could be targetable and are suitable for large scale production, and the size of transferred DNA is quite high[24]. It is known that lipid complexes overall show a higher toxicity than the complexing polymers although the doses were almost half the doses of polymers when used. Among lipids only LipfectAMINE exhibited high transfection efficiency (higher than any of the tested polymer)[25].

4.6 Ceramics

For appropriate differentiation and conduction of the bone via the delivery of the stem cells hydroxyapatite (HA), calcium phosphates and some other ceramics are considered as potential scaffolds. However, HA and calcium phosphates are not osteoinductive and are resorbed relatively slowly. To overcome these problems natural or synthetic biodegradable materials such as poly(lactic acid), poly(glycolic acid) and PLGA, as well as DegraPol-foam and Polyactive have been tested[5]. Biodegradable scaffolds provide the initial structure and stability for tissue formation but degrade as the tissue forms, providing room for matrix deposition and tissue growth. Despite theses attractive properties, polymers have one major disadvantage, their lack of mechanical competence.

4.7   RGD-Scaffolds

Recently the potential of human osteoprogenitor differentiation on RGD-coupled (arginine-glycine-aspartic acid) biodegradable scaffolds is being intensely studied. Yang have examined the attachment, proliferation, and differentiation of human bone marrow cells on modified PLA films and PLGA porous degradable scaffolds[26]. They observed a negligible adhesion, growth, and differentiation on the pristine PLA films, whereas cell attachment was enhanced on PLA films adsorbed with FN or coupled with the integrin adhesion motif, RGD. Extension of these studies to porous PLGA scaffolds suggests that biomaterial surfaces, which on their own do not support cell growth, can be modified to enhance human bone marrow cell growth, differentiation, and mineralization.

4.8   Hydrogels

Drug delivery techniques such as entrapment within a hydrogel matrix allowing growth factors to be released in a controlled fashion to aid the regenerating tissue have been one of the most promising approaches because hydrogels provide a highly water-filled environment for the fragile genetic material constructs. They are appealing as they avoid the use of organic solvents, and high processing temperatures (and therefore protein degradation). This strategy has been employed in many studies for bone tissue engineering via incorporation of Rh BMP-2[27], basic fibroblast growth factor[28] and vascular endothelial growth factor[29] into a hydrogel prior to in vivo implantation.

4.9   Foams

Supercritical fluid technology has evolved as a promising approach in the development of porous biodegradable scaffolds for tissue engineering. The absence of solvents and thermal processing makes this an attractive approach to growth factor incorporation. Howdle have demonstrated high protein ribonuclease loading into PLA foams that retained full activity on release over 3 months[30]. This technology could provide a simple one stem process to the difficulties of incorporating growth factors into a controlled release delivery system. The challenge in tissue engineering is the design of suitable scaffolds that incorporate and release appropriate combinations of signalling molecules to promote vascularization and osteoinduction with minimum inflamation at the site.

4.10 Depot Systems

The depot systems for delivery of macromolecules (eg. proteins) could provide continuous delivery after a single administration. Biodegradable implants of single procedure offer the advantage of no remove and microspheres, nanospheres or injectible gels allow for injection with a commercial needle or syringe. Several biodegradable matrices suitable for protein delivery have been studied and numerous examples with in vitro data have been published[4]. The administration site reaction to these matrices requires extensive examination to ensure that they are compatible with the site and the protein, therefore, pilot toxicology studies of the biodegradable matrix should be performed prior to development of the matrix for delivery.

4.11 Release Behavior

A further complicating factor is that different anatomical sites might require different kinetics of release for optimal performance. Also different animal species will have varying optimum release profiles.

5. GENE INSERTION MECHANISM

If gene insertion into the cell is performed outside the body the procedure is termed "ex vivo" or "cell therapy". If the gene is directly inserted into host cells inside the body, the procedure is termed the "in situ approach" and the vector can be considered the carrier. In general, plasmid DNA has fewer safety barriers than viral vector delivery but suffers from a lower overall transfection efficiency. Gene therapy has certain advantages over protein delivery, such as lower cost, potential longer expression of factors and a more physiological level of growth factor[6].

GAM (Gene Activated Matrix) was the first gene therapeutic approach designed specifically for tissue engineering applications. GAM consists of two ingredients: a plasmid DNA and a degradable structural matrix carrier.

The GAM matrix carrier serves as a scaffold that holds the DNA in situ until endogeneous wound healing fibroblasts arrive. Once transfected, fibroblasts in the carrier act as local in vivo bioreactors, secreting plasmid encoded proteins that augment tissue repair and regeneration. This is an unusual method of DNA delivery to cells. In traditional gene delivery the drug substance finds the target cells in a GAM, on the other hand the target cells find the DNA drug. In this system when collagen sponge GAM was used the in vivo transfection efficency was 20-50 % by semiquantitative assays [31].

6. POLYMERS

Polymers are versatile and malleable offer many advantageous options. Controlling the molecular weight, coupling to specific moities for targeting or molding into a specific shape and physical property are among such properties that enhance their usefulness. In order to obtain the best trasnfection efficiency with a polymer-DNA complex such factors should be considered and optimized as they strongly affect the overall result. The concentration of both species (polymer and DNA), ionic strength of the mixing solution, rate and order of the mixing process etc.

6.1 Polyanhydrides and Polyesters

The poly(anhydrides) and polyesters degrade by hydrolysis catalyzed by water and hydrogen ion. The mechanism of release from these systems is usually dependent on drug diffusion and polymer degradation. Major challanges for microsphere formulations of these polymers include the limitations in dose concentration due to drug loading constraints and the complexicity of the manufacturing process[4].

6.2 Polyethyleneimine (PEI)

Among the various synthetic vectors, poly(ethyleneimines) have shown particularly promising efficacy in transfections in cell culture as well as in a variety of applications in vivo[32].

PEI has the ability to complex even with large DNA molecules with high in vitro and in vivo transfection efficiency. One of the most important properties is the DNA protecting capacity against the nucleases and this is attributed to the high charge density of the polymer that enables the efficient complexation. However, PEI's high toxicity at high charge limits the use of this property to a certain degree. The proposed high transfection efficacy lies behind its structural specificy that enable a significant buffering capacity, so called "proton sponge" property. The Linear PEI (ExGen ™ 500) has recently been reported to have excellent transfection efficiency and lower toxicity owing to the cell cycle independent nuclear entry of the plasmid DNA.

6.3 Poly(L-Lysine)

Although poly(L-lysine) is taken up into cells with the same efficiency as PEI, its transfection efficiency is lower than that of PEI. This is thought to be due to the lack of endosomolysis properties that in turn prevent the escape of the polymer-DNA complex from the vesicles. However, co administration of endosomolytic agents like chloroquine may improve its efficiency.

6.4 Imidazole Containing Polymers

Polymers containing heterocyclic imidazole have shown promising transfection results. For example the modification of poly(L-lysine) with histidine showed significant improvements in gene expression most probably via mediating vesicular escape[33-36].

6.5 Chitosan

Chitosans are also capable of forming small stable DNA complexes that provide a better protection for the DNA against DNAse compared to PEI. They give the best results at an optimum molecular weight range (30-170 kDa). However, endosomal escape is their primary problem in the use.

6.6 Dendrimers

They are spherical, highly branched polymers that have similar structure to PEI in terms of high density of amines at the periphery of the molecule that enable efficient condensation of DNA leaving the inner amines for neutralization during the endolysosomal acidifaction, thus enabling the escape from the vesicle.

6.7 Sterically-Stabilized Complexes

Since the positive surface charge and aggregations are the main reasons for decreased circulation time and occurence of an unwanted distribution profile (accumulation in lungs and liver), covering the surface charge would potentially eliminate these problems. Thus attachment of hydrophilic polymers is a suggested method of steric stabilization. Polyethyleneglycol, Transferrin, poly (N-(2-hydroxypropyl)methacrylamide) are some of the polymers used for stabilization of the[37-40]. All of these molecules have shown increased efficiency while decreasing the side effcts like expression at unwanted sites at different levels.

7. PROBLEMS IN NUCLEIC ACID DELIVERY

To be able to deliver nucleic acids into the target cell where it would be expected to function properly, the complex system of the vector and the DNA has to pass through some stages/barriers successfuly[41]. The problems through out this route can occur either at the systemic or cellular level.

Systemic problems involve:

1. Passage through the endothelial barrier that is governed mainly by size of the molecule and, the permeability of the endothelial tissue at the site.

2. Unspecific interactions of the cationic surface charges of the complex with blood or endothelial elements (eg. albumin, complement factors, fibronectin). This results in a decrease in the circulation half life.

3. Gene expression at sites other than the target tissue. A number of targeting molecules are being sought to solve this problem. Besides active targeting the use of tissue specific promoters will also limit the gene expression at other tissues.

Cellular level problems involve:

1. Passage across the cell membrane problem for naked DNA can be overcome with polyplexes that can be internalized via endocytosis. This, however, creates another problem that is the enzymatic degradation by lysosomes that happens to be on the route of any endocytotic vesicle. A new approach for solving this problem is the use of a specific protein present in the genome of HIV virus, that mediate direct entry of the large molecules into the cells without endocytosis or even across the nuclear envelope.

2. The stage of the path for the release of vesicalized complex occurs is also highly important as hydrolytic enzymes or other lysosomal content may cause damage in cell leading to necrosis or apoptosis.

3. The transfer of DNA from cytosol to the nucleus and across the nuclear envelope is very inefficient. The mechanism of this route for plasmid DNA is also unclear. Thus the complexing agent has an important role in the total journey of the DNA until the last point, nucleus is reached. Increased mitotic activity in tumor cells might increase the efficiency of nuclear targeting in such cases.

8. CONCLUSION

Bioactive agents used for therapy or for other applications need to be available at the required concentrations at the sites of need. As is very well known, the conventional application routes are at times incapable of achieving this goal. Another handicap for the use of traditional methods is the fact that some bioactive agents are too labile or unstable to leave unprotected for long periods in the medium. This is especially important for tissue engineering applications involving growth factors and gene therapy applications that have higher potential for treatment of many diseases than the conventional methods. The most widely available forms for release applications involve micro- and nanoparticles (in capsule or sphere form), rods, fibers, membranes and foams. Among them foam is the most common carrier type for application of these delicate agents in tissue engineering. For the delivery of genetic material there is no predetermined structure and therefore the form that would give the highest protection and efficacy is chosen. As is indicated by the above survey currently very sophisticated methods of delivery are being developed and in the near future a high degree and rate of delivery of macromolecules will definitely be achieved.

REFERENCES

1. BIO, Biotechnology Industry Organization. Biotechnology in Perspective, 1990, "Gene therapy: an overview." Washington, D.C., Biotechnology Industry Organization, http://www.gene.com/ae/AB/IWT/Gene_Therapy_Overview.html.
2. Steiner, J., 2000/1, The genie in the test tube-from gene to gene therapy: part II . *Drug Discovery World* Winter: 55-61.
3. Guojun, L., 1996, www.cc.ndsu.nodak.edu/instruct/mcclean/plsc431/students/guojun.htm
4. Cleland, J.L., Daugherty, A., and Mrsny, R., 2001, Emerging protein delivery methods. *Current Opinion in Biotechnology* **12**, 212-219.
5. Rose, F.R.A., Oreffo, R.O.C., 2002, Bone tissue engineering: Hope vs hype. *Biochemical and Biophysical Research Communications* **292**: 1-7.
6. Li, H.R., and Woznet, J.M., 2001, Delivering on the promise of bone morphogenetic proteins. *Trends in Biotechnology* **19**, 255-265.
7. Musgrave, D. S., Bosch, P., Ghivizzani, S., Robbins, P. D., Evans, C. H., Huard, J., 1999, Adenovirus-mediated direct gene therapy with bone morphogenetic protein-2 produces bone. *Bone* **24**, 541-547.
8. Wivel, N., What is gene therapy. http://www. uphs.upenn.edu/ihgt.
9. Tanaka, S., 2002, Adenovirus vector-mediated gene transduction for the treatment of bone and joint destrution of rheumatoid arthritis, In *Tissue Engineering and Biodegradable Equivalents, Scientific and Clinical Applications.* (Lewandrowski, K.,. Wise, D.L, Trantolo, D.J,. Gresser, J.D, . Yaszemski, M.J, Altobelli, D.E. Eds.) Marcel Dekker, Inc., N, Y., pp. 467-482.

10. Madsen, S.K., and Mooney, D.J., 2000, Delivering DNA with polymer matrices: applications in tissue engineering and gene therapy. *PSTT* **3**, 381-384.
11. Baltzer, A., Lattermann, C., Whalen, J. D., Braunstein, S., Robbins, P.D., Evans, C. H, 1999, A gene therapy approach to accelerate bone healing. knee surg, *Sports Traumatol, Arthrosc.* **7**, 197-202.
12. Buyong-Soo, K., Mooney, D.J., 1998, Development of biocompatible synthetic extracellular matrices for tissue engineering. *Trends Biotechnol.* **16**, 197-237.
13. Beer, S., Hilfinger, J. M., Davidson, B. L., 1997, Extended release of adenovirus from polymer microspheres: potential use in gene therapy for brain tumors. *Advanced Drug Delivery Reviews* **27**, 59-66.
14. Partridge, K., Yang, X., Clarke, N.M.P., Okubo, Y., Bessho, K., Sebalt, W., Howdle, S. M., Shakesheff, K.M., Oreffo, R. O. C., 2002, Adenoviral BMP-2 gene transfer in mesenchymal stem cells: In vitro and in vivo bone formation on biodegradable polymer scaffolds. *Biochemical and Biophysical Research Communications* **292**, 114-152.
15. Laurencin, C.T., Attawia, M.A., Lu, L.Q., Borden, M.D., Lu, H.H., Gorum, W.J., Lieberman, J.R., 2001,Poly(lactide-co-glycolide)/hydroxiapatide delivery of BMP-2 producing cells: A regional gene therapy approach to bone regeneration. *Biomaterials* **22**, 1271-1277.
16. Koltover I., Wagner, K., Safinya C.R., 2000, DNA condensation in two dimensions. *Proc. Natl. Acad. Sci. USA* **97**, 14046-14051.
17. Şendil, D., Gürsel, İ., and Hasırcı, V., 2000, Preparation of PHBV foams and investigation of their potential for drug release, *Tr. J. Medical Sciences* **30**: 9-14.
18. Baran E.T, Ozer N, and Hasirci V., 2002, Poly(hydroxybutyrate-co-hydroxyvalerate) nanocapsules as enzyme carriers for cancer therapy: an in vitro study. *J Microencapsulation* **19**, 363-376.
19. Sendil, D., Wise, D.L., and Hasirci, V., 2002, Assessment of biodegradable controlled release rod systems for pain relief applications. *J. Biomaterial Science, Polymer Edition* **13**, 1-15.
20. Jeong, B., and Gutowska, A, 2002, Lessons from nature: stimuli-responsive polymers and their biomedical applications. *Trends in Biotechnology* **20**, 305-311.
21. Kabanov, A.V., 1999, Taking polycation gene delivery system from in vitro to in vivo. *Pharm. Sci. Tech. Today* **2**, 365-372.
22. Smedt, S. D., Demeester, J., and Hennink, W., 2000, Cationic polymer based gene delivery systems. *Pharm. Res.* **5**, 1425-1433
23. Kabanov, A.V., Lemieux, P., Vinogradov, S., and Alakhov, V, 2002, Pluronic block copolymers: novel functional molecules for gene therapy. *Advanced Drug Delivery Reviews* **54**, 223-233.
24. Zhdanov, R.I, Podobed, O.V. and Vlassov, V.V., 2002, Cationic lipid-DNA complexes-lipoplexes-for gene transfer and therapy. *Bioelectrochemistry* **58**, 53-64.
25. Gebhart, C.L., and Kabanov, A.V., 2001, Evaluation of polyplexes as gene transfer agents. *J. Controlled Release* **73**, 401-416.
26. Yang, X.B., Roach, H.I., Clarke, N.M.P., Howdle, S. M., Quirk, R., Shakesheff, K.M., and Oreffo, R.O.C., 2001, Human osteoprogenitor growth and differentiation on synthetic biodegradable structures after surface modification. *Bone* **29**, 523–531.
27. Itoh, S., Kikuchi, M., Takakuta, K., Koyama, Y., Matsumoto, H.N., Ichinose, S., Tanaka, J., Kawauchi, T., and Shinomiya, K, 2001, The biocompatibility and osteoconductive activity of a novel hydroxyapatite/collagencomposite biomaterial and its function as a carrier of rhBMP-2. *J. Biomed. Mater.Res.* **54**, 445-453.

28. Tabata, Y., 2000, The importance of drug delivery systems in tissue engineering, *Pharm.Sci.Tech.Today* **3**, 80-89.
29. Lee, K.Y., Peters, M.C., Anderson, K.W., Mooney, D.C., 2000, Controlled growth factor release from synthetic extracellular matrices. *Nature* **408**, 998-1000.
30. Howdle, S.M., Watson, M.S., Whitaker, M.J., Popov, V.K., Davies, M.C., Mandel, F.S., Wang, J.D., Shakesheff, K.M, 2001, Supercritical fluid mixing: Preparation of thermally sensitive polymer composites containing bioactive materials. *Chem. Commun.* **7**, 109-110.
31. Bonadio, J., 2000, Tissue engineering via local gene delivery: update and future prospects for enhancing the technology. *Advanced Drug Delivery Reviews* **44**, 185-194.
32. Kircheis, R., Wightman, L., and Wagner, E, 2001, Design and gene delivery activity of modified polyethylenimines. *Advanced Drug Delivery Reviews* **53**, 341-358.
33. Fajac, I., Allo, J.C, Souil, E., Merten, M., Pichon, C., Figarella, C., Monsigny, M., Briand, P., and Midoux, P., 2001, Histidylated polylysine as a synthetic vector for gene transfer into immortalized cystic fibrosis airway surface and airway gland. *Gene Med.* **2**, 99–101.
34. Benns, J.M., Choi, J.S., Mahato, R.I., Park, J.S., and Kim, S.W., 2000, pH-sensitive cationic polymer gene delivery vehicle: N-Ac-poly(L-histidine)-graft-poly(L-lysine) comb shaped polymer, *Bioconjug. Chem.* **11**, 637–645.
35. Midoux, P., and Monsigny, M., 1999, Efficient gene transfer by histidylated polylysine/pDNA complexes. *Bioconjug. Chem.* **10**, 406–411.
36. Putnam, D., Gentry, C.A., Pack, D.W., and Langer, R., 2001, Polymer-based gene delivery with low cytotoxicity by a unique balance of side-chain termini. *Proc. Natl. Acad. Sci. USA* **98**, 1200–1205.
37. Ogris, M., Brunner, S., Schuller, S., Kircheis, R., and Wagner, E., 1999, PEGylated DNA/transferrin-PEI complexes: Reduced interaction with blood components, extended circulation in blood and potential for systemic gene delivery. *Gene Ther.* **6**, 595-605.
38. Nguyen, H.K., Lemieux, P., Viogradov, S.V., Gebhart, C.L., Guerin, N., Paradis, G., Bronich, T.K., Alakhov V.Y, and Kabanov, A.V., 2000, Evaluation of polyether-polyethyleneimine graft copolymers as gene transfer agents. *Gene Ther.* **7**, 126-138.
39. Kircheis, R., Wightman, L., Schreiber, A., Robitza, B., Rossler, V., Kursa M., and Wagner, E, 2001, Polyethylenimine/DNA complexes shielded by transferrin target gene expression to tumors after systemic application, *Gene Ther.* **8**, 28-40.
40. Kopecek, J., Kopeckova, P., Minko, T., and Lu, Z., 2000, HPMA copolymer-anticancer drug conjugates: design, activity, and mechanism of action. *Eur. J. Pharm.Biopharm.* **50**, 61-81.
41. Merdan, T, Kopecek, J., and Kissel, T., 2002, Prospects for cationic polymers in gene and oligonucleotide therapy against cancer. *Advanced Drug Delivery Reviews* **54**, 715-758.

INTERLEUKIN 1 (IL-1) INDUCES THE ACTIVATION OF STAT3

Ahmet Arman[1,2] and Philip E. Auron[1]
[1]The New England Baptist Bone and Joint Institute, Harvard Medical School, 77 Avenue Louis Pasteur, Boston, MA 02115l, U.S.A.; [2]Environmental Engineering, Faculty of Engineering, Marmara University, Istanbul, Turkey

1. INTRODUCTION

Interleukin-1 (IL-1) is involved in a variety of immune system activities, such as acute phase response, fever and cartilage breakdown[1]. The acute phase response is a result of injury, virus or bacterial infection, all of which induce acute phase protein synthesis. Expression of the acute phase proteins is predominantly regulated by IL-1 and IL-6; however, the liver centrally regulates the acute-phase response by inducing the release of acute phase reactants (APRs)[2]. There are two classes of these acute phase reactants. IL-1 induces class 1 acute phase proteins, such as serum amyloid A and Δ_1 acid glycoprotein, synergistically, with or without IL-6[3]. However, class 2 APRs, including various anti-proteases and Δ_2-macroglobin[4], are induced only by IL-6. The promoters of some of the acute phase genes contain regulatory respond elements called acute phase response elements (APRE). APRE bind to transcription factors termed acute-phase response factor (AFRF) or to the signal transducer and activator of transcription 3, (Stat3)[5]. Additional types of regulatory elements found in promoters of APRs are CCAAT enhancer-binding protein (C/EBP) and nuclear factor-NB (NF-NB) binding elements that bind to C/EBP family of transcription factors such as NF-IL6, C/EBPΔ,

E, I[6] and NF-NB[7] respectively. IL-1 only activates NF-NB and C/EBP transcription factors[8]; however, IL-6 activates Stat3 molecules.

The question at hand is whether or not IL-1 activates Stat3 molecules involved in the regulation of the expression of acute phase genes. Previously, we reported that a novel, Stat-like factor (LIL-Stat), that is not Stat1, 2, 3, 4, or 5 [9], is activated by IL-1, LPS and IL-6. It has been reported that IL-1 and IL-6 activate Stat3 through regulation of the lipopolysaccharide-binding protein (LBP) gene, which is class 1 APR[10]. Also, it was reported that IL-1 activates the short form of Stat3 in clonal insulin secreting cells[11]. The sole goal of this paper is to report that IL-1 directly activates Stat3 by inhibiting the induction of class 1 acute phase 9 fibrinogen by NF-*k*B, which binds to the overlapping Stat3 site[12]. Also, It has been shown that LPS posttranslationally activates Stat3 [13].

STAT family transcription factors consist of at least 6 members: Stat 1, 2, 3, 4, 5, and 6[14]. The STAT proteins are activated by extracellular ligands like cytokines, growth factors, and hormones. They are tyrosine phosphorylated by JAK kinases and undergo serine phosphorylation by P38 MAPK[15]. Then, they enter the nucleus, bind to specific promoter of genes and activate transcription. One of the members of the STAT family, Stat3 is activated by IL-6 family cytokines (IL-6, leukemia inhibitory factor, oncostatin M), growth factors (EGF, PDGF), and hormones (GH)[16].

In this study, we showed that Stat3 is activated by IL-1 in transiently transfected Cos cells and Hep3B cells. EMSA experiments showed that Stat3 is antigenically related to C-terminal and the internal domain of Stat3 Δ but not to N-terminal Stat3. However, the western blotting results showed that Stat3, which had been immuneprecipitated at the C-terminal, was also recognized by N-terminal Stat3 antibody.

2.   MATERIALS AND METHODS

2.1   Oligonucleotides

High-affinity sis-inducible element (hSIE) oligonucleotides 5'-AGCTTG TGCATTTCCCGTAAATCTTGTCGTCGA-3', Lipopolysaccharide-IL-1 response element (LILRE) 5'-AGCTTATAAGAGGTTTCACTTCCTG GAGAGTCGA-3' and LILRE core 5'-AGCTTCACTTCCTGAGAGTCG A-3' were synthesized by Qiagen Operon Technology, CA. The other oligonucleotides, Δ_2-Macroglobin (MG), acute phase response element (APRE) 5'-GATCCTTCTGGGAATTCCTAGATC-3', mutant Δ_2-Macro-globin (MMG) 5'- GATCCTTCTGGGCCGTCCTAGATC-3', Gamma activation sequences (GAS) 5'-AAGTACTTTCAGTTTCATATTACTCTA-3' were purchased by Santa-Cruz Company, CA.

2.2 Transient Transfection Assay

Cos or Hep3B cells were seeded in 6 or 12 well plates and were grown about 60-80% confluent. Then, they were transfected with 0.5 µg of IL-1R and β gal, or pRL-TK reporter plasmids using 1.5 µl of fugene 6 transfectant reagent per ml (Boehringer Mannheim, Germany). After 48 hours, the cells were treated with or without IL-1 (2 ng/ml) and lysed for further experiments.

2.3 Cell Culture and Nuclear Extract

Cos and Hep3B cell lines were obtained from American Type Culture Collection (ATCC). Cos cells were grown in an incubator containing Dulbecco's modified Eagle's medium (DMEM), 10% fetal bovine serum (FBS), and a 5% CO_2 environment; however, Hep3B cells were grown in minimal essential medium supplemented with 10% FBS and 0.5% penicillin and streptomycin. The Hep3B cell line was seeded in 150 mm of petri dishes. The cells were washed three times with serum free medium and incubated with 3.55 mM cycloheximide for 1 hour. Then the cells were treated with or without IL-1 (20 ng/ml) for 15 min. The Nuclear extract was prepared as previously explained[9].

2.4 Electrophoretic Mobility Shift Assay (EMSA)

10 ng of APRE oligonucleotides (Santa Cruz) were labeled with T_4 Polynucleotide kinase (New England Biolabs, MA) containing γ-^{32}P-ATP at 6000 cpm/mmol (DuPont-NEN, MA). Incorporated nucleotides were purifies using a G-25 column (Pharmacia Corporation, NJ). 2-5 µg of nuclear extract was incubated with 20-30 000 cpm of labeled oligonucleotide in 1x binding buffer containing 10 mM tris-HCl (pH-7.5), 1mM EDTA, 4% glycerol, 40 mM NaCl and 1 mM β-mercaptoethanol with 200-1000 ng of poly dI-dC at room temperature for 15 min. Then the antibodies or cold oligonucleotides were added to the solution and the solution was incubated for an additional 15 min. DNA-protein complexes were resolved in 4.5 % TBE polyacrylamide gel.

2.5 Immunoblot

Hep3B cells were washed three times with serum free medium and were starved overnight. The cells were then treated with IL-1 (20 ng/ml) for 15 min and washed with PBS-PMSF 3 times. Then the cells were lysed with RIPA, or non-denaturing buffer, with 1mM of NaVanadate (Sigma, MO), 10 mg/ml of PMSF and proteinase inhibitor cocktails (Sigma, MO). Coimmunoprepicitations or immunoprepicitations were performed with suitable antibodies using cell lysates. The precipitated complexes were resolved by 7.5 % SDS-PAGE. Proteins were transferred to a Hybond-ECL membrane. The membrane was blocked with PBS/4 % milk or BSA and incubated with suitable antibodies. The membrane was developed with ECL (Amersham, IL) and visualized by exposure to X-ray film. Stat1 (E-23), Stat3-N terminal (H-190), Stat3-internal (K-15) and Stat3-C terminal (C-20) antibodies were purchased from Santa Cruz Company, California. The Phospho-Stat3 (705), Phospho-Stat3-(S727) and phospho-Stat3 (705), clone 9E12 were purchased from Upstate Biotechnology, NY.

3. RESULTS

3.1 IL-1 Induces Stat3 Activation

We determined the Stat3 activation by the electrophoretic mobility shift assay (EMSA). We examined the induction of Stat3 by IL-1 in the APRE-nuclear extract complex using specific Stat3 antibodies raised against N-terminal Stat3 (50-240), internal (626-640) and C-terminal Stat3 (750-769) in the EMSA system. Fig. 1 shows that internal Stat3 antibody specifically supershifted APRE-nuclear complex and this complex was abrogated by C-terminal Stat3 antibody. However, IL-1-induced APRE-nuclear complex was not affected by N-terminal Stat3 antibody or Stat1 antibody. These results indicates that IL-1 may induce isoform of Stat3.

Interleukin 1 (IL-1) Induces the Activation of Stat3 301

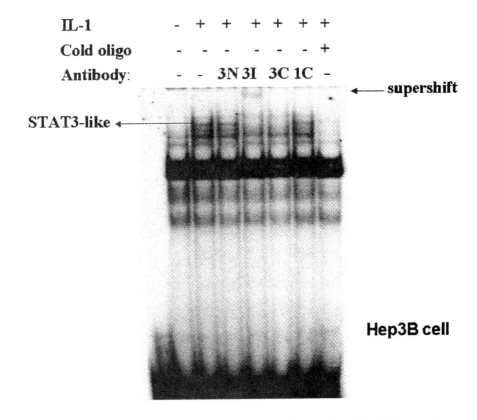

Figure 1. IL-1 induces protein-APRE complex and this complex (top band) is inhibited by C-terminal and Internal Stat3 antibodies but not N-terminal Stat3 or Stat1 antibodies. Hep3B cells were starved in serum free medium in presence of 3.55 mM cycloheximide and treated with or without IL-1 (20 ng/ml). They were then lysed and nuclear extract was prepared. 5-10 µg of nuclear extracts were treated with 20-30 000 cpm labeled APRE for 15 min and Stat3 antibodies including, Stat3 (H190), Stat3 (K-15), Stat3 (C-20) and Stat1 (E-23), were added to solution and incubated for 15 min more at room temperature. N refers N-terminal, I refers internal and C refers C-terminal.The samples were subjected to 7.5 % PAGE gel and the gel was dried and exposed to X-ray film overnight.

3.2 LILRE core, LILRE, hSIE, GAS and C/EBP Do Not Compete With α_2-Macroglobin Oligonucleotides

We further characterized IL-1 induced APRE-nuclear extract complex using several oligo competition experiments. Fig. 2 showed that oligonucleotides, hSIE, LILRE core, LILRE, GAS and C/EBP did not compete with IL-1-induced Stat3 or other complexes. Also, we checked the other oligonucleotides, Stat1, IRF-1, Stat5/6 and hSIE for IL-1 induced Stat3 and other complexes. The mutant APRE (MMG) (AAT->CCG), Stat1, IRF-

1 (Stat4), Sat5/Sat6 and hSIE did not compete IL-1-induced Stat3 and or IL-1 induced complexes (data not shown). However, wt APRE (MG), and IRF-1 (Stat4) competed with IL-1 induced Stat3 and the other complexes. Literature showed that IRF-1 can bind to all Stat transcription factors. These results show that IL-1 induced Stat3 does not show any relationship with other Stat molecules and C/EBP transcription factors.

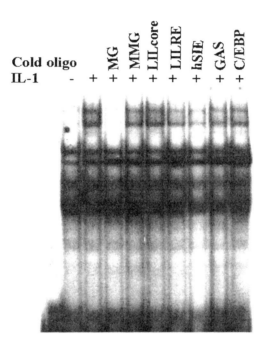

Figure 2. LILRE core, LILRE, hSIE, GAS and C/EBP do not compete with APRE oligonucleotides. The oligonucleotides sequences of LILRE core, LILRE, hSIE, GAS, C/EBP, and mutant APRE (MMG) (AAT->CCG) are shown in materials and methods. After 15 min incubation of nuclear extract with 20-30 000 cpm of labeled APRE (MG), the solutions were incubated with unlabelled competitor LILRE core, LILRE, hSIE, GAS and C/EBP oligonucleotides. The concentrations of unlabelled oligonucleotides are 100-fold molar excess over concentration of labeled oligonucleotides.

3.3 IL-1 Induced Tyrosine and Serine Phosphorylation of Stat3 in Transient Transfected Cos Cells

We checked whether IL-1 induces tyrosine and serine phosphorylation of Stat3. Transiently transfected Cos cells with IL-1R were starved overnight with serum free medium (DMEM) and were incubated with or without IL-1 (20ng/ml). Fig. 3a showed that Stat3 tyrosine phosphorylation is IL-1dependent, since Stat3 levels in lanes with or without IL-1-treatment were western blot the same. Also, we looked at serine phosphorylation of Stat3 using results, which showed that (Figure 3b) IL-1 induced serine phosphorylation of Stat3. All results showed that IL-1 induces serine and tyrosine phosphorylation of Stat3 in transiently transfected Cos cells.

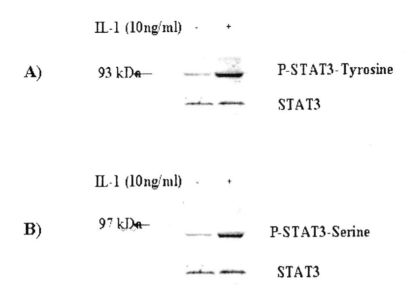

Figure 3. IL-1 induced tyrosine and serine phosphorylation of Stat3 in transient transfected Cos cells. Cos cells were transiently tranfected with IL-1R using Fugene 6. After 48 hours later, the cells were starved with serum free medium (DMEM). Then cells were were treated with or without IL-1 (20ng/ml). A) Blot was incubated with phosphotyrosine-Stat3 (705) (Upstate Biotechnology) and antibody was striped and incubated with c-terminal Stat3 (C-20) Santa Cruz . B) Blot was treated with phosphoserine-Stat3 (727) (Upstate Biotechnology) and antibody was removed from blot and filter was reblotted with C-terminal Stat3 (C-20).

3.4 IL-1 Induced Activation of Stat3 in Hep3B Cells

Cell lysates, both with and without IL-1 treatment, from overnight starved Hep3B cells were subjected to immunoprecipitation with C-terminal Stat3 antibody. This result revealed that tyrosine phosphorylation of Stat3 is IL-1 dependent (figure 4A). We also checked the Stat3 levels in the lanes with C-terminal Stat3 antibody and found that Stat3 levels were same (4B).

These results showed that immunoprecipitation with C-terminal Stat3 antibody gave IL-1 dependent Stat3 tyrosine phosphorylation. We further characterized IL-1-induced Stat3 in Hep3 cell lines using Stat3 N-terminal antibody. We striped antibodies from the filter and then the filter was re-probed with N-terminal Stat3 antibody (figure 4C). These results showed that Stat3-N antibody recognized IP-Stat3C. Also, immunoprecipitation was done by N-terminal Stat3 antibody and the filter was probed with C-terminal Stat3 antibody. This result indicated that C-terminal Stat3 antibody recognized the N-terminal Stat3 (data not shown). All these results may indicate that IL-1 induced Stat3 may be Stat3Δ.

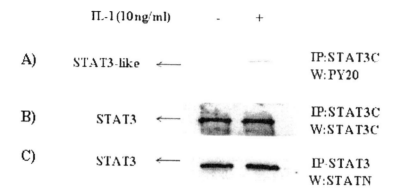

Figure 4. IL-1 induced tyrosine phosphorylation of Stat3 in Hep3B cell. Hep3B cells were starved in DMEM overnight and incubated either with or without IL-1 (20 ng/ml) for 15 min. The cells were lysed, homogenized, and immunoprecipitated with C-terminal Stat3 (C-20) or N-terminal Stat3 antibody from Santa Cruz. The immunocomplexes were resolved by 7.5%SDS-PAGE and immunoblotted. A is an immunoblot with phospho-Stat3 (Y705), B is an immunoblot with C-terminal Stat3, C is an immunoblot with N-terminal Stat3.

4. DISCUSSION

The IL-1 induced NF-ΝB, JNK, and P38 MAPK signal transduction pathways are thoroughly understood[17]; however, the IL-1-induced-JAK-STAT pathway remains quite poorly understood. Our group previously reported that a novel, Stat-like molecule, that is not Stat 1, 2, 3, 4, 5, or 6, is activated by IL-1, LPS and IL-6[9]. There is only one report showing that IL-1 induces the short form of acute phase respond factor (AFRF), (Stat3) in insulin secreting cells[11]. It has been reported that Stat3 bound to APRE[18], a palindrome motif (TTNAA) with a spacing of 4bp selectively has affinity to Stat3[19] and the high sis inducible element (hSIE) bound to Stat1 and Stat3[20]. Stat3 is activated with different cytokines, such as the IL-6 family, growth factors, and IL-2 and IL-10[16]. Two isoforms of Stat3 were observed in cells: Stat3 Δ and Stat3 E, an alternatively spliced form of Stat3. Stat3 E has a high affinity for DNA-binding, but lacks a transcriptional activation domain that may regulate the function of wt-Stat3. Stat3E is acting as a dominant-negative for transcriptional activation, but this response is dependant on cell type. Morton et al., (1999) reported that their characterized short form of Stat3 lacks the C terminal site that has transcriptional activity in insulin secreting cells[11]. We analyzed IL-1-induced Stat3 activation in the EMSA system. Our EMSA results, given either two or three bands, showed that the IL-1-induced APRE-protein complex is reproducible. The top band of the APRE-nuclear complex reacts with Stat3 C-terminal (C-20) and Stat3 internal (corresponding to SH2 domain) (K-15) antibodies (figure 2). However, Stat3 N-terminal (H-190) antibody did not react with the APRE-nuclear complex. All these results showed that IL-1 induced Stat3 may interact with another transcription factor in the APRE promoter to activate gene expression. Most probably, the N-terminal Stat3 antibody did not react with the APRE-Stat3 complex as a result of competitive inhibition by another transcription factor that interacts with the N-terminus of Stat3. Additionally, Tsukuda et al, (1996) did not detect a strong hSIE-nuclear complex when they used radiolabeled hSIE probe in IL-1-induced EL4 extract[9].

IL-1-induced nuclear extract induced bonding when APRE-probe was used. Antibody experiments showed that the top band antigenically related with Stat3; however, the bottom band was not understood. In order to characterize both bands, we did competitive experiments with different oligonucleotides. Interestingly, oligonucleotides for Stat3, hSIE, and SIE did not have affinity to APRE, except the IRF-1 sequences that bound to all Stat molecules. These results further prove that cooperative binding of Stat3 with unknown transcription factors is inhibiting competition from the unlabeled oligonucleotides.

The activation of Stats requires tyrosine phosphorylation. It has been shown that IFN-9 induces tyrosine phosphorylation of p91 and this phosphorylated form binds to the GAS element[21]. Also, p91 is tyrosine phosphorylated by many cytokines, (IL-6, CSF, IL-10, CNF) and growth factors (PDGF)[22, 16]. Serine phosphorylation of Stats is involved in the maximum activation of gene transcription. It has been reported that the mutation of the serine residue on Stat1 blocks serine phosphorylation, but has no effect on tyrosine phosphorylation or DNA binding. However, this mutation causes the reduction of transcription activation[23]. Our western blot analysis showed that Stat3 is phosphorylated on tyrosine and serine residues in an IL-1-dependant manner in transiently transfected Cos cells. Additionally, we showed that IL-1 induces Stat3 tyrosine phosphorylation in Hep3B cells. The pertinent question is which enzyme phosphorylates tyrosine and serine residues? Nearly all cytokine receptors lack intrinsic kinase activity, but it has been reported that non-tyrosine kinases, janus associated kinase (JAK) family, including JAK1, 2, 3, and tyk2, are involved in tyrosine phosphorylation[24]. The other cytokine receptors, such as the IL-6 family, LIF, and CNTF utilize gp130, associated with JAK1 and JAK2[25]. It is possible that the other tyrosine kinases may also be involved in the activation of Stat3. It has been reported that Stat3-DNA binding activity is altered by serine kinase inhibitor H7 and protein phosphatase 2[26].

ACKNOWLEDGEMENTS

This work was supported by NIH grants. Dr. Deborah L. Galson is acknowledged for her invaluable critical discussion, and advice. Special thanks to Mr. Dylan J Wirtz, Department of Internal Medicine, The Ohio State University, USA for the critical reading of the manuscript.

REFERENCES

1. Dinarello, C.A., 1996, Biological basis for Interleukin 1 in diseases. *Blood* **87**, 2095-2147.
2. Shen, X., Tian, Z., Holtzman, M.J., and Gao, B., 2000, Cross-talk between interleukin 1E and IL-6 signaling pathways: IL-1E selectively inhibits IL-6-activated signal transducer and activator of transcription factor 1 (STAT1) by a proteasome-dependent mechanism. *Biochem. J.* **352**, 913-919.
3. Wilson, D.R., Juan, T.S., Wilde, M.D., Fey, G.H., and Darlington, G.J., 1990, A 58-base-pair region of the human C3 gene confers synergistic inducibility by interleukin-1 and interleukin *Mol Cell Biol.* **10**, 6181-6191.
4. Hocke, G.,M., Barry, D., and Fey, G.H., 1992, Synergistic action of interleukin-6 and glucocorticoids is mediated by the interleukin-6 response element of the rat alpha 2 macroglobulin gene. *Mol Cell Biol.* **12**, 2282-94.
5. Wegenka, U.M., Lutticken, C., Buschmann, J., Yuan, J., Lottspeich., F., Muller-Esterl, W., Schindler, C., Roeb, E., Heinrich, P.C., and Horn, F., 1994, The interleukin-6-activated acute phase response factor is antigenically and functionally related to members of the signal transducer and activator of transcription (STAT) family. *Mol Cell Biol.* **14**, 3186-96.
6. Akira, S., Isshiki, H., Sugita, T., Tanabe, O., Kinoshita, S., Nishio, Y., Nakajima, T., Hirano, T., and Kishimoto, T., 1990, A nuclear factor for IL-6 expression (NF-IL6) is a member of a C/EBP family. *EMBO J.* **9**, 1897-906.
7. Rothwarf, D.M., and Karin, M., 1999, The NF-kappa E activation pathway: a paradigm in information transfer from membrane to nucleus. *Sci STKE* **5**, Review.

8. Auron P.E., 1998, The interleukin 1 receptor: ligand interactions and signal transduction. *Cytokine Growth Factor Rev.* **9**, 221-37.
9. Tsukada, J., Waterman, W.R., Koyama, Y., Webb, A.C., and Auron, P.E., 1996, A novel STAT-like factor mediates lipopolysaccharide, interleukin 1 (IL-1), and IL-6 signaling and recognizes a gamma interferon activation site-like element in the IL1E gene. *Mol Cell Biol.* **16**, 2183-94.
10. Schumann, R.R., Kirschning, C.J., Unbehaun, A., Aberle, H.P., Knope, H.P., Lamping, N., and Herrmann, F. 1996, The lipopolysaccharide-binding protein is a secretory class 1 acute-phase protein whose gene is transcriptionally activated by APRF/STAT/3 and other cytokine-inducible nuclear proteins. *Mol. Cell Biol.* **16**, 3490-503.
11. Morton, N.M., de Groot, R.P., and Emilsson, V., 1999, Interleukin-1E activates a short STAT-3 isoform in clonal insulin-secreting cells. *FEBS Lett.* **442**, 57-60.
12. Zhang, Z., and Fuller, G.M., 2000, Interleukin 1E inhibits interleukin 6-mediated rat 9 fibrinogen gene expression. *Hemostasis, Thrombosis Vasc. Biol.* **96**, 3466-3472.
13. Benkhart, E.M., Siedlar, M., Wedel, A., Werner, T., Ziegler-Heitbrock, H.W., 2000, Role of Stat3 in lipopolysaccharide-induced IL-10 gene expression. *J. Immunol.* **165**, 1612-7.
14. Bromberg, J., 2002, Stat proteins and oncogenesis. *J Clin Invest.* **109**, 1139-42.
15. Schindler, C., and Darnell, J.E., Jr., 1995, Transcriptional responses to polypeptide ligands: the JAK-STAT pathway. *Annu Rev Biochem.* **64**, 621-51. Review.
16. Akira, S., Nishio, Y., Inoue, M., Wang, X.J., Wei, S., Matsusaka, T., Yoshida, K., Sudo, T., Naruto, M., and Kishimoto, T.,1994, Molecular cloning of APRF, a novel IFN-stimulated gene factor 3 p91-related transcription factor involved in the gp130-mediated signaling pathway. *Cell* **77**, 63-71.
17. Kuno, K., and Matsushima, K., 1994, The IL-1 receptor signaling pathway. *J. Leukoc. Biol.*, **56**, 542-7. Review.
18. Yoo, J.Y., Wang, W., Desiderio, S., and Nathans, D., 2001, Synergistic activity of STAT3 and c-Jun at a specific array of DNA elements in the alpha 2-macroglobulin promoter. *J. Biol. Chem.* **276**, 26421-9.
19. Seidel, H.M., Milocco, L.H., Lamb, P., Darnell, J.E., Jr, Stein, R.B., and Rosen, J.,1995, Spacing of palindromic half sites as a determinant of selective STAT (signal transducers and activators of transcription) DNA binding and transcriptional activity. *Proc. Natl. Acad. Sci. USA* **92**, 3041-3045.
20. Wagner, B.J., Hayes, T.E., Hoban, C.J., and Cochran, B.H., 1990, The SIF binding element confers sis/PDGF inducibility onto the c-fos promoter. *EMBO J.* **9**, 4477-84.
21. David, M., 1995, Trancription factors in interferon signaling. *Pharm. Ther.* **65**, 149 161.
22. Zhong, Z., Wen, Z., and Darnell, J.E. Jr., 1994, Stat3:a stat family member activated by tyrosine phosphorylation in respons to EGF and IL-6. *Science* **264**, 95-98.
23. Schuringa, J.J., Schepers, H., Vellenga, E., and Kruijer, W., 2001, Ser727-dependent transcriptional activation by association of p300 with STAT3 upon IL-6 stimulation. *FEBS Lett.* **495**, 71-6.
24. Finidori, J., and Kelly, P.A., 1995, Cytokine receptor signalling through two novel families of transducer molecules: Janus kinases, and signal transducers and activators of transcription. *J. Endocrinol.* **147**, 11-23.
25. Wilks, A.F., and Oates, A.C., 1996, The JAK/STAT pathway. *Cancer Surv.* **27**, 139-63.
26. Boulton, T.G., Zhong, Z., Wen, Z., Darnell, J.E. Jr, Stahl, N., and Yancopoulos, G.D., 1995, STAT3 activation by cytokines utilizing gp130 and related transducers involves a secondary modification requiring an H7-sensitive kinase. *Proc. Natl. Acad. Sci. USA.* **92**, 6915-9.

THE USE OF ANTIBODIES IN DIAGNOSIS AND THERAPY OF CANCER

Aslı Muvaffak[1] and Nesrin Hasırcı[2]
[1]*Department of Biotechnology, Middle East Technical University, Ankara 06531 Turkey;*
[2]*Department of Chemistry, Middle East Technical University, Ankara 06531, Turkey*

1. INTRODUCTION

Immunology began as a study of the response of the living bodies to infections. Over the years, it has become progressively more basic, passing through phases of emphasis on serology, cellular immunology, molecular immunology and immunogenetics. Immunology has also grown to comprise many fields such as immunochemistry, immunopathology, immunopharmacology, allergy, clinical immunology, tumor immunology and transplantation. It has always provided an excellent mix of fundamental and applied sciences[1-2]. The development of monoclonal antibody (MoAb) technology by Köhler and Milstein[3] provided an enormous opportunity for examination of a range of issues, which previously seemed difficult to handle. MoAbs were used in immunocytopathology, radioimmunoassays, enzyme-linked immunosorbent assays, and flow cytometry *in vitro* and *in vivo* for diagnosis and immunotherapy of human disease.

Immunologic therapy in its broadest sense encompasses the treatment and prevention of a large number and variety of immunologic and nonimmunologic diseases. Historically, therapeutic immunology began in 1976, when Willian Jenner showed that an ancient viral scourge, smallpox, could be successfully prevented by immunization. Later, a new and lethal viral disease, acquired immune deficiency syndrome (AIDS), appeared and rapidly became a major worldwide public health problem. The causative virus, human immunodeficiency virus (HIV), infects the CD4 T cell, which is the central focus of the immune response itself. As the subject of widespread research by thousands of immunologists and other scientists, AIDS has generated an enormous expansion of our knowledge of human immunology; however, it has thus far eluded all attempts at successful treatment or prevention by immunization[5,6].

To better understand the mechanisms and clinical indications for the many forms of treatment, the immune system can be divided functionally into two categories: *the immune response* and *the inflammatory response*. Therapy directed at the immune response can be either antigen-specific or antigen-nonspecific. Some diseases require that the immune response be stimulated, whereas others require suppression. In therapy, these diverse goals now include chemically defined drugs obtained from natural sources such as fungal products, synthetic chemicals, specific antibodies, and many of the actual cellular and chemical components of the immune system itself. Genetic engineering, cloning techniques make available adequate quantities of virtually any cytokine, adhesion molecule, cell membrane molecule, or receptor in remarkably short time after their discovery. Increasingly, antibodies are being used as drugs because of their ability to target a particular structure within the body with great specificity. MoAb technology has largely supplanted the traditional use of serum gamma globulin from animals immunized with relevant antigen. Although this greatly increases specificity and eliminates the problems of allergic reactions to irrelevant serum proteins, the MoAb is itself antigenic and may in time become ineffective by neutralization or by an allergic reaction to it[2,4]. If the target cell death is the therapeutic goal, the MoAb has been coupled to a potent toxin such as ricin, diptheria toxin, or *Pseudomonas* exotoxin A. In fact the generation of human monoclonal antibodies (HuMoAbs) by Steinitz et al. in 1977 by using Epstein-Barr virus have provided useful information to develop encouraging therapies[7]. HuMoAbs were desirable for clinical applications because: a) HuMoAbs didn't develop any damage or response because of cross-species differences, as it was the case when mouse MoAbs were used; b) HuMoAbs can easily recognize tumor specific antigens that were masked in a mouse model. But, the production of HuMoAbs was limited because of the lack of known tumor specific antigens and the inability to sensitize human subjects with tumor preparations. Several other studies were conducted in order to develop the use of HuMoAbs, including the use of circulating antitumor antibodies from cancer patients [2, 8-10], lymphocytes from lymph nodes [9-11], peripheral blood lymphocytes[13], lymphocytes from malignant pleural effusions and spleen lymphocytes[12,13] of cancer patients. They have been used as the source of tumor specific B lymphocytes. These studies indicated the possibility of an ongoing humoral immune response in cancer patients toward tumor associated antigens.

One other way to overcome some of the complications arising by mouse MoAbs, is to prepare engineered MoAbs by using recombinant DNA technology. Use of recombinant MoAbs is an emerging therapeutic area[14]. MoAbs have been successfully used in cancer patients as both a diagnostic[15-18] and a therapeutic[19, 20] tools. It was shown that these MoAbs specifically localize neoplastic cells in different cancers. Indeed, reports support the use of MoAbs (e.g. rituximab) in cases of lymphomas showing resistance or relapse after antineoplastic chemotherapy, either alone or in combination with cytotoxic drugs[19].

1.1 Immunoglobulin Structure

Immunoglobulins (Igs) (which are antibodies) are the antigen-binding proteins present on *B-cell membrane* and secreted by plasma cells. Membrane bound Ab confers antigenic specificity on *B cells*; antigen-specific proliferation of B-cell clones depends on the interaction of membrane Ab and antigen. Selected antibodies circulate in the blood and serve as effectors of "humoral immunity" by searching out and neutralizing or eliminating antigens. Immunoglobulins (Figure 1) are actually built up of two types of polypeptide chains: "larger heavy chains" (M.Wt. 50-70 Kd) and "smaller light chains" (M.Wt. 23 Kd). Both the heavy and the light chains contain a variable (V) region consisted of 100-110 amino acids and which differs from one Ab to the other. The rest of the Ig molecule is composed of constant (C) regions (shown as N or O in light chains and Π, Δ, Γ, or H in heavy chains). The heavy chains of a given Ab molecule determines the class of that Ab: i.e. *IgM, IgG, IgA, IgD or IgE*. A single Ab molecule has two identical heavy chains and two identical light chains. In humans, there are two subclasses of Δ heavy chains and four subclasses of ϑ heavy chains; in mice there are four subclasses of ϑ heavy chains [5,6].

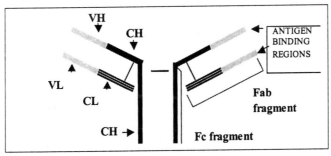

Figure 1. Immunoglobulin structure (**CH**: Constant Heavy, **CL**: Constant Light, **VH**: Variable Heavy, **VL**: Variable Light, **Fab**: Antigen-binding, **Fc**: Complement activation).

Studies of the Ig structure indicated that heavy and light chains were organized into domains, each containing 110 amino acid residues and an intrachain disulphide bond that formed a 60-aa loop. It is known that in humans 60% of the light chains are O and 40% are O, whereas in mice 95% of the light chains are N and only 5% are O. A single Ab molecule contains either N or O light chains, but never both[5,6]. Indeed, those O chains are classified into subtypes. In mice there are three subtypes, however in humans there are four subtypes. Single amino acid interchanges at two or three positions are responsible for the subtype differences.

Detailed analysis of the amino acid sequences of VL (light chain variable) and VH (heavy chain variable) domains revealed that the sequence variability was mainly present in several hypervariable (HV) regions. Three such hypervariable regions are present in each mouse and human heavy and light chain (constituting 15%-20% of the variable domain). The remainder of the VL and VH domains exhibit far less variation; these stretches are called as framework regions (FRs). Because the antigen-binding site is complementary to the structure of the epitope, the hypervariable regions are also called as complementarity-determinig regions (CDRs). The more conserved sequence of the framework regions generates the basic E pleated sheet structure of the VH and VL domains. The wide range of specificities exhibited by antibodies is a function of variations in the length and amino acid composition of the six hypervariable loops in each Fab fragment[4-6].

1.2 Antigen Determinants of Immunoglobulins

Antibodies are glycoproteins and they function as potent immunogens to induce an Ab response. Such anti-Ig antibodies are powerful tools for the study of the B-cell development and humoral immune responses. The "antigenic determinants", or "epitopes", on Ig molecules fall into three major categories: isotypic, allotypic and idiotypic determinants, which are located in characteristic portions of the molecule (Figure 1).

Isotypic determinants are C region determinants that collectively define each heavy chain class and subclass and each light chain type and subtype within a species. Each isotype is encoded by a separate C region gene, and all members of a species carry the same C region genes. Within a species, each normal individual will express all isotypes in their serum. Different species inherit different C region genes and therefore express different C region genes and therefore express different isotypes. Therefore, when an Ab from one species is injected into another species, the isotypic determinants will be recognized as foreign, inducing an Ab response to the isotypic determinants on the foreign Ab. Anti-isotype Ab is routinely used for research purposes to determine the class or subclass of serum Ab produced during an immune response or to characterize the class of membrane bound Ab present on B cells. Although all members of a species inherit the same set of isotype genes, multiple alleles exist for some of the genes. The amino acid differences, which are encoded by these alleles, comprise the allotypic determinants and occur in some, but not all members of a species.

In humans, allotypes have been characterized for all four IgG subclasses, for one IgA subclass, and for the N light chain. The gamma chain allotypes are referred to as Gm markers and 25 different Gm allotypes have been identified. For the two IgA subclasses, only the IgA2 subclass has 2 allotypes. The N light chain has three allotypes. Each of these allotypic determinants represents differences in one to four amino acids that are encoded by different alleles. Ab to allotypic determinants can be produced by injecting Abs from one member of a species into another member of the same species who carries different allotypic determinants. (Ab to allotypic determinants sometimes is produced by a mother during pregnancy in response to paternal allotypic determinants on the fetal Igs. Antibodies to allotypic determinants can also arise following a blood transfusion)[4-6].

The idiotypic determinants are generated by the conformation of the heavy and light chain V regions. Each individual antigenic determinant of the variable region is referred to as an idiotype. In some cases an idiotype may be the actual antigen-binding site, and in some cases an idiotype may comprise variable region sequences outside of the antigen binding site. Each Ab will present multiple idiotypes; the sum of the individual idiotypes is called the idiotype of the Ab. Because the antibodies produced by individual B cells derived from the same clone have identical variable chain sequences, they all have the same idiotype. Anti-idiotype Ab is produced by minimizing isotypic or allotypic differences, so that the idiotypic difference can be recognized. Often a homogeneous Ab such as myeloma protein or MoAb is used. Injection of such an Ab into a syngeneic recipient will result in the formation of anti-idiotype Ab to the idiotypic determinants.

Most *anti-idiotypic antibodies* utilized in the treatment of human lymphoid malignancies are directed towards *B cell immunoglobulin idiotypes*. Idiotypic MoAbs to Ig were used for the treatment of patients with B cell lymphomas[15]. One patient had an uninterrupted remission for more than 4 years after therapy. However, there were certain difficulties. During maturation, B cells use somatic hypermutation to increase their diversity. Thus, there is tremendous idiotypic heterogeneity within the B cell population, which permits some neoplastic B cells to escape the attack of an Ab directed toward an individual idiotype.

2. MONOCLONAL ANTIBODIES

Most antigens possess multiple epitopes and induce proliferation and differentiation of a variety of B cell clones. The resulting serum Abs are heterogeneous, comprising a mixture of Abs each specific for one epitope. Such as "polyclonal" Ab response facilitates the localization, phagocytosis, and complement-mediated lysis of antigen; it thus has clear advantages for the organism *in vivo*. Unfortunately, the Ab heterogeneity that increases immune protection *in vivo* often reduces the efficacy of an antiserum for various *in vitro* uses. For most research, diagnostic, and therapeutic purposes, MoAbs, derived from a single clone and thus specific for a single epitope, are preferable.

Georges Köhler and Cesar Milstein[3] devised a method for preparing MoAbs. By fusing a normal activated, Ab-producing B cell with a myeloma cell (a cancerous plasma cell), they were able to generate a hybrid cell, a hybridoma, that possessed the immortal growth properties of the myeloma cell and secreted the Ab produced by the B cell. Resulting hybridoma cells, which secrete large quantities of MoAb, can be cultured indefinitely.

2.1 Production of Monoclonal Antibodies

The production of a given monoclonal Ab involves three basic steps: 1) Generating B-cell hybridomas by fusing antigen-primed B cells and myeloma cells and selecting for fused clones, 2) Screening the resulting clones for those that secrete Ab with the desired antigenic specificity and, 3) Propagating the desired hybridomas. In the procedure of MoAb production, myeloma cells that are deficient in both, hypoxanthine guanine phosphoriobosyl transferase (HGPRT$^-$) and immunoglobulin (Ig$^-$), are used as one fusion partner[5,6]. These cells, which contribute immortal-growth properties to the fused cells, cannot grow in HAT (Hypoxanthine, Aminopterin and Thymidine) medium or secrete Ab. The other fusion partner is made up of spleen cells, which contain primed B cells that are HGPRT$^+$ and Ig$^+$. Because unfused spleen cells are terminally differentiated cells and thus only capable of limited growth *in vitro*, they do not need to carry a selection gene.

In the process, the aliquots are cultured in wells containing HAT medium, after the cell fusion step. Some wells may contain small clusters of viable cells after 7-10 days where each cluster represents clonal expansion of a hybridoma. Single cells from these cultures are transferred and cultured in separate wells, subclones derived from single cells are then screened for the presence of Ab and Ab-positive clones, subcultured at low cell densities to ensure clonal purity in each well [3,5,6]. The obtained pure clones of Ab-secreting hybridomas must be screened for the desired antigenic specificity. The supernatant of each hybridoma culture contains its secreted Ab and can be assayed for a particular antigenic specificity in various ways. Two of the most common screening techniques are ELISA and RIA.

The production of HuMoAbs has a number of technical difficulties. The most important is the difficulty of obtaining antigen-primed B cells in humans equivalent to the mouse spleen cells. Human hybridomas must be prepared from human peripheral blood, which contains few activated B cells in an immune response. It is possible to obtain B cells primed to the antigens in accepted vaccines, but human volunteers cannot be immunized with the range of antigens that can be given to mice or other animals. To overcome this difficulty, cultured human cells can be primed with antigen *in vitro*. However, the *in vitro* system cannot mimic the normal microenvironment of lymphoid tissue. One way to avoid the need for *in vitro* priming of human B cells is to incorporate genes encoding human Ab within mice. SCID- human mice contain human B and T cells. Following immunization of these mice, activated human B cells can be isolated from the spleen and used to produce HuMoAbs. GenPharm International used another approach and has knocked out the heavy and light chain genes within mice and then introduced yeast artificial chromosomes engineered with large DNA sequences containing heavy and light chain genes. The resulting transgenic mice produce human Abs exclusively[5,6]. Another difficulty in producing HuMoAbs has been the lack of human myeloma cells that exhibit immortal growth, are susceptible to HAT selection, and do not secrete Ab. As an alternative to conferring immortality on human B cells through fusion to myeloma cells, normal human B lymphocytes can be transformed with Epstein-Barr virus (EBV), some of the B cells acquire the immortal growth properties of a transformed cell while continuing to secrete Ab. Cloning of such primed, transformed cells has permitted production of HuMoAbs.

2.2 Engineered Monoclonal Antibodies

When mouse MoAbs are introduced into humans they are recognized as foreign and evoke an Ab response. The induced human anti-mouse Ab quickly reduces the effectiveness of the mouse MoAb by clearing it from the bloodstream. In addition, circulating complexes of mouse and human Abs can cause allergic reactions. In some cases the buildup of these complexes in organs such as the kidney can cause serious and even life threatening reactions. Because of these reactions, the use of mouse MoAbs for clinical purposes in humans was limited. Clearly, one way to overcome at least some of these complications is to use HuMoAbs. Since then researchers have begun engineering MoAbs using recombinant DNA technology[11-14, 20-23, 26, 28].

One approach to engineering an Ab is to clone recombinant DNA containing the promoter, leader and V region sequences from a mouse Ab gene and the C region exons from a human Ab gene (Figure 2). The Ab encoded by such a recombinant gene is a "mouse-human chimera", known as a "humanized Ab". Its antigenic specificity is determined by the V region and derived from the mouse DNA. Its isotype is determined by the C region and derived from the human DNA as shown in Figure 3. Because human genes encode their C regions, these chimeric Abs have fewer mouse antigenic determinants and are far less immunogenic than mouse MoAbs when administered to humans. Another advantage of a chimeric Ab is that it retains the biological effector functions of the human Ab and is more likely to trigger complement activation or Fc receptor binding[5, 21, 22]. In order to produce chimeric mouse-human MoAbs (Figure 3-b), chimeric mouse-human heavy- and light-chain expression vectors can be produced and transfected into Ab⁻ myeloma cells. Culture in amphicillin medium selects for transfected myeloma cells, which secrete the chimeric Ab[1, 5, 6].

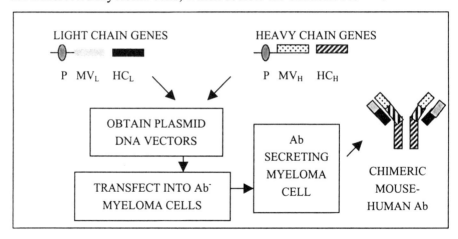

Figure 2. Production of chimeric mouse-human MoAbs (**P**: Promoter, **M**: Mouse, **H**: Human, V_L: Variable Light, C_L: Constant Light, V_h: Variable Heavy, C_h: Constant Heavy).

Heteroconjugates (Figure 4-a) are hybrids of two different Ab molecules. Various heteroconjugates have been designed in which one half of the Ab has specificity for a tumor and the other half has specificity for a surface molecule on an immune effector cell, such as an NK cell, an activated macrophage, or a cytotoxic T lymphocyte (CTL). The heteroconjugate thus serves to cross-link the immune effector cell to the tumor. Some heteroconjugates have been designed to activate the immune effector cell when it is cross-linked to the tumor cell so that it begins to mediate the destruction of the tumor cell.

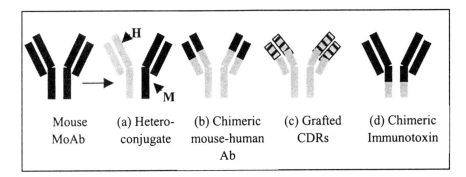

Figure 3. Chimeric and hybrid MoAbs engineered by recombinant DNA technology (**H**: Human (gray), **M**: Mouse (black)).

Wong et al.[21] used chimeric T84.66 (cT84.66), which was a high affinity IgG1 MoAb against carcinoembryonic antigen (CEA) and evaluated the tumor targeting properties, biodistribution, pharmacokinetics and immunogeneicity of ^{111}I-labelled cT84.66. cT84.66 is a genetically engineered human/murine chimeric IgG, with high affinity and specificity to carcinoembryonic antigen (CEA). Patients were administered a single intravenous dose and it was observed that, cT84.66 demonstrated tumor targeting that was comparable to that of other radiolabelled intact anti-CEA MoAbs. Its immunogenicity after single administration was lower than murine MoAbs. These properties make cT84.66 or a lower molecular weight derivative attractive for further evaluation as an imaging agent. Wong et al.[22] also evaluated the toxicities, biodistribution, pharmacokinetics, tumor targeting, immunogenicity, and organ and tumor absorbed dose estimates of cT84.66 and represented further improving in the therapeutic potential of this agent through refinements in the characteristics of the Ab and the treatment strategies. Average tumor doses when compared with red marrow doses indicated a favorable therapeutic ratio.

2.3 CDR -Grafted Chimeric Monoclonal Antibodies

Chimeric antibodies containing less regions, only "mouse CDRs", from mouse antibodies have been developed in order reduce the negative effects in humans (Figure 4-c). In this approach, the CDRs of a mouse Ab are grafted to human framework regions to construct a variable region retaining the human E-strand framework. These Abs are less immunogenic in humans than humanized Abs containing the entire mouse V region. Since the CDRs compose the antigen-binding site, some CDR-grafted Abs retain their ability to bind antigen. Often, however, CDR-grafted Abs exhibit reduced binding affinity. In some cases, this can be corrected by introducing small mutations in the framework region that induce small changes in the three-dimensional configuration of the CDRs resulting in improved Ab affinity. CDR-grafted antibodies have many potential therapeutic uses (Table 1).

Table 1. Therapeutic Uses for CDR-Grafted Antibodies

TARGET ANTIGEN	CLINICAL POTENTIAL
Cdw52 (surface molecule on leukocytes)	Lymphoma, systematic vasculitis, rhematoid arthritis
CD3 (T-cell marker)	Organ transplantation
CD4 (T-cell marker)	Organ transplantation, rhemateuid arthritis, Chron's disease
Receptor for interleukin-2	Leukemias and lymphomas, organ transplantation, graft-versus host disease
Tumor necrosis factor Δ	Septic shock
Human immunodeficiency virus (HIV)	AIDS
Rous sarcoma virus (RSV)	Respiratory syncytial virus infection
Herpes simplex virus (HSV)	Neonatal, ocular, and genital herpes infection
Receptor for human epidermal growth factor (EGF)	Cancer
Placental alkaline phosphatase	Cancer
Carcinoembryonic antigen	Cancer

Clinical remission was reported in two patients with non-Hodgkin's lymphoma who received daily injections of the CDR grafted MoAb specific for a cell membrane antigen on the lymphoma cells[28]. Different chimeric MoAbs for the treatment of cancer in humans were prepared. Presta et al [23] aimed to humanize the muMoAb (murine monoclonal Ab) VEGF (vascular endothelial growth factor) A.4.6.1. The murine anti-human VEGF MoAb A.4.6.1 has been shown to potently suppress angiogenesis and growth in a variety of human tumor cell lines transplanted in nude mice and also to inhibit neovascularization. They transferred the six CDRs from muMoAb VEGF A.4.6.1 to consensus human framework. Seven framework residues in the humanized variable heavy domain (VH) domain and one framework residue in the humanized variable light (VL) domain were changed from human to murine to achieve binding equivalent to muMoAb VEGF A.4.6.1.

Chimeric MoAbs that function as immunotoxins (Figure 4-d) can also be prepared. In this case, the terminal constant region domain in a tumor specific MoAb is replaced with toxin chains. Because these immunotoxins lack the terminal Fc domain, they are not able to bind to cells bearing Fc receptors. These immunotoxins could bind only to tumor cells, making them more efficient as a therapeutic reagent [5,6].

2.4 Monoclonal Antibodies From Ig-Gene Libraries

Another approach for generating MoAbs employs the polymerase chain reaction (PCR) to amplify the DNA encoding Ab heavy chain and light chain Fab fragments from hybridoma cells or plasma cells. A promoter region and EcoRI site is added to the amplified sequences, and the resulting constructs are inserted into bacteriophage lambda (O), yielding separate heavy and light chain libraries. Cleavage with EcoRI and random joining of the heavy and light chain genes yield numerous novel heavy-light constructs. This procedure generates an enormous diversity of Ab specificities; clones containing these random combinations of H+L chains can be rapidly screened for those secreting Ab to a particular antigen. For example, in one study a million clones were screened in just two days, with over 100 clones being identified that produced Ab specific for the desired antigen. The technique has the potential of producing an enormous repertoire of Ab specificities without the limitations of antigen priming and hybridoma technology that currently complicate the production of MoAbs [4-6].

3. MONOCLONAL ANTIBODIES IN DIAGNOSIS AND THERAPY OF CANCER

Monoclonal antibodies have been applied clinically to the diagnosis and therapy of an array of human disorders, including cancer and infectious diseases and have been used for the modulation of immune responses. MoAb-mediated therapy has been revolutionized by advances such as the definition of cell surface structures on abnormal cells as targets for effective MoAb action, genetic engineering to create less immunogenic and more effective MoAbs, and the arming of such Abs with toxins or radionuclides to enhance their effector function [1, 2, 21, 22, 27, 29].

3.1 Cell Surface Cancer Antigens

Tumor antigens are cellular proteins that give rise to peptides presented with MHC (Major Histocompatibility Complex) molecules. Typically, these antigens have been identified by their ability to induce antigen-specific CTLs. Tumor antigens must be capable of inducing either humoral or cell mediated immune response. The presence of tumor antigens that elicit a cell mediated response has been demonstrated by the rejection of tumors transplanted into syngeneic recipients. Since then they are named as transplantation antigens. The relevant tumor antigens fall into two groups, named as tumor-specific transplantation antigens and tumor association transplantation antigens.

Tumor specific transplantation antigens (TSTAs) are unique to tumor cells and do not occur on normal cells in the body. Cytosolic processing of genetically altered proteins give rise to novel peptides that are presented with class 1 MHC molecules, including a cell-mediated response by CTLs. According to the formation of these novel peptides, TSTAs have two types; chemically or physically induced ones and virally induced tumors. The majority of tumor association transplantation antigens (TATAs) are not unique to tumor cells, but are also present on normal cells. They are grouped as oncofetal tumor antigens, oncogene protein products and TATAs on human melanomas. Oncofetal tumor antigens are normally found on 2 to 6 months old fetuses and also can be found in some normal adults in trace amounts and in some non-cancerous disease states. So the presence of these oncofetal antigens is not diagnostic for tumors, but rather serves to monitor tumor growth. Two types are CEA and AFP [4-6]. Carcino embryonic antigen (CEA) is a glycoprotein found on gastrointestinal and liver cells of 2 to 6 months old fetuses. CEA is widely used to monitor tumor growth after colorectal surgeries. For example, 90% patients with advanced colorectal cancer and 50 % patients with early colorectal cancer have increased levels of CEA in their serum [11, 21, 22]. Elevated alpha fetoprotein (AFP) levels are found in a majority of patients with liver cancer [5,6].

The increased levels of the oncogene product can be recognized by the immune system as a tumor associated antigen. For example, human breast cancer cells exhibit elevated expression of the oncogene encoded Neu-protein (a growth factor receptor) whereas normal adult cells express only trace amounts of Neu protein. Because of this difference in Neu level, anti Neu MoAbs can recognize and selectively eliminate breast cancer cells without damaging normal cells. Single point mutations in ras proto-oncogene have been recorded in human colorectal cancers, in more than 90% of pancreatic carcinomas, in acute myelogenous leukemia and in preleukemic syndromes [2,4-6].

Goi et al.[24] demonstrated that there were dramatic decreases of DCC (deleted in colorectal carcinoma) protein as well as its mRNA in colon cancer tissues. Furthermore, the clinical significance of the reduction of DCC expression in the diagnosis and treatment of colorectal cancer patients was investigated. As a consequence, the researchers have established a DCC-specific MoAb by using a GST-DCC fusion protein for immunization. This MoAb proved to be very useful in Western immunoblot, flow cytometry and immunohistostaining. As expected, DCC protein was scarcely detectable in human cancer cell lines, except for some haemotopoietic lines. Colon cancer tissues from patients were also negative or they expressed at a very low level. On the other hand, normal colonic tissues and adenoma tissues showed almost equivalent intensities of DCC bands in immunoblots. These results indicated that DCC may play an important role as a tumor-suppressor gene and the down regulation or defect of the gene may trigger the progression of colon cancers from adenomas[24].

Several growth factors and growth factor receptors expressed at high levels can serve as tumor associated antigens. A variety of tumor cells express epidermal growth factor (EGF) receptor at levels 100 times greater than that in normal cells [1,2,5]. Transferrin growth factor, TGF, serves as a tumor associated antigen and it is designated as p97, which aids in the transport of Fe into the cells. Normally, cells express less than 8000 molecules of p97, but melanoma cells express 50.000-500.000 molecules of p97 per cell. A recombinant vaccina virus has been prepared carrying the p97 cloned gene. When this vaccine was injected into mice, it induced both humoral and cell-mediated immune responses which protected the mice against live melanoma cells expressing the p97 antigen. These results highlight the importance of identifying tumor antigen as potential targets of tumor immunotherapy [1-2].

TATAs on Human Melanomas are expressed on a significant proportion of human melanoma tumors as well as on a number of other human tumors. It might be possible to produce a tumor vaccine expressing the shared antigen for the treatment of number of these tumors (Table 2).

Table 2. TATAs Expressed on Human Melanoma Cells

TATAs Expressed on Human Cells	Percent Expression & Locations
MAGE-1	40 % of human melanomas
GAGE-1,2, BAGE, MAGE-1,3	75% of human melanomas
MAGE-1,2,3	Melanomas, glioma cells, breast tumors, non small cell lung tumors and head and head or neck carcinomas

3.2 Diagnosis of Cancer by Monoclonal Antibodies

Radiolabelled MoAbs were commonly used in diagnosis of cancer. Horak et al.[25] evaluated the specificity, toxicity and efficacy of ^{212}Pb in nude mice bearing the SK-OV-3 human ovarian tumor cell line expressing the

HER2/neu proto-oncogene. It was shown that the rate of growth of small SK-OV-3 tumors were modestly inhibited. However, tumor growth was not inhibited in mice bearing larger SK-OV-3 tumors by the administration of a single dose. As a result, ^{212}Pb -AE1 as a radiolabelled MoAb may be of only modest value in the therapy of bulk solid tumors due to the short physical half-life of ^{212}Pb and time required to achieve a useful tumor to normal tissue ratio of radionuclide after administration. However, the radiolabelled MoAb may be useful in therapy of tumors in the adjuvant setting.

Mariani et al.[26] explored the tumor targeting potential of radiolabelled MoAb BC-1 in cancer patients It was suggested that high expression of oncofetal protein during neoangiogenesis induced by cancer provides the biological basis for specific accumulation of radioactivity in the tumor mass. The results indicated the diagnostic potential of MoAbTc-99m-BC-1 for immunoscintigraphy in cancer patients.

Biassoni et al.[27] showed the use of techneticum (Tc)-99m- labeled SM3 MoAb for evaluating the preoperatively axillary lymph node involvement in patients with breast cancer. They showed that planar images were insufficiently sensitive for the detection of involvement impalpable or small axillary lymph nodes, and Tc-99m-labelled-SM3 appears a promising technique for the imaging of the axilla.

3.3 Monoclonal Antibody Therapy of Cancer

Treatment approaches using chemotherapy and radiotherapy have increased host toxicity to obtain antitumor activity. The development of MoAbs provided hope that tumor targeted therapy would one day play a role in the treatment of cancer. Indeed, promising results have been presented in several areas; however, these treatments have often proved technically difficult, produced disappointing efficacy, and were often not broadly applicable to patients with a given malignancy.

Maloney et al.[28] used IDEC-C2B8, a chimeric MoAb directed against B-cell specific antigen CD20 for the treatment on non-Hodgkin's lymphoma (NHL). The MoAb mediates complement and Ab-dependent cell mediated cytotoxicity and has direct antiproliferative effects against malignant B cell lines *in vitro*. Results were found to be comparable with the results obtained with standard chemotherapy, and thus IDEC-C2B8 showed a safety profile.

Another strategy for MoAb therapy of Lymphoma was also shown in literature[29,30]. It was suggested that bacterial DNA and synthetic oligodeoxynucleotides containing the CpG motif (CpG ODN) can activate immune cell subsets, including natural killer cells and macrophages. CpG ODN activated murine splenocytes induced lysis of tumor targets more effectively than unactivated splenocytes. *In vivo*, CpG ODN alone had no effect on survival of mice with lymphoma cells. 95% of mice treated with MoAb alone developed tumor compared with 20% of mice treated with Ab and CpG ODN. A single dose of CpG ODN appeared to be as effective as multiple doses of interleukin-2 at inhibiting tumor growth when combined with antitumor MoAb. As a consequence, immunostimulatory CpG ODN can enhance Ab dependent cellular cytotoxicity and can act as a source for potential immunotherapeutic reagents in cancer.

4. CONCLUSIONS

The target therapy developed at the turn of century was based on the idea that "a drug will attack its target without damaging any other tissues". The use of antibodies was considered as a way to selectively deliver the anticancer drugs. Modern advances in the field of immunotherapy hold the promise of providing the clinical oncologist with new tools to fight cancer. Various MoAb based strategies, which are currently under investigation, have provided useful means to develop better diagnostic and therapeutic approaches for cancer. MoAb based immunotherapies showed a particular emphasis on target antigens, MoAb design and potential applications in diagnosis and therapy of cancer. However, those early trials with MoAb therapy for solid tumor oncology met with limited success due to difficulty in MoAb design and production, the development of host immunological responses against murine MoAb, target antigen selection, and poor MoAb pharmacokinetics and tumor tissue penetration. Recent advances in the fields of immunology and oncology have provided ways to circumvent these obstacles. Today MoAb based strategies have proved to be useful and effective for cancer diagnosis and therapy. The field of MoAb based immunotherapy continues to evolve. New discoveries in this area of cancer therapy show promise for the future.

ACKNOWLEDGEMENTS

The work was supported by TUBITAK and DPT-METU-AFP Grants.

REFERENCES

1. Waldmann, T.A., 1991, Monoclonal antibodies in diagnosis and therapy. *Science* **252**, 1657-1662.
2. Old, L. J., 1996, Immunotherapy of cancer. *Scientific American.* **Sep'96**, 136-143.

3. Köhler, G., and Milstein, C., 1975, Continuous culture of fused cells secreting antibody of predefined specificity. *Nature* **256**, 495.
4. Abbas, A.K., Lichtman, A.H., and Pober, J.S., 2000, *Cellular and Molecular Immunology*, W.B. Saunders Co.
5. William, E.P. (Editor), 1998, *Fundamental Immunology*, Lippincott Williams & Wilkins Publishers.
6. Steties, D.P., Abba, I.T., and Tristam, G.P., 1994, *Basic and Clinical Immunology*. Appleton & Lange, Stanford.
7. Steinitz, M., Klein, G., Koskimies, S., and Makel, O., 1977, EB Virus induced B lymphocyte cell lines producing specific antibody. *Nature* **269**, 420-422.
8. Pfreundschuk, M., Shiku, H., and Takahashi, T. *et al.*, 1978, Serological analysis of cell surface antigens of malignant human brain tumors. *Proc. Natl. Acad. Sci. USA* **75**, 5122-5126.
9. Meda, R., Shiku, H., and Pfreundschuh, M. *et al.*, 1979, Serological analysis of cell surface antigens of human renal cancer defined by autologoius typing. *J. Exp. Med.* **150**, 5564-5579.
10. Huth, J.F., Gupta, R.K., Eilber, G.R., and Morton, D.L., 1984, A prospective post operative evaluation of urinary tumor associated antigens in sarcoma patients. *Cancer* **53**, 1306-1310.
11. Koda, K., Glassyand, M.C., and Chang, H.R., 1990, Generation of human monoclonal antibodies against colon cancer. *Arch Surg* **125**, 1591-1597.
12. Vollmers, H.P., O'Connar, R.O., Muller, J., Kirchner, T., and Muller-Hemelink, H.K., 1989, SC-1, A functional human monoclonal antibody against autologous stomach carcinoma cells. *Cancer Res.* **49**, 2471-2476.
13. Cote, R.J., Morrissey, D.M., Houghton, A.N., Beattie, E.J., Oettgen, H.F., and Old, L.J., 1983, Generation of human monoclonal antibodies reactive with cellular antigens. *Proc. Natl. Acad. Sci. USA* **80**, 2026-2030.
14. Zhang, W., Marzilli, L.A., Rouse, J.C., and Czupryn, M.J., 2002, Complete disulfide bond assignment of a recombinant immunoglobulin G4 monoclonal antibody. *Anal. Biochem.* **311**(1), 1-9.
15. Wang, C., Amato, D., Rabah, R., Zheng, J., and Fernandes, B., 2002, Differentiation of monoclonal B lymphocytosis of undetermined significance (MLUS) and chronic lymphocytic leukemia (CLL) with weak CD5 expression from CD5(-) CLL. *Leuk. Res.* **26**(12), 1125-1129.
16. Harkins, L., Volk, A.L., Samanta, M., Mikolaenko, I., Britt, W.J., Bland, and K.I., Cobbs C.S., 2002, Specific localisation of human cytomegalovirus nucleic acids and proteins in human colorectal cancer. *Lancet* **360**(9345), 1557-1563.
17. Rhee, D., Wenig, B.M., and Smith, R.V., 2002, The significance of immunohistochemically demonstrated nodal micrometastases in patients with squamous cell carcinoma of the head and neck. *Laryngoscope* **112**(11), 1970-1974.
18. DiGiovanna, M.P., Chu, P., Davison, T.L., Howe, C.,L., Carter, D., Claus, E.B, and Stern, D.F., 2002, Active signaling by HER-2/neu in a subpopulation of HER-2/neu-overexpressing ductal carcinoma in situ: Clinicopathological correlates. *Cancer Res.* **62**(22), 6667-6673.
19. Viguier, M., Bachelez, H., Brice, P., Rivet, J., and Dubertret, L., 2002, Cutaneous B-cell lymphoma treatment with rituximab: two cases. *Ann Dermatol Venerol.* **129**(10), 1152-1155.
20. Palapattu, G.S., and Reiter, R.E., 2002, Monoclonal antibody therapy for genitourinary oncology: promise for the future. *J. Urol.* **168**(6), 2615-2623.

21. Wong, J.Y.C., Thomas, G.E., Yamauchi, D., Williams, L.E., Odom-Maryon, T.L., Liu, A., Esteban, J.M., Neumaier, M., Dresse, S., Wu, A.M., Primus, F.J., Shively, J.E., and Raubitschek, A.A., 1997, Clinical evaluation of Indium-111-labelled chimeric anti-CEA MoAb. *J. Nuclear Med.* **38**, 1951-1959.
22. Wong, J.Y.C., Chu, D.Z., Yamauchi, D.M., Williams, L.E., Liu, A., Wilczynski, S., Wu, A.M., Shively, J.E., Doroshow, J.H., and Raubitschek, A.A., 2000, A phase I radioimmunotherapy trial evaluating 90yttrium-labeled anti-carcinoembryonic antigen (CEA) chimeric T84.66 in patients with metastatic CEA-producing malignancies. *Clin Cancer Res.* **6**(10), 3855-63.
23. Presta, L.G., Chen, H., O'Connor, S.J., Chisholm, V., Meng, Y.G., Krummen, L., Winkler, M., and Ferrara, N., 1997, Humanization of an anti-vascular endothelial growth factor monoclonal antibody for the therapy of solid tumors and other disorders. *Cancer Research* **57**, 4593-4599.
24. Goi, T., Yamaguchi, A., Nakagawara, G., Urano, T., Shiku, H. and Furukawa, K., 1997, Reduced expression of deleted colorectal carcinoma (DCC) protein in established colon cancers. *Br. J. Cancer* **77**(3), 466-471.
25. Horak, E., Hartman, F., Garmestani, K., Wu, C., Brechbiel, M., Gansow, O. A., Landolfi, N. F., and Walmann, T. A., 1997, Radioimmunotherapy targeting of HER2/neeu oncoprotein on ovarian tumor using lead-121-DOTA-AE1. *The J. Nuclear Med.* **38**, 1944-1950.
26. Mariani, G., Lasku, A., Pau, A., Villa, G., Motta, C., Calcano, G., Taddei, G. Z., Castellani, P., Syrigos, K., Dorcaratto, A., Epenetos, A. A., Zardi, L., and Viale, G. A., 1997, A pilot pharmacokinetic and immunoscintigraphic study with the technetium-99m-labeled monoclonal antibody BC-1 directed against oncofetal fibronectin in patients with brain tumors. *Cancer Suppl.* **80**, 2484-2489.
27. Biassoni, L., Granowska, M., Caroll, M.J., Mather, S. J., Howell, R., Ellison, D., MacNeil, F. A., Wells, C. A., Carpenter, R., and Britton, K. E., 1998, 99m Tc-labelled sm3 in the preoperative evaluation of axillary lymph nodes and primary breast cancer with change detection statistical processing as an aid to tumor detection. *Br. J. Cancer* **77**(1), 131-138.
28. Maloney, D.G., Lopez, A. J. G., White, C.A., Bodkin, D., Schilder, R. J., Neidhart, J.A., Janakiraman, N., Foon, K. A., Liles Dallaire, B. K., Wey, K., Royston, I., Davis, T., and Levy, R., 1997, IDEC-C2B8 (Rituximab) Anti-CD20 monoclonal antibody therapy in patients with relapsed low-grade non-Hodgkin's lymphoma. *Blood* **90**, 2188-2195.
29. Van Der Bruggen, P., Zhang, Y., Chaux, P., Stroobant, V., Panichelli, C., Schultz, E.S., Chapiro, J., Van Den Eynde, B.J., Brasseur, F, and Boon, T., 2002, Tumor-specific shared antigenic peptides recognized by human T cells. *Immunol. Rev.* **188**(1), 51-64.
30. Wooldridge, J., Ballas, E. Z, Krieg, A. M., and Weiner, G. J., 1997, Immunostimulatory oligodeoxynucleotides containing CpG motifs enhance the efficacy of monoclonal antibody therapy of lymphoma. *Blood* **89**, 2994-2998.

DETECTION OF PHAGE DISPLAYED PEPTIDES WITH BLOCKING ABILITY IN VASCULAR ENDOTHELIAL GROWTH FACTOR (VEGF) MODEL

Berrin Erdağ[1], B.Koray Balcıoğlu[1], Aslı Kumbasar[1], and Beyazıt Çırakoğlu[1,2]

[1]*The Scientific and Technical Research Council of Turkey (TUBITAK), Research Institute for Genetic Engineering and Biotechnology, Gebze, Kocaeli, Turkey;* [2]*Marmara University, School of Medicine, Haydarpasa, İstanbul, Turkey*

1. INTRODUCTION

Vascular endothelial growth factor (VEGF) is a prime regulator of angiogenesis, vasculogenesis and vascular permeability[1-2]. Structurally VEGF is a homodimeric protein in which the monomers are linked by a pair of disulfide bonds[3-4]. Six isoforms of VEGF which have 121, 145, 165, 183, 189 or 206 residues in each monomer are expressed in humans[5]. These isoforms of VEGF appear by a different splicing process. $VEGF_{165}$ is the predominant molecular species, but transcripts encoding $VEGF_{189}$ are also commonly found in cells expressing the VEGF gene[6]. High levels of VEGF expression have been found in several types of human tumor[7-8]. In animal models, overexpression of VEGF has been showed to enhance tumor growth whereas suppression of VEGF inhibited tumor growth in several types of tumor [9-10-11].

VEGF has been characterized as a mitogen for vascular endothelial cells derived from arteries, veins and lymphatics[12-13]; however mitogenic effects of VEGF on a few non-endothelial cell types; such as retinal pigment epithelial cells[14] pancreatic duct cells[15] and Schwann cells[16] have been also reported.

Recent studies have shown that the interaction of VEGF with its receptors plays an important role in a number of pathological events like tumor development. Two tyrosine kinase receptors have been identified for which VEGF acts as a high affinity ligand : an *fms*-like tyrosine kinase-1 (flt-1 or VEGFR-1)[17] and kinase domain receptor (KDR/flk-1 or VEGFR-2)[18]. Although VEGFR-1 binds to VEGF with 50 fold higher affinity than VEGFR-2[17], most of the VEGF mitogenic properties are mediated by interaction with VEGFR-2[19-20-21].

Phage displayed peptide library system contains a library of variants of a peptide expressed on the outside of a phage virion, while the genetic material encoding each variant residues is on the inside[22]. Clones specifically binding to a target molecule can be selected by consecutive cycles of *in vitro* selection process called biopanning and *in vivo* amplification[23]. The screening of phage display libraries is a powerful technique for identifying peptides mimicking protein surfaces[24-25-26]. In recent year, new agonists and antagonists for cell membrane receptors have been identified successfully using phage displayed peptides[27-28].

In this study, we attempted to obtain peptides that block binding of VEGF to its receptor. First, we screened phage displayed 7 mer random library against recombinant human vascular endothelial growth factor (rhVEGF$_{165}$) to obtain peptides that bind VEGF. Second, VEGF binding peptides were tested with competition cell enzyme linked immunosorbant assay (ELISA). Thus, we tried to obtain peptides blocking the interaction between the VEGF molecule and its receptors.

2. MATERIALS AND METHODS

2.1 Library Screening with rh VEGF$_{165}$

Biopanning was adapted from Ph.D-7 kit standard procedure (New England BioLabs, Beverly, M.A.). Libraries were selected using 75 mm x 12 mm immunotubes (Nunc, Maxisorb) coated overnight at 4°C with 0.5 ml of 0.5µg/ml rhVEGF (NCI;Rockville,USA). Four rounds of selection were performed with a specific elution of bound phages in pH: 2.2 acidic buffer. To analyze the selected clones, overnight cultures of *Escherichia coli* (strain TG1) were diluted 1:100, infected with single clones, grown for 4.5 hours with shaking at 37°C and the culture supernatant containing phage particles was harvested. This phage stock was used to perform ELISA binding assays.

2.2 Phage ELISA

Phages binding to VEGF were detected by phage ELISA method. 96 well plates were coated with 0.5µg/ml VEGF or 0.5µg/ml BSA in coating buffer (0.1M NaHCO$_3$ pH: 8.6) overnight at 4°C and blocked with PBS containing 1% BSA. Phage solution (10^{10}pfu) mixed with PBS, 1 %BSA was added to the wells and assayed as described in the procedure of Pharmacia phage detection module.

2.3 Cell Culture

Human umbilical vein endothelial cells (HUVEC) were purified and cultured using a modification of the procedure described by Jaffe *et al.* (29). Briefly, untraumatized umbilical cord segments were cannulated and flushed with Buffer K (10 mM Hepes pH 7.3, 140 mM NaCl, 4 mM KCl, 11 mM D-Glucose). Cells were isolated by incubating umbilical veins with 0.05% Collagenase/Dispase (Roche Molecular Biochemicals) at 37°C for 10 min Cords were then flushed with 50ml Medium 199, the cell pellet centrifuged and washed in Medium 199. Cells were maintained in Medium 199 containing 20 % fetal bovine serum, 20mM Hepes pH:7.4, penicillin (100 u/ml) streptomycin (100 µg/ml) and heparin (5 u/ml), in tissue culture plates preincubated with human plasma fibronectin (40 µg/ml Biological Industries). On the day of the experiment, HUVEC were isolated by trypinisation, resuspended in 1% BSA, and 0.05% NaN$_3$ containing PBS and counted using a hemocytometer.

2.4 Whole Cell ELISA with HUVEC in Suspension

The blocking effect of phage displayed peptides were tested by whole cell ELISA with HUVEC in suspension. Cell ELISA method was performed using a modification of the procedures described by Roush[30] and Hoogenboom[31]. 96 well microtiter plates were coated with 10µg/ml BSA and left overnight at 4°C. Next day, 10^5 cells were incubated with VEGF (0.2 µg/ml) in a final volume of 0.2 ml per well. After one hour cells were washed three times with 1 % BSA containing PBS, 10^{11} phages were added to each well and incubated, for one hour at room temperature. At the end of the incubation wells were washed three times with PBS containing 1% BSA. The amount of bound phages was detected with peroxidase conjugated anti-M13 phage serum (Pharmacia Bioteh, Uppsale, Sweden).

3. RESULTS

In order to find rhVEGF binding peptides, a random 7 mer peptide library composed of 2×10^9 independent clones was screened by biopanning against immobilized rhVEGF. After four rounds of selection, the number of phages that bind rhVEGF increased 10^3 fold. The results of these biopanning experiments are summarized in Table 1.

Table 1. Phages Numbers in Biopanning Reaction

Panning number	Phage Quantity Input Pfu/ml	Phage Quantity Output Pfu/ml
1.	2×10^{11}	8×10^4
2.	1×10^{11}	1×10^5
3.	3×10^{11}	1×10^7
4.	1×10^{11}	2×10^7

At the end of the selection, 106 clones were isolated. The binding of each selected clone to VEGF was tested by phage ELISA. 80 clones showed affinity for the VEGF molecule (Fig.1). 51 of the positives clones, with an ELISA signal higher than OD_{405}: 0.4, were tested with cell ELISA to find peptides that are able to block the interaction between the VEGF molecule and its receptor on HUVEC.

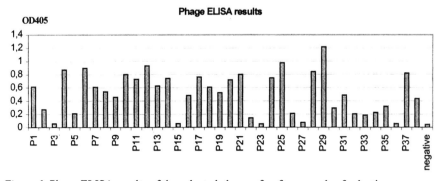

Figure 1. Phage ELISA results of the selected clones after four rounds of selection.

ELISA signals were detectable only for phage concentrations $> 10^{10}$/ml (data not shown). In this study, we tested our peptide clones using two parallel strategies. In the first strategy, clones were screened using HUVEC preincubated with VEGF. In the second strategy, phage particles were preincubated with VEGF. At the end of the incubation, phages were added to wells containing cells. 48 clones, tested by cell ELISA gave positive results, three peptide clones, EB55, EB10, E2 did not (Fig.2).

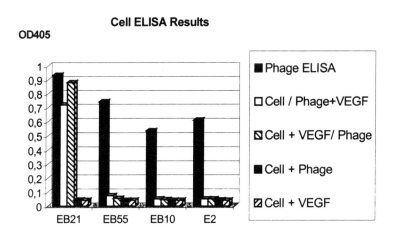

Figure 2. Cell ELISA results.

4. CONCLUSION

Screening phage displayed random peptide libraries represents a powerful means of identifying peptide ligands for targets of interest[32]. Random peptide libraries displayed on phage have been used in a number applications[33], including epitope mapping[34-35], mapping protein-protein contacts[36] and identification of peptide mimics of non-peptide ligands[37].

In this study, random 7 mer peptide library was screened against recombinant human $VEGF_{165}$. The previous studies have shown that VEGF is involved in numerous pathological conditions[38-39-40]. Overexpression of VEGF in tumors correlates with microvessel density and poor prognosis. Tumor growth has been inhibited by blocking the VEGF pathway, which is initiated by the specific interaction of VEGF with its receptors. Therefore, VEGF antagonists preventing this interaction might play an important role in the effective treatment of tumors as well as pathogenic vascularization in general. In animals, blockade of the VEGF pathway has been achieved by blocking antibodies targeted against VEGF[41] or its receptors[42], soluble decoy receptors that prevent VEGF from binding to its normal receptors, and small molecule inhibitors of the VEGF receptors. There are only limited examples of direct screening of peptide libraries with a cellular receptor, the main difficulty being the removal of clones that bind non-specific determinants.

In this case, a peptide library was screened against VEGF. This method was an indirect way to isolate peptides antagonistic for VEGF-VEGF receptor interactions. We obtained 80 clones that showed binding affinity to VEGF by phage ELISA. When 51 of these clones were tested by cell ELISA, all but 3 peptide clones tested positive after preincubation with VEGF. This result suggested that peptides of these clones could bind VEGF in the region of VEGF receptor binding site. In this context, our target is to determine the peptide sequences of these groups and after the synthesizing these peptides, investigate their ability to inhibit angiogenesis by cell proliferation assays.

ACKNOWLEDGEMENTS

This work was supported by a grant from TUBITAK Health Science Research Group project (SBAG-MAM-1, 102S005). We thank National Cancer Institute Biological Resources Branch (Rockville, MD, USA) for the generous gift of rhVEGF$_{165}$ and Aydın Bahar for technical assistance.

REFERENCES

1. Klagsbrun, M., and Soker, S., 1993, VEGF/VPF: the angiogenic factor found? *Curr. Biol*, **3**, 699-702.
2. Ferrara, N., and Davis Smith, T., 1997, The biology of vascular endothelial factor. *Endocrine Rev.,* **18**, 4-25.
3. Muller, Y.A., Li, B., Christinger, H.W., Wells, J. A., Cunningham, B.C. and de Vos, A.M., 1997, Vascular endothelial growth factor: crystal structure and functional mapping of the kinase domain receptor binding site. *Proc. Natl. Acad. Sci. USA,* **94**, 7192-7197.
4. Muller, Y.A., Christinger, H.W., Keyt, B.A., and de Vos, A.M., 1997, The crystal structure of vascular endothelial growth factor (VEGF) refined to 1.93 Å resolution: multiple copy flexibility and receptor binding. *Structure* **5**, 1325-1338.
5. Ferrara, N., 2001, Role of vascular endothelial growth factor in regulation of physiological angiogenesis. *Am. J. Physiol. Cell Physiol.* **280**, 1358-1366.
6. Pepper, M.S., Montesono, R., Mandrioto, S.S., Orci, L., and Vassolli, J.D., 1996, Angiogenesis a paradigm for balanced extracellular proteolysis during cell migration and morphogenesis. *Enzyme Protein* **49**, 138-162.
7. Chow N.H., Hsu P.I.Lin, X.Z., Hong, H.B., Chan S.H., Chang, K.S., Huang S.W., Su, I.J., 1997, Expression of vascular endothelial growth factor, in normal liver and hepatocellular carcinoma: on immunohistochemical study. *Hum. Pathol.* **28**, 698-703.
8. Samoto K., Ikezaki K., Oro, M., Shoro T., Kohno, K., Kuwano M., and Fukui M, 1995, Expression of vascular endothelial growth factor and its possible relation with neovascularization in human brain tumors. *Cancer Rev.* **55**, 1189-1193.

9. Takahashi A., Kitadai Y, Bucana CD, Cleary KR., and Ellis LM., 1995, Expression of vascular endothelial growth factor and its receptor, KDR, correlates with vascularity, metastasis and proliferation of human colon cancer. *Cancer Res.* **55**, 3964-3968
10. Potgens, A.S., von Altera, M.C., Lubsen, M.H., Ruter, D.J, and de Wool, R.M., 1996, Analysis of the tumor vasculature and metastatic behavior of xenografts of human melanoma cell lines transfected with vascular permeability factor. *Am. J. Pathol.* **148**, 1203-1217.
11. Kim, K.J., Li, B., Winer, J., Armanini, M., Gillett, N., Philips, H.S., and Ferrara, N., 1993, Inhibition of vascular endothelial growth factor induced angiogenesis suppresses tumor growth *in vivo*. *Nature* **362**, 841-844.
12. Ferrara, N., and Davis-Smith, T., 1997, The biology of vascular endothelial growth factor. *Endocr. Rev.* **18**, 4-25.
13. Plouet, J., Scholling, J., and Gospodarowicz, D., 1989, Isolation and characterization of a newly identified endothelial cell mitogen produced by At T20 cells. *EMBO J.* **8**, 3801-3808.
14. Guerrin, M., Moukadirs, H., Chollet, P., Moro, f., Dutt, K., Malecaze, F., and Plouet, J., 1995, Vasculotropin/ vascular endothelial growth factor is an autocrine growth factor for human retinal pigment epithelial cells cultured *in vitro*. *J. Cell. Physiol.* **164**, 385-394.
15. Oberg-Welsh, C., Sandler, S., Andersson, A., and Welsh, M., 1997, Effects of vascular growth factor on pancreatic duct cell replication and the insulin production of fetal islet-like cell clusters *in vitro*. *Mol. Cell Endocrinol.* **126**, 125-132.
16. Sondell, M., Lundborg, G., and Konje, M., 1999, Vascular endothelial growth factor has neurotrophic activity and stimulates axonal outgrowth, enhancing cell survival and Schwann cell proliferation in the peripheral nervous system. *J. Neurosci.* **19**, 5731-5740.
17. de Veries, C., Escobedo, J.A., Hero, H., Houck, K., Ferrara, N., and Williams, L.T., 1992, The fms-like tyrosine kinase, areceptor for vascular endothelial growth factor. *Science* **255**, 989-991.
18. Ternon, B.I., Dougher-Vermozen, M., Carrion, M.E., Dimitrov, P., Armellino, D.C., Gospodarowicz, D., and Bohler, P., 1992, Identification of KDR tyrosine kinase as a receptor for a vascular endothelial cell growth factor. *Biochem. Biophys. Rev. Commun.* **187**, 1579-1586.
19. Konno, S., Oku, N., Abe, M., Tero, Y., Ito, M., Shitara, K., Tabaya, K., Shibuye, M., and Soto, Y., 2000, Roles of two VEGF receptors, flt and KDR, in the signal transduction of VEGF effects in human vascular endothelial cells. *Oncogene* **19**, 2138-2146.
20. Yoshiji, H., Kuriyama, S., Hicklin, D., Huber, J., Yoshii, J., Miyamoto, Y., Kawata, M., Ikezaka, Y., Maktani, T., Tsujinoue, H., and Fukui H., 1999, KDR/Flk-1 is a major regulator of vascular endothelial growth factor – induced tumor development and angiogenesis in murine hepatocellular carcinoma cells. *Hepatology* **30**, 1179-1186.
21. Ferrara, M., 2000, VEGF: an update on biological and therapeutic aspects. *Curr. Opin. Biotechnol.* **11**, 617-624.
22. Smith, G.P., 1988 Filamentous fusion phages: Novel expression vectors that display cloned antigens on the virion surface. *Science* **228**, 1315-1317.
23. Parmley, S.F. and Smith, G.P., 1988, Antibody selectable filamentous fd phage vectors: Affinity purification of target genes. *Gene* **73**, 305-318.
24. Scott, J.K., and Smith, G.P., 1990, Searching for peptide ligands with an epitope library. *Science* **249**, 386-390.
25. Arop, W., Pasqualine, R., and Ruoslohi, E., 1998, Cancer treatment by targeted drug delivery to tumor vasculature in a mouse model. *Science* **279**, 377-380.

26. Fukumoto, T., Torigoe, N., Kawabota, S., Murakami, M., Uede, T., Mishi, T., Ito, Y., and Sugmura, K., 1998, Peptides mimics of the CTLA4- binding domain stimulate T-cell proliferation. *Nat. Biotechnol.* **16**, 267-270.
27. Binetruy-Tournoire, R., Demongel, C., Mulavaud, B., Vassy, R., Rouyre, S., Kraemer, M., Plouet, J., Derbin, C., Perret, G., and Maize, J.C., 2000, Identification of a peptide blocking vascular endothelial growth factor (VEGF) mediated angiogenesis. *EMBO J.* **19**, 1527-1533.
28. Asai, T., Magatsuka, M., Kuromi, K., Yamakawa, S., Kurohane, K., Ogino, K., Tanaka, M., Taki, T. and Oku, N., 2002, Suppression of tumor growth by novel peptides homing to tumor-derived new blood vessels. *FEBS Letters* **510**, 206-210
29. Jaffe, E.A., Nachmann, R.L., Becker, C.G., and Minick, C.R., 1973, Culture of human endothelial cells from umbilical veins. Identification by morphologic and immunologic criteria. *J. Clin. Invest.* **52**, 2745-2756.
30. Rousch M., Lutgerink J.T., Coote J., de Bruine A., Arends J.W., and Hoogenboom, H.R., 1998, Somatostatin displayed on filamentous phage as a receptor-specific ago. *Br. J. Pharmacol.* **125**(1), 5-16.
31. Hoogenboom, H.R., Lutgerink, J.T., Pelsers, M.M., Roush, M.J., Coote, J., Van Neer, N., De Bruine, A., Van Nieuwenhoven, F.A., Glatz, J.F., and Arends, J.W., 1999, Selection-dominant and nonaccessible epitopes on cell-surface receptors revealed by cell-panning with a large phage antibody library. *Eur. J. Biochem.* **260**(3), 774-84.
32. Smith, G.P., 1985, Filamentous fusion phage: novel expression vectors that display cloned antigens on the viron surface. *Science* **228**, 1315-1317.
33. Zwick, M., Shen, J., and Scott, J., 1998, Phage displayed peptide libraries. *Curr. Opin. Biotechnol.* **9**(4), 427-436.
34. Scott, J.K., and Smith, G.P., 1990, Searching for peptide ligands with an epitope library. *Science* **249**, 386-390.
35. Felici, F., Castagnoli, L., Musacchio, A., Jappelli, R., and Cesareni, G., 1991, Selection of antibody ligands from a large library of oligopeptides expressed on a multivalent exposition vector. *J. Mol. Biol.* **222**, 301-310.
36. Hong, S.S., and Boulanger, P., 1995, Protein ligands of the human adenovirus type 2 outer capsid identified by biopanning of a phage-displayed peptide library on separate domains of wild-type and mutant penton capsomers. *EMBO J.* **14**(19), 4714-4727.
37. Scott, J.K., Loganathan, D., Easley, R.B., Gong X., and Goldstein, I.J., 1992, A family of concanavalin A-binding peptides from a hexapeptide epitope library. *Proc. Natl. Acad. Sci. US,* **89**, 5398-5402.
38. Berse, B., Brown, L.F., van De Water, L., Dvorak, H.F., and Senger D.R., 1992, Vascular permeability factor (vascular endothelial growth factor) gene is expressed differentially in normal tissues, macrophages, and tumors. *Mol.Biol. Cell*, **3**, 211-220.
39. Miura, H., Miyazaki, T., Kuroda, M., Oka, T., Mochinow, R.., Kodama, T., Shibuya, M., et al., 1997, Increased expression of vascular endothelial growth factor in human hepatocellular carcinoma. *J. Hepatol.* **27**, 854-861.
40. Yoshiyi, H., Gomez, D.E., Shibuya, M., and Thorgeirsson, U.P., 1996, Expression of vascular endothelial growth factor, its receptor, and other angiogenic factors in human breast. *Cancer Rev.* **56**, 2013-2016.
41. Asano, M., Yukita, A., Matsumoto, T., Kondo, S., and Suzuki, H., 1995, Inhibition of tumor growth and metastasis by an immunoneutralizing monoclonal antibody to human VEGF/ vascular permeability factor 121. *Cancer Res.* **55**, 5296-5301.
42. Fong, T.A., Shawver, L.K., Sun, L., Tang, C., App, H., Powell, T.J., Kim, Y.H. et al., 1999, SU5416 is potent and selective inhibitor of the vascular endothelial growth factor receptor(flk-1/KDR) that inhibits tyrosine kinase catalysis, tumor vascularization, and growth of multiple tumor types. *Cancer Res.* **59**, 99-106.

INDEX

Acute phase genes	298
Adhesive glycoproteins	172
Adult stem cells	35
Albumin production	60
Alginate-poly(L-lysine)	60
AlloDerm®	130
Allogeneic cells	2
Alpha-1-antitrypsin	267
Alpha-fetoprotein	127
Alzheimer's disease	53, 97
Amino acid sequences	180
Ammonia plasma	170
Amphiphilic block copolymers	191
Angiogenesis	61, 168, 327
Angiogenic factors	61
Angiopoietins	62
Animal models	269
Animal welfare	268
Antibody	309
Antigen presenting cells	20
Apheresis	110
Apligraf®	130
Apoptosis	169
Artificial vascular substitutes	180
Autologous stem cells	112
Basement membrane	167
Beta cells	17
Beta-sheet structures	149
Bilirubin conjugates	59
Bioactive agents	279
Bioactive materials	236
Bioactive prosthesis	172
Biocompatibility	60, 203, 235, 283
Biodegradability	235
Biodegradable polymers	59, 180, 191
Biological substitutes	57
Biomaterials	58, 171, 247
Biopanning	330
Bio-surface engineering	155
Blastocyst	11, 49
Blood flow	166
Blood vessel	7, 171
Bone marrow	19, 35, 47, 223
Bone marrow cell line	17
Bone morphogenetic proteins (BMP)s	236, 281
Bone formation (remodelling)	201, 218, 247, 283
Bovine serum albumin	171
Brain cells	97
Calcification	16
Calcium alginate	171
Cancer antigens	319
Capillary ingrowth	172
Cardiogenesis	15
Cardiomyocytes	14, 41
Cardiovascular diseases	180
Cardiovascular substitutes	4
Carrier matrix	201, 281
Cartilage	237
Cationic lipids	288
Cell adhesion	59, 184, 191, 203
Cell culture	121, 139, 329

Cell cycle	271	DNA biomarkers	129
Cell line	11, 33	DNA isolation	132, 139
Cell expansion	160	DNA point mutation	137
Cell morphology	251	DNA transfer	265
Cell proliferation	226	Dopaminergic neurons	15
Cell reprogramming	38	Ectoderm	29
Cell signalling	166	Elastin	221
Cell spheroid	60	Embryo transfer	18
Cell technology	4	Embryoid body	13, 30, 52
Cellular biomarker	130, 141	Embryonal carcinoma	12
Cellulose acetate	203	Embryonic development	57
Central nervous system	15, 97	Embryonic liver development	120
Ceramics	288	Embryonic stem cells	5, 11, 28, 48, 115, 265
CD34+ cells	107		
Chemotherapeutic drugs	114	Encapsulation	60
Chimaera	265	Endoderm	29, 119
Chimeric antibody	317	Endogenous promoter	268
Chitin	203	Endolumbar transplantation	101
Chitosan	60, 203, 255	Endothelial cells	17, 165, 179
Chitosan-glycerol phosphate	287	Endothelialization	165
Chondrogenesis	122, 228	Engineered implants	1
Cirrhosis	65	Engraftment	108
Cloning	265	Epidermal autograft	130
Co-culture models	60	Epidermal growth factor (EGF)	240
Collagen	60, 131, 170, 221, 284	Epigastric groin fascia	258
Collagen-poly(propylene)	62	Epilepsy	97
Colony-stimulating factor (CSF)	48	Epithelial cells	41
Computer-assisted modelling (CAM)	207	Erythropoietin	267
		Ethics	18, 27, 48
Congenital liver diseases	115	*Ex vivo* gene therapy	281
Connective tissue	221	Extracellular matrix	58, 131, 166, 236
Construct technology	4	Feeder cells	50
Controlled release	171, 279	Fertilization	29
Cord blood stem cells	48	Fetal cell transplantation	98
Cryopreserved embryo	33	Fetal porcine hepatocytes	62
Cystic fibrosis	115, 267	Fetal tissue	98
Cytochrome P450	60, 127	Fiber bonding	203
Cytokines	42, 120, 167	Fibrin	170
Cytotoxic chemotherapy	109	Fibroblast growth factor- acidic (FGF-a)	120
De novo liver	58		
De-differentiation	52	Fibroblast growth factor- basic (FGF-b)	62, 168, 240, 281
Degenerative disorder	50, 97		
Demineralized bone particles	236	Fibronectin	168, 236
Dermagraft®	130	Fibrosis	256
Dermal equivalent	2	Flow bioreactor	60
Diabetes mellitus	53, 69, 255	Fluorescent *in situ* hybridization	137
Differentiation	14, 121, 171	Foam	285

Index 337

Free radicals	129	Hybrid genotype	19
Fused deposition modelling	203	Hybrid scaffold	235
Gene-activated matrix	290	Hydrogel hollow fiber	60
Gene delivery	161	Hydrogel	289
Gene expression	161	Hyperacute rejection	270
Gene silencing	265	Hypocellular marrow	109
Gene targeting	265, 251	Hypoxia	255
Genetic damage	137	Ig-gene libraries	319
Genome	265	Immobilization	170, 217, 256
Genomic DNA	272	Immune system activities	6, 20, 266, 282, 297, 310
Germ cells	11, 29		
Germ layers	18	Immunogenicity	258
Germline	241	Immunoglobulins	267, 311
Glia	14	Immunoisolation	255
Glucose stimulation	260	Immunologic therapy	309
Glycosaminoglycan	60, 236	Immunosuppression	20, 60, 69
Granulocyte	107	Implant industry	1
Growth factor	48, 119, 171, 213	*In vitro* differentiation	11
Growth hormone	267	*In vitro* fertilization	18
Gunn rat	59	Inflammatory response	129, 286
Haematopoietic precursors	17	*In situ* polymerization	210
Haemocompatibility	170	Insulin	69, 258
Heart	7	Insulin-like growth factor	267
Heart valve	7	Integra®	130
HeLa cells	132	Integrins	166, 188
Hematologic malignancy	107	Interleukin 1 (IL-1)	297
Hematopoiesis	40	Interleukin 6 (IL-6)	120
Hematopoietic lineage	47	Internal calibration standards	142
Hematopoietic stem cells	35, 47, 107	International reference standards	130
Hemorrhagic apoplexy	97	Ischaemic apoplexy	97
Hep3B cells	298	Ischaemic injury	15
Heparan sulphate	169	Islet of Langerhans	69, 255
Heparin	167	Islet transplantation	69
Hepatic differentiation	120	Keratin	221
Hepatic oval cells	64	Kidney	7
Hepatic precursors	123	Knock-out mice	268
Hepatic stellate cells	64	Lactoferrin	267
Hepatic stem cells	127	Laminar structures	285
Hepatocyte	17, 119	Leukapheresis	110
Hepatocyte engraftment	119	Leukemia inhibition factor (LIF)	12
Hepatocyte growth	58	Lipopolysaccharide-binding protein	298
Hepatocyte growth factor (HGF)	120	Liver	7, 41
		Liver organogenesis	65, 120
Hepatocyte-specific gene	127	Liver organoid	62
Hepatotrophic stimulation	61	Liver tissue engineering	57
Homologous recombination	272	Liver-specific function	127
Humoral immunity	311	Lysis-resistant cells	111

Localized delivery	171, 281	Nuclear transfer	265
Major histocompatibility	31, 295	Oligodendrocytes	15
Medical products	139	Optimal mobilization yield	109
Membrane lamination	203	Organogenesis	57
Mesenchymal stem cells	19, 39, 50, 119, 223	Organ transplant	7
Mesoderm	29	Orthopaedic tissue engineering	4, 223
Metabolic liver diseases	65	Osteoarthritis	16, 53, 222
Metabolic organ	57	Osteoblast	14, 247, 283, 259
Microcapsule	285	Osteoclast	247
Micro-cellular polymer	248	Osteogenesis	16, 122, 223, 239
Microporosity	212	Osteopontin expression	225
Microsphere	171, 256, 285	Osteoporosis	16
Microvascular bed	61	Osteoprogenitor cells	283
Molecular lego	149	Osteosarcoma cells	224
Molecular self-assembly	147	Oxidative DNA damage	129
Monoclonal antibody	309	p53 gene	137
Multi-lineage differentiation	122	Pancreas	7, 41
Multiple myeloma	109	Pancreas transplantation	69
Multiple sclerosis	97	Pancreatic islets	69, 225
Multipotency	28	Parkinson's disease	53, 97, 115
Muscular dystrophy	115	Particulate leaching	203
Myelination defects	15	PEO-peptide derivatives	194
Myeloablative chemoradiotherapy	107	Peptide-containing polymers	186
Myeloma	108	Peptide nanotube	147
Myoblast	40	Peptide scaffold	147
Myocardium	15	Peripheral blood	47, 111
Nanocapsule	285	Peri-transplant morbidity	112
Nanofiber	147	pH sensitive polymers	288
Nanosphere	285	Phage displayed peptides	327
Nonovesicle	147	Pharmaceutical industry	130
Natural materials	201	Pharmaceutical proteins	267
Neo-intima	165, 172	Phase separation/inversion	203
Neonatal fibroblasts	129, 131	PLA/PEO block copolymers	179, 192
Neonatal keratinocytes	129	Plasticity	36, 47
Neovascularization	61, 256	Platelet	107
Nerve regeneration	130	Platelet derived growth factor (PDGF)	62, 240
Neural cells	14, 41	PLGA-hydroxyapatite	284
Neural injury	161	Pluripotency	13, 28, 50
Neurogenesis	14	Policies	34
Neurohumoral regulation	98	Poly(α-amino acid)	192
Neurological diseases	98	Poly(caprolactone) (PCL)	203
Neurons	14	Poly(ethylene imine) (PEI)	288
Neurosphere	15	Poly(ethylene oxide) (PEO)	60, 179
Neutrophil	107	Poly(ethylene teraphtalate) (PET)	165
Non-viral vectors	282	Poly(glycolic acid) (PGA)	59, 235
		Poly(HIPE)	248

Index

Poly(lactic acid) (PLA)   59, 179, 203, 235
Poly(lactic acid-co-glycolic acid) (PLGA)   171, 235, 255, 283
Poly(L-lysine)   288
Polymer biomaterials   58, 192
Polymer-DNA complex   291
Polymer film   183
Polymeric microparticles   209
Poly(plex)es   288
Poly(propyl acrylic acid)   288
Poly(tetrafluoroethylene) (PTFE)   165
Porcine endogenous retrovirus (PERV)   270
Preimplantation embryo   18
Primary brain cell culture   99
Pro-active surface   166
Progenitor cell   17, 37, 107, 161
Proliferation   168, 203
Pro-nuclear injection   265
Proteoglycan   167
Pseudo-aneurysm   165
Putative liver stem cell   62
Random peptide library   331
Recipient-immune system   39
Re-differentiation   52
Refractory disease   109
Regenerative medicine   12, 27, 53
Regulatory issues   53
Religion   33
Reproductive cloning   30, 53
Resistance gene   268
Retrovirus   282
RGD   170
Scaffold   58, 201, 247, 255, 283
Sclerosis   97
Selectin   167
Senescence   271
Serum-free medium   15
Signalling pathways   15, 304
Skin   130
Skin cancer   137
Skin substitute (equivalent)   2, 130, 221
Small intestine submucosa (SIS)   236
Solid tumor   107
Solvent casting   203
Somatic cell nuclear transfer   53

Somatic cells   265
Spinal cord injury   53
Spontaneous fusion   19
Starch-based polymers   206
Stat3 molecules   298
Stem cell factor (SCF)   120
Stem cell plasticity   51
Stem cell therapy (transplantation)   21, 27, 107
Stem cells   28, 57, 119, 223
Stroke   115
Structural tissue   57
Submyeloablative mobilization chemotherapy   112
Substratum   166
Subventricular zone   20
Superovulation   18
Surface chemistry   203
Surface roughness   60
Surfactant peptides   153
Synthetic dermal matrix   130
Target locus   273
T-cells   20
Telomere   271
Teratoma   30
TestSkin II®   131, 140
Therapeutic cloning   33, 53
Thermoplastic proteins   216
Three-dimensional (3D) printing   203
Thrombosis   165
Tissue-engineered bone   237
Tissue-engineered skin   129, 137
Tissue factory   32
Tissue ingrowth   236
Tissue regeneration (repair)   115, 130, 138, 168
Totipotency   28
Transcription factors   298
Trans-differentiation   39
Transfected cells   273, 298
Transforming growth factor-E (TGF-E)   62, 240
Transgenesis   265
Transgenic livestock   265
Transgenic mice   265
Transient transfection   299
Transplantation   1, 30, 107, 258

Tumorigenesis	20	VEGF-binding peptides	330
Tumor-specific monoclonal antibodies	114	Ventricular subependyma	20
		Viral infection	20
Unipotency	28	Viral vector	282
Vascular endothelial cell growth factor (VEGF)	62, 168, 240, 256, 281, 327	Vitronectin	168
		White blood cells	110
		Wound healing	61, 130, 171
Vascular endothelial cells	4	Xenoantigen	270
Vascular graft	166	Xenosupport systems	12
Vascular network	61	Xenotransplantation	270
Vascular permeability	327	Y chromosome	137
Vascular prostheses	165	Z-DNA	149
Vascular smooth muscle cells	165		
Vasculogenesis	169, 327		